KU-289-231

Horizons in Medicine

number **19**

Edited by
Professor David Lomas
Department of Medicine, University of Cambridge

West Sussex Health Libraries
COPY NUMBER 2081645

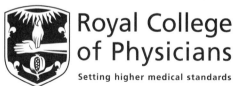

Royal College
of Physicians
Setting higher medical standards

Acknowledgement

The Royal College of Physicians acknowledges with thanks a grant from the Haymills Trust and the contribution of The Lavenham Press towards the cost of printing this book.

The Royal College of Physicians of London

The Royal College of Physicians plays a leading role in the delivery of high quality patient care by setting standards of medical practice and promoting clinical excellence. We provide physicians in the UK and overseas with education, training and support throughout their careers. As an independent body representing over 20,000 Fellows and Members worldwide, we advise and work with government, the public, patients and other professions to improve health and healthcare.

Citation of this book: Royal College of Physicians. *Horizons in medicine*, volume 19. London: RCP, 2007.

Front cover photograph:
TOM BARRICK, CHRIS CLARK, SGHMS/SCIENCE PHOTO LIBRARY
Brain pathways. Coloured 3-dimensional magnetic resonance imaging scan of the white matter pathways of the brain, side view.

Royal College of Physicians of London
11 St Andrews Place, London NW1 4LE

Registered Charity No. 210508

Copyright © 2007 Royal College of Physicians of London
All rights reserved. No part of this publication may be reproduced in any form (including photocopying or storing it in any medium by electronic means and whether or not transiently or incidentally to some other use of this publication) without the written permission of the copyright owner. Applications for the copyright owner's written permission to reproduce any part of this publication should be addressed to the publisher.

ISBN: 978-1-86016-312-8

Typeset by Dan-Set Graphics, Telford, Shropshire
Printed in Great Britain by The Lavenham Press Ltd, Suffolk

British Library Cataloguing in Publication Data
A catalogue record of this book is available from the British Library

Editor's introduction

This nineteenth volume of *Horizons in Medicine* represents the contributions to the 2007 Advanced Medicine Conference. It is a credit to the College that it wishes to showcase this important meeting through the publication of the *Horizons* series. It is a great honour to be asked to organise the Advanced Medicine Conference but also a daunting task. I attempted to provide a mix of cutting-edge basic science with important lessons in clinical practice. Often the two were combined as a testament to the exciting era in which we live. It is particularly satisfying when novel understandings in the molecular mechanisms of disease can be translated through to new therapeutic opportunities and changes in patient care. This is particularly so for the amyloidoses and myeloproliferative disorders but also for inherited skin disorders and asthma.

Not all new discoveries have to be based on molecular mechanisms, and great improvements in patient care come from large randomised trials in cardiovascular disease, pleural effusion, and osteoporosis. It was exciting to hear about new developments in the treatment of the vasculitides and, interestingly, that John F Kennedy was one of the first patients with Addison's disease to receive a perioperative infusion of hydrocortisone for spinal surgery while he was a senator.

These presentations were mixed with important updates on emerging infectious diseases such as bird flu as well as the more established HIV and diseases of the returning traveller. There were practical demonstrations on how to interpret thyroid function tests and manage patients with acute renal failure. I introduced radiology into this year's programme and was delighted to hear about the latest advances in imaging of the lungs, the endocrine system, and oncological disease. The highlights of the Advanced Medicine Conference are the named lectures, and this year was no exception. Peter Goadsby used the Croonian Lecture to address one of the most common medical disorders, headache, while Tom Solomon used the Linacre Lecture to review his excellent work on Japanese encephalitis.

The Advanced Medicine Conference is a success only because of the attendance and participation of the audience. It was wonderful to see a mix of scientists and clinicians being enthused by new discoveries in clinical medicine. Finally, I am grateful to Jo Summers, Anne McSweeney, and the team in the Conference Department for organising the meeting and to Hannah Thompson and Jemma Lough for managing the manuscripts. None of this would have been possible without them!

DAVID LOMAS
Cambridge 2007

Contributors

DAVID H ADAMS *Professor of Hepatology, Liver Research Group, Institute for Biomedical Research, Wolfson Drive, University of Birmingham, Edgbaston, Birmingham B15 2TT*

DWOMOA ADU *Consultant Physician, Department of Nephrology, Queen Elizabeth Hospital, Edgbaston, Birmingham B15 2TH*

EBAA AL-OZAIRI *Newcastle Diabetes Centre, Newcastle upon Tyne NE4 6BE*

RICHARD ANDREWS *Consultant Ophthalmologist, Moorfields Eye Hospital, 162 City Road, London EC1V 2PD*

JANE F APPERLEY *Department of Haematology, Imperial College, Hammersmith Hospital, Du Cane Road, London W12 0NN*

WIEBKE ARLT *Professor of Medicine, MRC Senior Clinical Fellow, Division of Medical Sciences, Institute of Biomedical Research, Rm 233, University of Birmingham, Birmingham B15 2TT*

TIPU Z AZIZ *Department of Neurosurgery, Department of Neurosurgery Level 3, West Wing, John Radcliffe Hospital, Headley Way, Headington, Oxford OX3 9DU*

PAUL BOWNESS *Reader in Immunology and Consultant Rheumatologist, MRC Human Immunology Unit, Weatherall Institute of Molecular Medicine, John Radcliffe Hospital, Oxford OX3 9DS and Nuffield Orthopaedic Centre, Windmill Road, Headington, Oxford OX3 7LD*

EDWARD J CETTI *Clinical Research Fellow, Royal Brompton Hospital, Sydney Street, London SW3 6NP*

ANTONI CHAN *ARC Clinical Research Fellow, MRC Human Immunology Unit, Weatherall Institute of Molecular Medicine, John Radcliffe Hospital, Oxford OX3 9DS*

JULIET COMPSTON *Professor of Bone Medicine, School of Clinical Medicine, University of Cambridge, Addenbrooke's Hospital, Hills Road, Cambridge CB2 2QQ*

TIMOTHY M COX *Professor of Medicine, University of Cambridge, Honorary Consultant Physician, University of Cambridge Teaching Hospitals NHS Foundation Trust, Level 5, Addenbrooke's Hospital, Cambridge CB2 2QQ*

ROBERT JO DAVIES *Reader and Consultant in Respiratory Medicine, Oxford Centre for Respiratory Medicine, Churchill Hospital Site, Oxford Radcliffe Hospital, Headington, Oxford OX3 7LJ*

ANAND DEVARAJ *Fellow in Thoracic Imaging, Department of Radiology, Royal Brompton Hospital, Sydney Street, London SW3 6NP*

JONATHAN CW EDWARDS *Professor in Connective Tissue Medicine, University College London, Room 118, Windeyer Building, Cleveland St, London W1T 4JF*

JOHN FIRTH *Consultant Physician and Nephrologist, Cambridge University Hospitals NHS Foundation Trust, Addenbrooke's Hospital, Cambridge CB2 8QQ*

ANDREW FREEDMAN *Senior Lecturer in Infectious Diseases, Honorary Consultant Physician, Cardiff University School of Medicine, Heath Park, Cardiff CF14 4XN*

PETER S FRIEDMANN *Professor of Dermatology, University of Southampton, Dermatopharmacology Unit, Level F South Block (825), Southampton General Hospital, Tremona Road, Southampton SO16 6YD*

DUNCAN M GEDDES *Professor of Respiratory Medicine, Royal Brompton Hospital, Sydney Street, London SW3 6NP*

ANTHONY H GERSHLICK *Department of Cardiology, University Hospitals of Leicester, Groby Road, Leicester LE3 9QP*

ALEXANDER GIMSON *Consultant Physician and Hepatologist, Cambridge University Hospital Foundation NHS Trust, Cambridge CB2 2QQ*

PETER J GOADSBY *Headache Group, Institute of Neurology, The National Hospital for Neurology and Neurosurgery, Queen Square, London; Department of Neurology University of California, San Francisco, California, USA*

ANTHONY R GREEN *University of Cambridge, Department of Haematology, Cambridge Institute for Medical Research, Hills Road, Cambridge CB2 0XY*

MARK GURNELL *University Lecturer in Endocrinology & Honorary Consultant Physician, University of Cambridge, Department of Medicine, Level 5, Box 157, Addenbrooke's Hospital, Cambridge CB2 2QQ*

DAVID M HANSELL *Professor of Thoracic Imaging, Department of Radiology, Royal Brompton Hospital, Sydney Street, London SW3 6NP*

PHILIP N HAWKINS *National Amyloidosis Centre, Department of Medicine, Royal Free and University College Medical School, Royal Free Hospital, Rowland Hill Street, London NW3 2PF*

BRENDAN HEALY *Specialist Registrar in Infectious Diseases/Microbiology, NPHS Wales Cardiff (Microbiology Department), University Hospital of Wales, Heath Park, Cardiff CF14 4XW*

STEPHEN T HOLGATE *Professor of Immunopharmacology, Allergy and Inflammation Research, Division of Infection, Inflammation and Repair, School of Medicine, Southampton General Hospital, Tremona Road, Southampton SO16 6YD*

PHILIP HOME *Professor of Diabetes Medicine and Consultant Physician, SCMS-Diabetes, The Medical School, Framlington Place, Newcastle upon Tyne NE2 4HH*

BRIAN HUNTLY *Department of Haematology, Imperial College, Hammersmith Hospital, London W12 0NN*

KIMME L HYRICH *Honorary Rheumatology Consultant, Manchester Royal Infirmary; Clinical Lecturer, ARC Epidemiology Unit, Stopford Building, University of Manchester, Oxford Road, Manchester M13 9PT*

DOW-MU KOH *Senior Lecturer and Honorary Consultant, Cancer Research UK, Clinical Magnetic Resonance Group, Institute of Cancer Research and Department of Radiology, Royal Marsden Hospital, Downs Road, Sutton SM2 5PT*

SIMON KOLLNBERGER *ARC Career Development Fellow, MRC Human Immunology Unit, Weatherall Institute of Molecular Medicine, John Radcliffe Hospital, Oxford OX3 9DS*

MARIA J LEANDRO *Consultant Rheumatologist and Honorary Senior Lecturer, University College London, Room 118, Windeyer Building, Cleveland St, London W1T 4JF*

DAVID LOMAS, *Wellcome Trust/MRC Building, Hills Road, Cambridge CB2 2XY*

JOHN A MCGRATH *Professor of Molecular Dermatology, Genetic Skin Disease Group, St John's Institute of Dermatology, Division of Genetics and Molecular Medicine, St Thomas' Hospital, Lambeth Palace Road, London SE1 7EH*

PUJA MEHTA *Department of Haematology, Imperial College, Hammersmith Hospital, London W12 0NN*

NICHOLAS W MORRELL *University Reader in Respiratory Medicine, University of Cambridge School of Clinical Medicine, Department of Medicine, Box 157, Addenbrooke's Hospital, Hills Road, Cambridge CB2 2QQ*

CHRISTOPHER J MOWATT *Specialist Registrar in Anaesthesia and Intensive Care Medicine, Honorary Lecturer, Department of Anaesthesia and Intensive Care, University Hospital Birmingham, Birmingham B15 2TT*

KATHRYN L NASH *Specialist Registrar in Hepatology, Hepatobiliary & Liver Transplant Unit, Addenbrooke's Hospital, Hills Road, Cambridge CB2 2QQ*

ALBERT CM ONG *Reader in Nephrology/Honorary Consultant Nephrologist, Academic Nephrology Unit, Sheffield Kidney Institute, The Henry Wellcome Laboratories for Medical Research, School of Medicine and Biomedical Sciences, University of Sheffield, Beech Hill Road, Sheffield S10 2RX*

YE HTUN OO *Clinical Research Fellow, Liver Research Group, Institute for Biomedical Research, Wolfson Drive, University of Birmingham, Edgbaston, Birmingham B15 2TT*

MILES PARKES *Consultant Gastroenterologist, IBD Genetics Research Group, Addenbrooke's Hospital, Cambridge CB2 2OQ*

NAJIB M RAHMAN *Specialist Registrar and MRC Training Fellow, Oxford Centre for Respiratory Medicine, Oxford Centre for Respiratory Medicine, Churchill Hospital Site, Oxford Radcliffe Hospital, Headington, Oxford OX3 7LJ*

STEPHEN D RYDER *Consultant Hepatologist, Queens Medical Centre Campus, Nottingham University Hospitals NHS Trust, Derby Road, Nottingham NG7 2UH*

TOM SOLOMON *Professor of Neurology, and MRC Senior Clinical Fellow, Viral Brain Infections Group, University of Liverpool, Walton Centre for Neurology and Neurosurgery, Liverpool L9 7LJ*

IAIN STEPHENSON *Senior Clinical Lecturer and Consultant in Infectious Diseases, University Hospitals of Leicester, Leicester Royal Infirmary, Leicester LE1 5WW*

NICOLA HILARY STRICKLAND *Consultant Radiologist, Hammersmith Hospitals NHS Trust; Honorary Senior Lecturer, Imperial College School of Medicine, London W12 0HS*

WAI Y TSE *Consultant Physician and Honorary Senior Lecturer, Department of Nephrology, Derriford Hospital, Derriford Road, Plymouth PL6 8DH*

ANGELA VINCENT *Professor of Neuroimmunology, Department of Clinical Neurology, University of Oxford, Oxford OX3 9DS*

DAVID A WARRELL *Emeritus Professor of Tropical Medicine, University of Oxford, Nuffield Department of Clinical Medicine, John Radcliffe Hospital, Headington, Oxford OX3 9DU*

Contents

HAEMATOLOGY

SKIN AND BONES

RENAL DISEASE

RHEUMATOLOGY

HEPATOLOGY/GASTROENTEROLOGY

CROONIAN LECTURE

LINACRE LECTURE

Cardiology

Pulmonary hypertension

Nicholas W Morrell

☐ INTRODUCTION

Pulmonary arterial hypertension (PAH) is defined as an elevation of the mean pulmonary arterial pressure above 25 mmHg at rest or above 30 mmHg as a result of exercise. A number of clinical conditions can increase pulmonary arterial pressure, and these have been categorised by international consensus on the basis of clinical and pathological features into the classification shown in Table 1. Our understanding of the pathobiology of PAH has increased dramatically over the past few years, with a subsequent improvement in the treatment of the condition. We now have practical and targeted therapies that improve symptoms and survival in patients with PAH. Identification in 2000 of the genetic mutation that underlies familial PAH has led to a better understanding of this enigmatic condition and paved the way for new and more effective approaches to treatment. This article will

Table 1 Venice classification of pulmonary hypertension, 2003.

Group	Classification
I	• Pulmonary arterial hypertension (PAH) • Idiopathic PAH (IPAH) • Familial PAH (FPAH) • Associated with (APAH): – Connective tissue disease – Congenital systemic-to-pulmonary shunts – Portal hypertension – HIV infection – Drugs and toxins – Other (thyroid disorders, glycogen storage disease, Gaucher's disease, hereditary haemorrhagic telangiectasia, haemoglobinopathies, myeloproliferative disorders, splenectomy) • Associated with significant venous or capillary involvement – Pulmonary veno-occlusive disease (PVOD) – Pulmonary capillary haemangiomatosis (PCH) • Persistent pulmonary hypertension of the newborn (PPHN)
II	• Pulmonary hypertension associated with left heart diseases
III	• Pulmonary hypertension associated with respiratory diseases and/or hypoxaemia (including chronic obstructive pulmonary disease)
IV	• Pulmonary hypertension due to chronic thrombotic and/or embolic disease
V	• Miscellaneous group – for example, sarcoidosis, histiocytosis X, and lymphangiomatosis

focus on two forms of PAH: that caused by chronic thromboembolism and the idiopathic/familial form of the disease.

□ CHRONIC THROMBOEMBOLIC PULMONARY HYPERTENSION

Chronic thromboembolic pulmonary hypertension (CTEPH) occurs when a clot fails to resolve completely after an acute pulmonary embolic event. The rate of resolution of clots after acute pulmonary embolism varies and is longer in patients with pre-existing cardiopulmonary disease, but normal perfusion should be restored by 4–6 weeks after the acute event. To some extent, the rate of resolution depends on the initial clot burden or the size of the acute pulmonary embolism.

If the clot fails to resolve, it becomes organised before it can be completely fibrinolysed. The organised thrombus is incorporated into the wall of the pulmonary artery, becomes covered by endothelial cells and forms a false intima. The organised material occludes the vascular lumen, which increases pulmonary vascular resistance and leads to pulmonary hypertension. Depending on the extent of the obstruction to blood flow, the increased right ventricular preload ultimately may lead to right ventricular failure. Clinically, the patient may present with persistent symptoms of dyspnoea after an acute embolic event and despite anticoagulation. Up to 60% of patients with CTEPH will have a prior documented episode of previous venous thromboembolism, although some patients may present with gradually worsening dyspnoea in the absence of acute events. The true prevalence of CTEPH is hard to ascertain, because it is not usually sought in patients who are recovering from acute pulmonary embolism (PE), but it almost certainly is underdiagnosed.

One well-designed study found that 4% of patients with a history of acute PE had a persistent elevation of pulmonary arterial pressure after two years.[1] Evidence also shows that those with a higher initial clot burden (massive PE) are more likely to develop CTEPH than those with minor PE. The more widespread use of thrombolysis for acute PE is often assumed to reduce the prevalence of CTEPH, but no data at present support this view. It is of note that some of the classic risk factors for acute deep vein thrombosis (DVT)/PE are not found with increased frequency in the population that develops CTEPH. For example, the factor V Leiden polymorphism, which leads to activated protein C resistance and is found with high prevalence in the population of patients with acute DVT, is not overrepresented in patients with CTEPH.[2] The prevalence of protein C and S deficiency is increased in patients with CTEPH, although these conditions account for a small minority of patients. In addition, some 10% of patients with CTEPH may have circulating antiphospholipid antibodies. Recent research points to a deficiency in the ability to fibrinolyse established clots as a predisposing factor.

A potentially curable form of PAH

Pulmonary endarterectomy (PEA) is a surgical procedure during which organised thrombi are removed from the proximal pulmonary arteries. The procedure is a major operation that usually requires the patient to undergo repeated cycles of cardiopulmonary bypass with cerebral cooling. This ensures a bloodless field of view for the surgeon, who can then enter the left and right main pulmonary arteries via arteriotomy. The aim is to identify a dissection plane along the base of the false intima and to dissect distally as far as possible. It is often possible to remove organised material as far distally as segmental pulmonary arteries. With successful clearance of proximal clots, the pulmonary vascular resistance can fall dramatically postoperatively, and near normalisation of resistance can be achieved in the long term. Patients then are maintained on warfarin and have an inferior vena cava filter sited prior to the operation. Long-term survival is often excellent after a successful procedure. The operation itself carries some risk, and perioperative mortality varies between 7% and 20% depending on the experience of the centre. In the United Kingdom, Papworth Hospital undertakes approximately 60 such operations per year and is the only centre at present to be designated for this procedure by the National Specialist Commissioning Advisory Group.

There are two main aspects to patient selection for this procedure. Comorbidities are important predictors of perioperative mortality and require careful assessment. A further important consideration is the distribution of the disease, as organised clots need to be anatomically accessible to the surgeon. If the organised material is predominantly of a distal distribution within the pulmonary arteries – that is, involves subsegmental vessels – there is a high risk that pulmonary vascular resistance will not decrease after the procedure and that the patient will be left with significant pulmonary hypertension.

The presurgical work-up of patients referred with a suspected diagnosis of CTEPH requires a multidisciplinary approach involving surgeons, physicians, and radiologists. Imaging plays a key role in determining whether a patient is suitable for surgery.[3] Computed tomographic pulmonary angiography with modern multi-slice scanners is a rapid and non-invasive technique that can provide several important pieces of information in the assessment of patients with suspected CTEPH. Computed tomography (CT) can assess the presence of any associated lung disease or tumours. Most importantly, a computed tomographic pulmonary angiogram gives an accurate assessment of the extent of proximal organised clots. Although occlusion of very small arteries cannot be visualised directly in the case of predominantly distal disease, the characteristic appearance of 'mosaic perfusion' suggests the presence of peripheral disease. Computed tomography can also reveal the extent of right ventricular hypertrophy and dilatation, although this is probably best seen by magnetic resonance (MR) imaging. Three-dimensional reconstruction of the two-dimensional CT and MR images can help decide whether the distribution of disease is suitable for PEA. The use of a combination of these techniques means that the more invasive traditional pulmonary angiogram can be avoided in most patients. In the series at Papworth Hospital, approximately 60% of cases of CTEPH are potentially suitable for surgery. Of the patients who are not suitable for surgical management, most may be suitable for targeted therapy with the new pharmacological agents described below. In summary, all patients with proved pulmonary hypertension should undergo careful assessment for the presence of CTEPH, as it represents a potentially curable form of pulmonary hypertension.

☐ ADVANCES IN THE TREATMENT OF IDIOPATHIC PULMONARY ARTERIAL HYPERTENSION

Idiopathic PAH (formerly known as primary pulmonary hypertension) is a devastating condition that, without treatment, leads to death from right heart failure within three years of diagnosis. Ten years ago, most patients diagnosed with idiopathic PAH were given palliative care only. The past few years, however, have witnessed the development of a range of interventions that have improved exercise limitation, quality of life, and probably survival in this condition.

Anticoagulation with warfarin has been a mainstay of treatment since retrospective studies suggested a beneficial effect on survival. The rationale was the frequent finding at autopsy of microthrombi within small pulmonary arteries, which were thought to represent *in situ* thrombosis. No prospective studies have been undertaken to confirm this, but most centres continue to anticoagulate patients with severe pulmonary hypertension. High-dose calcium channel blockers, such as diltiazem, have also been shown to have dramatic effects on survival in a small minority of patients with idiopathic PAH.[4] We now know that patients who respond to calcium channel blockers also demonstrate a marked reduction in pulmonary vascular resistance in response to an acute trial of a vasodilator, such as inhaled nitric oxide (NO), and a vasodilator trial forms part of the recommended work-up of patients with idiopathic PAH. Some 5% or fewer of patients will be responders and may represent a distinct clinical phenotype of PAH. Overuse of calcium channel blockers in non-responders may worsen survival through the negative inotropic effects of these agents.

A large body of evidence supports the view that an imbalance exists between endogenous vasodilators and vasoconstrictors in patients with PAH.[5] For example, patients with PAH have increased circulating levels and local production of lung endothelin-1 and serotonin. In addition, good evidence supports a deficiency of endothelial prostacyclin and production of nitric oxide. The earliest approach to replacement therapy was continuous infusions of prostacyclin. Prostacyclin has a half-life of around two minutes and must be freshly prepared every day for infusion by the patient. The patient remains connected to a portable infusion pump via a tunnelled Hickman line and remains in hospital over the first few days of dose-titration. Frequent side-effects of flushing, headache, flu-like symptoms and jaw pain usually subside over a few days. Problems with infusion failure can lead to rebound severe pulmonary hypertension, and line-related infections are problematic. Controlled trials of intravenous prostacyclin have confirmed beneficial effects on exercise tolerance and pulmonary haemodynamics.[6] Long-term data suggest a beneficial effect on survival. Newer formulations of prostanoids have attempted to overcome the problems associated with continuous infusion. The prostacyclin analogue iloprost is much more stable than prostacyclin and can be given intravenously or by regular nebulisation. Treprostinil is also very stable and can be given by subcutaneous infusion, although pain at the site of infusion often limits dose escalation. An oral prostanoid not available in the West, beraprost, was used in Japan, but use of this drug is limited by gastrointestinal side-effects. Intravenous prostacyclin remains the drug of first choice in patients with severe right ventricular failure at presentation.

The orally active endothelin (ET) receptor antagonist bosentan is licensed for the treatment of severe pulmonary hypertension (New York Heart Association classes 3 and 4). The seminal trial of bosentan was the largest controlled trial published to date in patients with PAH and showed beneficial effects on pulmonary haemodynamics, exercise tolerance, and time to clinical worsening.[7] About 10% of patients develop clinically significant increases in hepatic transaminases, which are usually reversible on cessation of the drug. Otherwise, the drug is well tolerated. Bosentan is a non-selective ET_A/ET_B receptor antagonist. Further ET_A selective antagonists are now in clinical use, including sitaxsentan and ambrisentan, although no evidence to date shows superior efficacy. These drugs may be particularly useful in patients who develop hepatic dysfunction on bosentan.

Although replacement of NO via the inhaled route is feasible, it is cumbersome and inconvenient. Nitric oxide exerts its effects on pulmonary vascular smooth muscle cells by stimulating soluble guanylyl cyclase and increasing intracellular levels of cyclic guanosine monophosphate (cGMP). The cGMP is hydrolysed by phosphodiesterases, which limits cellular accumulation. The availability of cGMP-specific (type 5) phosphodiesterase inhibitors such as sildenafil provides an alternative approach to overcoming deficiency of NO. Sildenafil is now licensed in the UK for the treatment of severe PAH and has similar efficacy to the endothelin receptor antagonists.[8] Sildenafil is given three times a day for PAH. Newer type 5 phosphodiesterases are becoming available with longer half-lives and once daily administration, but the results of trials with these agents are awaited.

Further experimental treatments are on the horizon for patients with PAH. Vasoactive intestinal polypeptide (VIP) works by elevating cyclic adenosine monophosphate (cAMP) in cells, rather like prostacyclin, and is undergoing evaluation. Drugs that inhibit the action or uptake of serotonin are also being investigated as potential treatments. Receptor tyrosine kinase inhibitors (new agents used to treat some forms of cancer) are also being used in clinical trials for patients with PAH.

☐ RECENT ADVANCES IN OUR UNDERSTANDING OF THE PATHOBIOLOGY OF FAMILIAL PAH

The aetiology of severe unexplained pulmonary hypertension remained a mystery until a few years ago. Reports of a causal association between appetite suppressant drugs and the occurrence of severe pulmonary hypertension provided some insight into pathogenesis; however, identification of the gene that underlies the familial form of PAH in 2000 provided a firm basis for mechanistic studies.[9,10] About 10% of patients with idiopathic PAH have an affected relative. In affected families, the disease segregates in an autosomal dominant pattern, with often markedly reduced penetrance. True estimates of penetrance are yet to be reported – and probably will vary with the nature of the underlying mutation – but, on average, penetrance is of the order of 20–30%.[11] Many patients who carry the disease gene thus will not manifest clinical PAH. After localisation of the disease gene to the long arm of chromosome 2 (2q33), two independent groups identified heterozygous germline mutations in the bone morphogenetic protein type 2 receptor (BMPR-2) – a receptor for the transforming growth factor (TGF)-β superfamily – in patients with familial PAH.[9,10] Mutations in the *BMPR2* gene have been found in about 70% of families.[12] In addition, up to 25% of patients with apparently sporadic idiopathic PAH have also been found to harbour similar mutations. At least a proportion of these are examples of familial PAH in which the condition has not manifested in relatives because of low penetrance, whereas others are examples of *de novo* mutations. To date, some 144 distinct mutations have been identified in 210 independent patients with familial PAH.[12]

About 30% of mutations are missense mutations that occur in highly conserved amino acids with predictable effects on receptor function. For example, many involve the serine-threonine kinase domain of the BMPR-2 receptor or the extracellular ligand binding domain. Most (approximately 70%) of the *BMPR-2* coding mutations are frame shift and nonsense mutations, however – many of which would be expected to produce a transcript susceptible to nonsense-mediated mRNA decay. Haplo-insufficiency for BMPR-2 thus represents the predominant molecular mechanism to underlie inherited predisposition to familial PAH. Further genetic analysis is revealing an increasing number of families in which a mutation in *BMPR-2* is implicated, including the identification of gene deletions and rearrangements. The genetics of familial PAH and mutations of *BMPR-2* was recently reviewed in detail.[12]

REFERENCES

1 Pengo V, Lensing AW, Prins MH *et al.* Incidence of chronic thromboembolic pulmonary hypertension after pulmonary embolism. *N Engl J Med* 2004;350:2257–64.

2 Wolf M, Boyer-Neumann C, Parent F *et al.* Thrombotic risk factors in pulmonary hypertension. *Eur Respir J* 2000;15:395–9.

3 Coulden R. State-of-the-art imaging techniques in chronic thromboembolic pulmonary hypertension. *Proc Am Thorac Soc* 2006;3:577–83.

4 Rich S, Kaufmann E, Levy PS. The effect of high doses of calcium-channel blockers on survival in primary pulmonary hypertension. *N Engl J Med* 1992;327:76–81.

5 Humbert M, Morrell NW, Archer SL *et al.* Cellular and molecular pathobiology of pulmonary arterial hypertension. *J Am Coll Cardiol* 2004;43(12 Suppl 1):13S–24S.

6 Barst RJ, Rubin LJ, McGoon MD *et al.* Survival in primary pulmonary hypertension with long-term continuous intravenous prostacyclin. *Ann Intern Med* 1994;121:409–15.

7 Rubin LJ, Badesch DB, Barst RJ *et al.* Bosentan therapy for pulmonary arterial hypertension. *N Engl J Med* 2002;346:896–903.

8 Galie N, Ghofrani HA, Torbicki A *et al.* Sildenafil citrate therapy for pulmonary arterial hypertension. *N Engl J Med* 2005;353:2148–57.

9 Lane KB, Machado RD, Pauciulo MW *et al.* Heterozygous germ-line mutations in BMPR2, encoding a TGF-β receptor, cause familial primary pulmonary hypertension. *Nat Genet* 2000;26:81–4.

10 Deng Z, Morse JH, Slager SL *et al.* Familial primary pulmonary hypertension (gene PPH1) is caused by mutations in the bone morphogenetic protein receptor-II gene. *Am J Hum Genet* 2000;67:737–44.

11 Newman JH, Trembath RC, Morse JA *et al.* Genetic basis of pulmonary arterial hypertension: current understanding and future directions. *J Am Coll Cardiol* 2004; 43(12 Suppl S):33S–9S.

12 Machado RD, Aldred MA, James V *et al.* Mutations of the TGF-beta type II receptor BMPR2 in pulmonary arterial hypertension. *Hum Mutat* 2006;27:121–32.

Contemporary management of acute myocardial infarction

Anthony H Gershlick

□ BACKGROUND

More than 150,000 patients are hospitalised in the United Kingdom (UK) each year for acute ST elevation myocardial infarction (STEMI). The 'open artery' hypothesis suggests that in order to improve patient outcome in the short, medium and longer term the priority should be to establish reperfusion and attain a patent infarct-related artery as soon as possible. This important objective has been highlighted as an aim in the *National service framework for coronary heart disease.* Current evidence supports two therapeutic options for such patients: thrombolytic treatment or percutaneous coronary intervention (PCI). Most patients in the UK currently receive in-hospital thrombolysis. This paper discusses the advantages and disadvantages of the two therapeutic approaches and describes ongoing trials.

□ THROMBOLYSIS

Evidence shows true benefit from thrombolytic treatment. More than 100,000 patients have been randomised in large clinical trials that have tested thrombolytic agents against controls or other thrombolytic agents. The results were summarised by the Fibrinolytic Therapy Trialists Collaborative Group.[1] The overall relative risk reduction in 35-day mortality with treatment was 18%, and the mortality at this point was reduced from about 13% in controls to about 8–9% in those who received treatment. This rate has been confirmed in recent European registry data. The beneficial effect of thrombolytic treatment is seen in those patients who present within 12 hours of the onset of symptoms – irrespective of age, sex, history of hypertension or diabetes, or previous myocardial infarction (MI).[1] It is clear that the earlier patients are treated the better: after 12 hours, there seems to be only a small and statistically uncertain benefit. The Late Assessment of Thrombolytic Efficacy (LATE) trial, for example, clearly showed a lack of benefit for treatment started more than 12 hours after the onset of symptoms.

Fibrin-specific thrombolytics, such as tissue-type plasminogen activator (tPA) and reteplase, theoretically should be more effective at opening coronary arteries than streptokinase (SK). This theory is supported by a number of angiographic studies, which showed a higher percentage of patients with patent arteries after treatment with tPA than with SK (about 70% versus about 35%).[2] The Global Utilization of Streptokinase and Tissue plasminogen activator for Occluded coronary arteries (GUSTO) trial, in which standard SK was compared with a more aggressive regimen, showed a small but significant mortality benefit with tPA (6.3% versus 7.3%). Although there was an excess of strokes with this accelerated regimen (0.72% for tPA versus 0.54% for SK), there was still a benefit in favour of tPA (6.9 % versus 7.8 %) when deaths and strokes were combined.

In the UK, fibrin-specific thrombolytics are increasingly being used first line when lytic treatment is chosen as the option for reperfusion.

Problems with thrombolysis

The open artery theory suggests that short-term and long-term outcomes after STEMI are determined predominantly by the extent and quality of patency obtained after attempted reperfusion; however, the maintenance of optimal patency is also critical. A number of studies have shown that long-term outcomes correlate with flow rates defined by the thrombolysis in myocardial infarction (TIMI) grading scheme as seen at the 90-minute angiogram.[3] For example, data from the angiographic arm of the GUSTO trial showed that patients with TIMI grade 0 flow (ie complete occlusion) at the 90-minute angiogram had a 30-day mortality of 8.4% compared with only 4% for those with TIMI grade 3 (ie normal flow).[4] Unfortunately, even contemporary thrombolytic treatment is able to produce TIMI grade 3 flow in <60% of patients treated with the most effective lytic (accelerated tPA). Adjunctive treatment with antiplatelet agents may improve early vessel patency,[5] and agents such as clopidogrel, which in a recent trial was shown to increase TIMI flow when used in combination with thrombolysis and aspirin compared with controls,[6] are likely to become standard adjunctive treatments in STEMI – as they have become in non-STEMI.

The second limitation of current thrombolytic regimens is the potential for vessel reocclusion. This is a time-related phenomenon that with lytic may reach 30% by three months. Reasons for reocclusion include re-release of thrombin, residual prothrombogenic plaque, and activation of coagulation factors V and VIII by plasmin. Patients with reoccluded vessels have a significantly higher clinical event rate at one year, and furthermore the event rate at three years is 73% in those who reocclude compared with 33% in those whose infarct-related artery is patent at three months. Therefore, lack of full efficacy when lytics are the first-line reperfusion therapy thus revolves around the dual issues of immediate and maintained patency. On the plus side, it is generally a safe, easily, administered, and readily available treatment that requires no specialised training for its initiation. Importantly, most patients present to hospitals where lytics are easily available and triage and audit policies are in place for its administration, which may not be the case for primary angioplasty.

Pre-hospital thrombolysis

As 'speed of re-perfusion equals muscle salvage equals outcome', it follows that the sooner a vessel can be opened the better, and thus the sooner any reperfusion treatment that could open a vessel can be given, the better. A number of investigators have assessed whether or not there is any advantage in giving thrombolysis before a patient arrives at hospital. Early trials in the development of thrombolytic treatment introduced this concept of 'time is muscle', which is supported by data that showed that benefits (eg reduction in mortality) gained from thrombolytic treatment become less evident over time – even within the first six hours. If this were true, it would seem logical to try to give a thrombolytic before the patient arrives at hospital, as long as the staff have adequate training and there is concurrent audit of outcome. Studies have indicated that the time the patient takes to call for help (pain-to-call time) and the time taken for the hospital to treat could account for about one hour each. As there seems little that can shorten the pain-to-call time apart from societal education, taking the lytic to the patient rather than waiting for the patient to arrive at the hospital, which compounds the delay, seems logical. However, this is not to say that we should not emphasise to potential patients the need to call for help as quickly as possible. Trials suggest that pre-hospital thrombolysis clearly results in a reduction in treatment time. In the Myocardial Infarction Triage and Intervention (MITI) trial, initiation of treatment before arrival in hospital reduced the period from onset of symptoms to treatment by a mean of 33 minutes. Significantly, more patients who received pre-hospital thrombolysis had resolution of pain (7% versus 23%), but there was no difference in the combined trial endpoint or in mortality (5.7% versus 8.1%). This was not the case, however, for those patients who received treatment very soon after the onset of pain (<70 minutes), who had significantly better outcomes (mortality 1.2% versus 8.7%, infarct size 4.9% versus 11.2%, and ejection fraction 53% versus 49%).

The European Myocardial Infarction Project (EMIP) group showed a saving in the time to treatment of 55 minutes when thrombolytic was administered before the patient arrived at the hospital, and there was a trend to overall mortality benefit, with a significant reduction in cardiac mortality (9.7% versus 11.1% and 8.3% versus 9.8% – a relative reduction of 17%). Morrison's meta-analysis of pooled data on pre-hospital thrombolysis from six trials (n=6434) showed that all-cause mortality was reduced significantly with pre-hospital thrombolysis compared with administration in hospital (odds ratio 0.83, 95% confidence interval 0.70 to 0.98).[2] Pre-hospital thrombolysis given by paramedics is included in the national service framework's recommendations, with reteplase (given as two bolus intravenous injections) or tenecteplase (given as a single bolus) being the agents of choice.

☐ PRIMARY ANGIOPLASTY

The big challenge to thrombolysis is primary PCI, in which balloon angioplasty and stenting are used to open the artery, and keep it open, at the time of presentation. This option is believed by many, but not all, to be superior even to optimal lysis. A number of studies have shown that the long-term outcome is better than lysis if this procedure is carried out within three hours of the onset of pain (and within 90 minutes of the patient arriving at hospital) and the artery is opened successfully (TIMI grade 3 flow is obtained in 80–97% of cases). Although reocclusion of the artery remains a problem with thrombolytic treatment, this is much less common with PCI. At 3–6 months after primary PCI, the rate of vessel patency is between 87% and 91%. Pooled data from the various trials that compared primary PCI with thrombolysis show a highly significant absolute short-term mortality benefit in favour of primary PCI of 2% and a reinfarction rate of 4% (both $p<0.001$).[7] With such marked advantages, it thus would seem logical to provide primary PCI to all patients who present with STEMI.

Problems with primary PCI

There are, however, difficulties with some of the data. The small numbers of patients in the trials used in Keeley *et al*'s meta-analysis[7] results in wide confidence intervals, and all the studies in this meta-analysis compared primary PCI with in-hospital thrombolysis. Critically, it may be difficult in the real world to achieve the time requirements to administer primary PCI effectively and according to the European and American guidelines on primary PCI (symptom-to-balloon time <180 minutes; door-to-balloon time <90 minutes).[8] In addition, the interventional centre and operator volume should be 'high' according to the guidelines (although this is not clearly defined), and, where appropriate, adjunctive treatment (eg glycoprotein IIb/IIIa inhibitors) should be used at the time. Ideally, 24/7 availability to primary PCI should be established in those centres undertaking it.

The biggest problem with routine interventional treatment for STEMI in the UK (and in other countries including the US) is the mismatch between availability of intervention facilities and the availability of reperfusion options at the hospitals at which patients would normally present – that is, non-interventional centres. One suggestion is that if PCI is particularly efficacious, patients with STEMI should be directed towards hospitals with interventional facilities rather than to the emergency department at the local hospital. They would bypass the non-interventional hospital. Once there, of course, this could mean that the ambulances are in the wrong places. Resource allocation, the European working time directive, and the need to increase staffing significantly are all issues that need to be considered in the establishment of a primary PCI service that is available 24 hours and seven days a week.

What if a patient turns up at a hospital without interventional facilities? In the DANish trial in Acute Myocardial Infarction (DANAMI)-2 and the PRimary Angioplasty in patients transferred from General community hospitals to specialized PTCA Units with or without Emergency thrombolysis (PRAGUE) study,[6,9] patients with STEMI seemed to have a better outcome when treated with primary PCI than with thrombolysis, even when they presented to their local hospital and were then transferred to an interventional centre – and this can be done with very low journey risks. Indeed, this is standard policy in parts of Europe. There are real problems with these studies, however, including the fact that the endpoints were measured only at 30 days and that the significant benefit was seen in recurrence of acute MI rather than mortality. Furthermore, the acceptable length of delay in getting the patient from the local centre to the interventional centre before any benefit from primary PCI over lysis is lost is unclear. A trial in the UK (TRANSPORT–AMI) is planned and designed to test whether or not there is any circumstance with respect to time in which it is better to give local thrombolysis rather than transfer the patient for primary PCI. Alternatively, and also not without problems, there are options to allow patients to receive primary PCI as soon as possible and within the guideline-recommended timeframes. These include establishing interventional facilities in district general hospitals to make them interventional centres. However, interventional units are required to undertake a minimum number of cases, and adhere to guidelines on the number of operators before primary PCI (or indeed any PCI) can be regarded as safe and optimal for patients.

The Department of Health National Infarct Angioplasty Project Pilots (NIAPP) group is currently testing the feasibility of setting up a primary PCI service in the UK. Early indications are positive.

Facilitated PCI

Some commentators advocate the administration of thrombolytic treatment (usually a half dose) before PCI and on the journey to receive PCI for STEMI ('facilitated PCI') to combine the early benefits of thrombolysis with the intermediate benefits of PCI. The Assessment of the Safety and Efficacy of a New Treatment Strategy for Acute Myocardial Infarction (ASSENT)-4 study, for a multitude of reasons, showed that the combination of lytic and *early* (immediate on arrival) angiography with follow-on PCI was a worse option than primary PCI alone – almost certainly because of the lack of benefit over risk when all patients (even those who had successful lysis) underwent early PCI rather than waiting to see who needed the PCI because thrombolytic administration had not led to successful reperfusion (rescue PCI). A meta-analysis that includes this and other currently available trials of facilitated PCI was published recently and supported the contention that primary PCI is a better option than facilitated PCI.[10] The results of the First International New Intravascular Rigid-Flex Endovascular Stent Study (FINESS), in which patients receive one half dose of upstream lysis and/or potent antiplatelet treatment, is awaited, but 'facilitated PCI' is currently out of favour.

Rescue PCI

It is now clear that if thrombolysis is given as first-line reperfusion therapy but does not result in reperfusion, so-called 'rescue PCI' is mandatory. In the Rapid Early Action for Coronary Treatment (REACT) trial,[11] which was based in the UK, the hazard ratios for rescue PCI compared with repeat lytic or conservative treatment alone were 0.45 ($p=0.002$) and 0.47 ($p=0.004$). The definition used to determine 'failure of lytic' in this trial was failure of the pre-lytic maximal ST segment elevation to resolve by more than 50% on the electrocardiograph (ECG) undertaken 90 minutes after thrombolysis. Thus, all patients should have an ECG at 90 minutes, and where the ECG indicates failure, the nearest interventionist should be contacted and, if necessary, the patient should be transferred for rescue PCI. Doing nothing or giving a repeat dose of lytic now is regarded to provide much less favourable outcome options for patients.

Recent data also suggest that even those with successful thrombolysis should have a pre-discharge angiogram and a follow-on PCI if evidence shows poor infarct-related artery TIMI flow or residual underlying stenosis.[12] Uptake of this second strategy in the UK is only patchy at the moment, although rescue PCI for failure is used widely now.

Studies that need to be completed

We still do not really know whether primary PCI is better than pre-hospital lysis. The Comparison of Angioplasty and Prehospital Thrombolysis In acute Myocardial infarction (CAPTIM) study suggested that results with these strategies were comparable, but this study was discontinued early and there was no mandated rescue PCI.[13] The STrategic Reperfusion Early After Myocardial infarction (STREAM) trial, due to start in January 2008, is designed to test optimal primary PCI against optimal (pre-hospital) lysis and is more about the complete strategy of managing patients with AMI. This European and Canadian study, which is planned to include significant input from paramedics in the UK, will randomise patients to receive primary PCI or pre-hospital lysis.

Those randomised to primary PCI will undergo direct transfer to the nearest interventional centre, with aspirin and clopidogrel being given in the ambulance. Patients randomised to receive pre-hospital lysis will receive the randomised lytic, again with aspirin and clopidogrel, as well as age-adjusted low molecular weight heparin, all given in the ambulance. Those who have an ECG that does not resolve to >50% at 90 minutes (estimated to be about 30% of patients) will be transferred for immediate rescue PCI as per the REACT trial; those with successful lysis will undergo in-patient angiography, with transfer if necessary. Cost efficacy will be an important part of this study. Assessment of whether the logistics of managing STEMI can be improved without loss of benefit will be an important apect of this comparison.

We still need to know whether local thrombolysis given early can be as good as transfer for primary PCI, and this is an aim of the TRANSPORT–AMI trial.

Cost-effectiveness comparisons of alternative strategies is mandatory.

□ SUMMARY

An open artery in patients with STEMI is clearly the key to improved outcome in the short, medium and long term. The practicality of routine thrombolysis is offset by the less than optimal arterial patency rates achieved. Some data show that pre-hospital thrombolysis saves time and may improve outcome, so thrombolysis should be time mandated. If lysis is given but fails (<50% ST segment resolution at 90 minutes), rescue PCI is mandated. Repeat lysis does no good and may lead to excess important bleeding.

Primary PCI achieves a higher arterial patency rate and, by dealing with the underlying stenosis, reduces the risk of longer term reocclusion, particularly when associated with stenting. However, logistical problems and resource issues limit its application in the UK at the present time – although its use is increasing every month. Some of the practical obstacles include access to interventional centres, which are not readily available to most patients who present with STEMI.

No randomised trials have compared the clinical outcomes of pre-hospital lysis and primary PCI in patients who present with STEMI. The comparative clinical and cost effectiveness are therefore unknown and need to be investigated in the context of NHS ambulance and hospital services

☐ AUTHOR'S INTERESTS

The author is a co-principal investigator on the STREAM study and principal investigator on the TRANSPORT–AMI trial.

REFERENCES

1 Fibrinolytic Therapy Trialists' (FTT) Collaborative Group. Indications for fibrinolytic therapy in suspected acute myocardial infarction: collaborative overview of early mortality and major morbidity results from all randomised trials of more than 1000 patients. *Lancet* 1994;343:311–22.

2 Stringer KA. TIMI grade flow, mortality, and the GUSTO-III trial. *Pharmacotherapy* 1998; 18:699–705.

3 The GUSTO Angiographic Investigators. The effects of tissue plasminogen activator, streptokinase, or both on coronary-artery patency, ventricular function, and survival after acute myocardial infarction. *N Engl J Med* 1993;329:1615–22.

4 Sabatine MS, Morrow DA, Montalescot G *et al.* Angiographic and clinical outcomes in patients receiving low-molecular-weight heparin versus unfractionated heparin in ST-elevation myocardial infarction treated with fibrinolytics in the CLARITY-TIMI 28 Trial. *Circulation* 2005;112:3846–54.

5 Morrison LJ, Verbeek PR, McDonald AC *et al.* Mortality and prehospital thrombolysis for acute myocardial infarction: a meta-analysis. *JAMA* 2000;283:2686–92.

6 Keeley EC, Boura JA, Grines CL. Primary angioplasty versus intravenous thrombolytic therapy for acute myocardial infarction: a quantitative review of 23 randomised trials. *Lancet* 2003;361:13–20.

7 Cannon CP, Gibson CM, Lambrew CT *et al.* Relationship of symptom-onset-to-balloon time and door-to-balloon time with mortality in patients undergoing angioplasty for acute myocardial infarction. *JAMA* 2000;283;2941–7.

8 Andersen HR, Nielsen TT, Rasmussen K *et al.* A comparison of coronary angioplasty with fibrinolytic therapy in acute myocardial infarction. *N Engl J Med* 2003;349:733–42.

9 Perez de Arenaza D, Taneja AK, Flather M. Long distance transport for primary angioplasty vs immediate thrombolysis in acute myocardial infarction (PRAGUE-2 trial). *Eur Heart J* 2003;24:1798.

10 Keeley EC, Boura JA, Grines CL. Comparison of primary and facilitated percutaneous coronary interventions for ST-elevation myocardial infarction: quantitative review of randomised trials. *Lancet* 2006;367:579–88.

11 Gershlick AH, Stephens-Lloyd A, Hughes S *et al.* Rescue angioplasty after failed thrombolytic therapy for acute myocardial infarction. *N Engl J Med* 2005;353:2758–68.

12 Fernandez-Aviles F, Alonso JJ, Pena G *et al.* Primary angioplasty vs. early routine post-fibrinolysis angioplasty for acute myocardial infarction with ST-segment elevation: the GRACIA 2 non-inferiority, randomized, controlled trial. *Eur Heart J* 2007;28:949–60.

13 Bonnefoy E, Lapostolle F, Leizorovicz A *et al.* Primary angioplasty versus prehospital fibrinolysis in acute myocardial infarction: a randomised study. *Lancet* 2002;360:825–9.

☐ CARDIOLOGY SELF-ASSESSMENT QUESTIONS

Pulmonary hypertension

1 Chronic thromboembolic pulmonary hypertension is:
- (a) Associated with failure of a clot to resolve completely after acute pulmonary embolism
- (b) Treated by thrombolysis
- (c) Potentially treated by pulmonary endarterectomy
- (d) Responsive to calcium channel blockers
- (e) Usually diagnosed by computed tomographic pulmonary angiography

2 Idiopathic pulmonary arterial hypertension is:
- (a) Familial in about 10% of cases
- (b) Only treatable by heart–lung transplantation
- (c) Caused by underlying lung disease
- (d) Responsive to treatment with sildenafil
- (e) A rare condition that affects 1–2 people per million population per year

3 Familial pulmonary arterial hypertension is:
- (a) Caused by mutations in thrombotic pathways
- (b) Caused by mutations in the bone morphogenetic protein type II receptor
- (c) Associated with complete disease gene penetrance
- (d) Associated with a worse prognosis than idiopathic disease
- (e) An autosomal dominant condition

Contemporary management of acute myocardial infarction

1 Pre-hospital thrombolysis:
- (a) Has been shown to be superior to primary percutaneous coronary intervention (PCI)
- (b) Requires a doctor to be in the ambulance
- (c) Reduces the time from symptoms to treatment
- (d) Is one of the aims of the national service framework
- (e) Avoids the need for rescue PCI

2 Transfer of a patient from their presenting hospital to a tertiary centre for primary PCI:
- (a) Has been proved to be beneficial irrespective of time delay
- (b) Carries significant risks related to the journey
- (c) Can be obviated by placing facilities for PCI in every district general hospital
- (d) Is common in the United Kingdom (UK)
- (e) May depend on logistics in relation to the ambulance service

3 Facilitated PCI:

(a) In fact, actually means there need to be facilities available for PCI
(b) Makes good sense
(c) Has been proved to be better than primary PCI
(d) Has been tested in the Assessment of the Safety and Efficacy of a New Treatment Strategy for Acute Myocardial Infarction (ASSENT)-4 trial
(e) Is part of standard procedure in the UK

4 The need for rescue PCI:

(a) Is determined by the presence of chest pain
(b) Is suggested by a post-lysis electrocardiograph (ECG) undertaken within 20 minutes
(c) Is better than conservative management or repeat lysis
(d) Is evident if the ECG shows >50% resolution of maximal ST segment elevation
(e) If met, overrides the need to treat patients with primary PCI

Respiratory medicine

New treatments for severe asthma in relation to pathophysiology

Stephen T Holgate

Asthma is a disorder in which the conducting airways contract too much and too easily spontaneously and on exposure to a wide range of stimuli. The prevalence of asthma has increased worldwide, and currently 5.1 million people are affected in the United Kingdom (UK). Asthma is responsible for 1500 avoidable deaths, 20 million lost working days, and symptoms that cost £2.5 billion per annum. Despite the availability of guidelines for management, current treatment is failing to control symptoms for more than half of people with asthma. Around 10% of patients with asthma have severe disease that remains symptomatic despite optimal treatment, and the management of these people accounts for 50% of the health costs of this disease, thereby identifying a clear unmet clinical need. The UK has the highest prevalence of asthma in the world – in adults and children – which highlights the importance of new treatments.

Research over the last two decades has clearly established that airway inflammation involving the T helper (Th) 2 subset of T lymphocytes orchestrates an inflammatory response in the airways of patients with asthma (Fig 1[1]). This is characterised by activation of mast cells, which results in the secretion of a wide range of preformed and newly generated inflammatory mediators and the selective recruitment of eosinophils and basophils from CD34+ precursors in the bone marrow via the circulation and CD34+ progenitor cells already present in the lung.[2] Switching of B lymphocytes to produce immunoglobulin (Ig) E occurs under the influence of the Th2 cytokines interleukin (IL) 4 and IL-13 produced by Th2 cells and mast cells. A second important component of chronic asthma is an increase in the amount and contractility of airways smooth muscle, which accounts for most of the variable airflow obstruction but, in addition, is an important source of proinflammatory mediators, cytokines, and chemokines that help support the inflammatory response (Fig 2). An increase in the population of mast cells and T lymphocytes between the bundles of airway smooth muscle in patients with asthma is likely to contribute to altered function of this muscle by interacting with specific mediators released by mast cells, such as the rapidly acting autacoid mediators histamine and prostaglandin D_2 and the cysteinyl leukotrienes LTC_4, LTD_4, and LTE_4 (previously known as SRS-A). Mast cells at this location are of a connective tissue subtype (that is, they are dependent on stem cell factor rather than T cell cytokines for survival) and release a range of cytokines and chemokines, including the classic Th2 cytokines IL-3, IL-4, IL-5, IL-9, IL-13, and granulocyte–macrophage colony-stimulating factor (GM-CSF), which are encoded by a cluster of genes on chromosome 5q31-34, together with the chemokines monocyte chemotactic protein (MCP)-3, RANTES, and eotaxins. Eosinophils at this site and elsewhere in the airway wall release basic proteins from their granules – such as major basic protein (MBP), eosinophil cationic protein (ECP), and eosinophil peroxidase – and are also important sources of tissue-damaging reactive oxygen, prostaglandins, and cysteinyl leukotrienes.

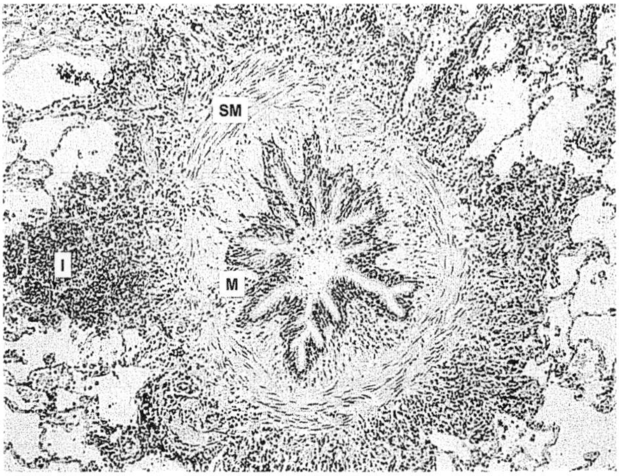

Fig 1 Cross section of an asthmatic airway showing a mixture of inflammation (I) and remodelling with deposition of matrix (M) and increased smooth muscle (SM). Reproduced from Holgate *et al* with permission of Elsevier.[1]

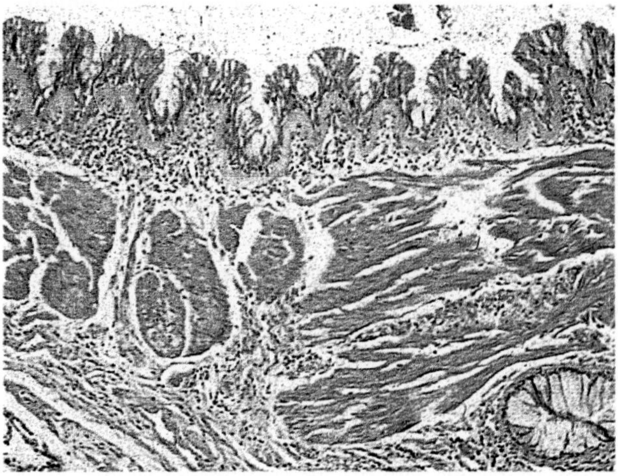

Fig 2 Cross section of part of a large airway from a patient who died during an asthma attack. Note the presence of a mucus plug, goblet cell metaplasia, submucosal and adventitial inflammation, thickening of the reticular basement membrane, smooth muscle hypertrophy and hyperplasia, and airway wall fibrosis.

In addition to having altered function, the amount of airway smooth muscle increases in patients with asthma. The mechanisms behind the hyperplasia and hypertrophy of the spiral bundles of airway smooth muscle in patients with asthma is not known, but it is highly likely to relate to an increase in the production of growth factors known to proliferate and mature smooth muscle, such as platelet-derived growth factors (PDGFs), insulin-like growth factors (IGFs), transforming growth factor (TGF)-β_1, and TGF-β_2, which are produced by immune, inflammatory, and structural cells.[3]

A third important component of asthma that is increasingly being recognised is remodelling of the airway wall, in which proteoglycans and collagen are laid down partly in response to the chronic inflammation and partly in response to epithelial damage and aberrant repair (a chronic wound scenario).[4] When the airway epithelium is injured, it is unable to repair itself efficiently, which leads to the secondary production of a range of growth factors, including TGF-βs, PDGFs, fibroblast growth factor (FGF)-1, FGF-2, and IGFs. These factors interact with fibroblasts, which causes them to proliferate and differentiate into myofibroblasts and possibly then into airway smooth muscle.[5]

Activation of the epithelium and underlying mesenchyme in patients with chronic asthma recapitulates some of the events that occur during branching morphogenesis of the foetal lung, which has led to the concept that the epithelial mesenchymal trophic unit becomes reactivated in patients with asthma (Fig 3[4]). The epithelium is unable to repair efficiently because the basal cells fail to enter the cell cycle as a result of the increased expression and nuclear translocation of cell cyclase inhibitors such as $P21^{waf}$. With respect to the origins of asthma (most cases of which occur in early childhood), the identification of susceptibility genes such as DPP10, GPR154, ETS-2, ETS-3, MUC8, HLA-G, SPINK 5, filaggrin, and PCDH-1 by positional cloning (which makes no assumption about the function of genes before their discovery) and their preferential expression in the airway epithelium point to a central role for the

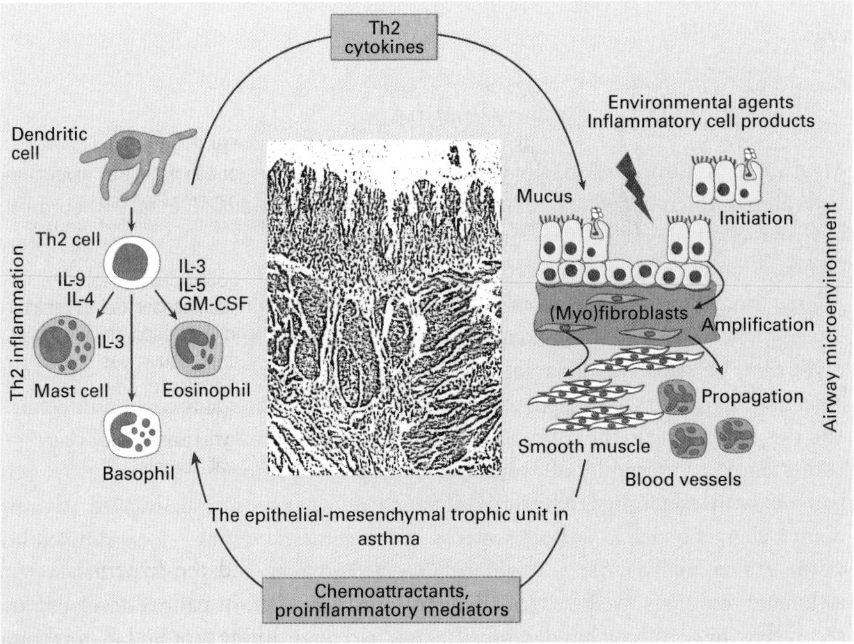

Fig 3 Schematic representation of cross talk between airway inflammation and remodelling in asthma, with reactivation of the epithelial mesenchymal trophic unit that is involved in branching morphogenesis in foetal development of the lung. GM-CSF = granulocyte–macrophage colony-stimulating factor; Ig = immunoglobulin; IL = interleukin. Reproduced from Davies *et al* with permission of Elsevier.[4]

epithelium in the origin and progression of this disease.[6] Remodelling of the airways also involves proliferation of microvessels under the influence of vascular endothelial growth factors (VEGFs) produced by the epithelium and inflammatory cells,[7] as well as an increase in the neural network driven by the production of neurotrophins such as nerve growth factor (NGF) by epithelial and inflammatory cells.

□ CURRENT TREATMENTS FOR ASTHMA

The concept of asthma as a combination of chronic airway inflammation and remodelling provides the basis for the use of inhaled (and oral) corticosteroids to control disease and inhaled β_2 adrenoceptor agonists to relieve acute attacks by relaxing the airway smooth muscle. As the disease becomes more severe and chronic, combination treatment with inhaled corticosteroids and long-acting β_2 adrenoceptor agonists (LABAs) taken twice daily (in the case of fluticasone and salmeterol) or as required (in the case of formoterol and budesonide) produces good control of asthma for many patients throughout the day and night but is totally dependent on good adherence with treatment.[8] Although such combination treatment is highly effective at controlling asthma in most patients, the introduction of inhaled corticosteroids in young children genetically at risk of developing asthma (or once asthma has become established in schoolchildren) has little effect on the natural history of the disease despite controlling inflammation and the resultant symptoms, which suggests that airway inflammation is a consequence rather than the primary cause of asthma.[9]

□ HOW IMPORTANT IS ALLERGY IN ASTHMA?

Most cases of asthma, especially those with onset in early childhood, are associated with atopy, which is defined as an enhanced ability to produce IgE against common environmental allergens. The recently published results of a 13-year longitudinal investigation in children from a community based study in Germany (the Multicenter Allergy Study (MAS)) has shown that atopy has little influence on the occurrence of intermittent or persistent wheezing in the first five years of life but becomes a powerful driver for persistent asthma into childhood after that time.[10] Much childhood wheezing up to the school-age years is driven largely by intercurrent viral infections, and this could explain the concept of 'growing out of asthma' during school years and adolescence as immunity to common respiratory pathogens develops. In most patients with established 'allergic' asthma, therefore, exposure to inhaled environmental allergens such as are encountered in the domestic setting – for example, dust mites and animal dander – might be expected to play a key role in driving the asthmatic response. Avoidance of allergens – primary (before asthma develops) and secondary (once asthma has developed) – has had no or little effect on the expression of asthma, however, which might have been expected to be the case if allergens and atopy were the principal driving causes of the disease. Prevention probably requires a combination of interventions instigated early in life in infants and children genetically at risk, including during pregnancy.[11]

THE EPITHELIUM AND INNATE IMMUNITY AT THE INTERFACE OF PATHOGENESIS

Although up to 40% of the population has atopy, only 5–7% develops persistent asthma, which raises the interesting question as to what characteristic(s) of patients with asthma leads to expression of atopy in the lower airways.[12] One possibility is that the epithelium is primarily abnormal in failing to serve as an adequate barrier. Some evidence for this has come from morphological studies, which showed that defective tight junctions would serve to increase epithelial permeability to environmental agents. The epithelium is also defective in its ability to generate the defensive cytokines interferon (IFN)-β and IFN-λ when patients with asthma are infected with common cold viruses such as rhinovirus.[13] The epithelial damage that occurs with viral infection during exacerbations could also contribute to the ongoing epithelial injury and possibly to the origins of this disease.[14] The International Study of Allergy and Asthma in Children (ISAAC) failed to demonstrate an association for the large intercountry differences in the prevalence of asthma or its rising trends in certain counties with changes in allergen load.[15]

Increasing evidence suggests that altered innate immunity that influences the polarisation of T lymphocytes towards a Th1, Th2, or possibly the newly recognised Th17 phenotype may have an important role in the origins of allergy and possibly asthma. The identification of a large number of pattern recognition receptors that are able to shape the adaptive immune response to environmental insult on epithelial and dendritic cells may provide a molecular mechanism by which the altered environment with reduced exposure to microorganisms encountered in the Western world could lead to polarisation of the immune response more towards a Th2 rather than Th1 phenotype.[16] These pattern recognition receptors, which include toll-like receptors (TLRs), respond to products from microorganisms, including viral double-stranded RNA (TLR-3), viral DNA (TLR-2), CpG repeats in bacterial DNA (TLR-9), lipopolysaccharide and lipoteichoic acid from bacterial cell walls (TLR-4), and chitin from fungi (mannose-binding receptors). The recent discovery that activation of these receptors on epithelial cells in the airways is able to generate the cytokine thymic stromal lymphopoeitin (TSLP), which has the capacity to deviate dendritic cell-driven Th2-cell differentiation,[17] has provided an important new link between activation of the epithelium and the subsequent Th2 response within the airways, which does not necessarily require the presence of allergen (Fig 4).[18] Evidence that mast cells are also able to generate TSLP in the presence of the pleiotrophic cytokines IL-1β and tumour necrosis factor alpha (TNF-α) provides another source for maintenance of the mast cell- and eosinophil-mediated inflammation that characterises chronic asthma.

THE TREATMENT OF SEVERE ASTHMA

Although treatment with inhaled corticosteroids and short- and long-acting β_2 adrenoceptor agonists is of great benefit to a large proportion of patients with asthma, recent patient-based surveys have shown that many patients' asthma is not adequately controlled with this treatment. For example, Partridge *et al* showed that

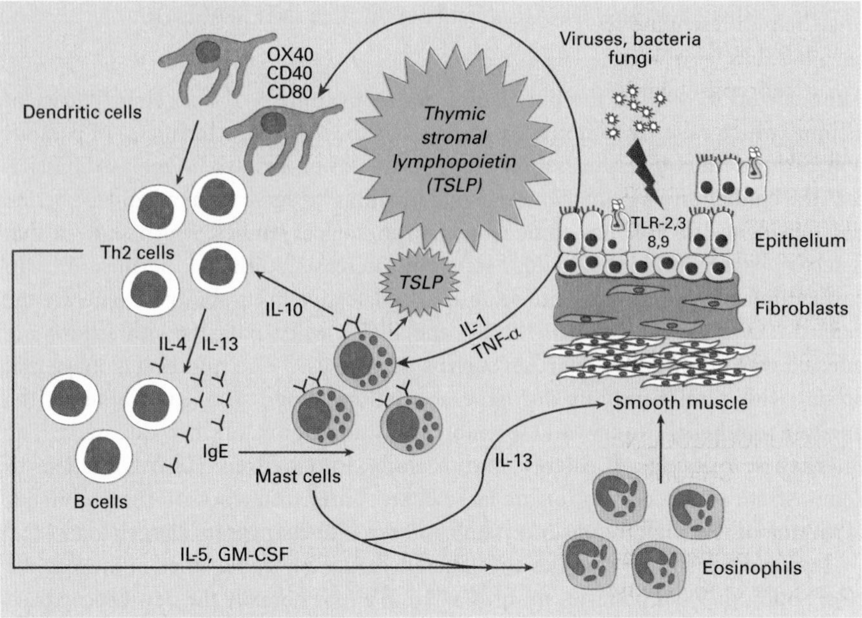

Fig 4 Proposed central role played by thymic stromal lymphopoietin (TSLP) secreted by epithelial cells and mast cells in supporting a Th2-type inflammatory response in asthma. GM-CSF = granulocyte–macrophage colony-stimulating factor; Ig = immunoglobulin; IL = interleukin; TLR = toll-like receptor; TNF = tumour necrosis factor. Reproduced from Holgate with permission of Elsevier.[18]

asthma is well controlled according to a standardised and validated asthma control questionnaire in only 28% of patients in a large European population, which means that 72% of patients have uncontrolled or inadequately controlled disease.[19] The reason for this less than optimal response to modern inhaled drugs most frequently relates to patients not wishing to take these drugs on a regular basis for fear of side-effects, of acquisition of treatment tolerance, or that aspects of their asthma are insensitive to these treatments.

In patients with chronic asthma, one important factor is the presence of comorbidities, especially chronic rhinitis, sinusitis, atopic dermatitis, and gastro-oesophageal reflux. It is important, therefore, that these comorbidities are recognised in the management of patients with asthma. For example, adequate treatment of chronic rhinosinusitis has been shown to have a beneficial effect on the clinical expression of asthma and vice versa. Provocation of the nose by allergens in patients with rhinitis aggravates asthma, while the opposite is true for lower airways challenge.

The addition of cysteinyl leukotriene receptor antagonists (LTRAs) such as montelukast has been shown to add some benefit to treatment with inhaled corticosteroids, but this treatment is not effective in all patients. An advantage of montelukast is that it can be taken orally once daily and, because it is systemically bioavailable, it is thus able to beneficially affect the upper and lower airways. Recent genetic studies have suggested that some patients are more responsive to oral LTRAs because of polymorphic variations in the leukotriene generating pathway or cysteinyl leukotriene receptors, which raises the possibility that pharmacogenetics may help differentiate responders from non-responders in the future.[20] Pharmacogenetics has also identified variations in responses to short- and long-acting β_2 adrenoceptor agonists, particularly in patients with the Arg16Arg genotype that predicts reduced responsiveness to bronchodilators.[20] At present, genetic profiling of patients' therapeutic responses has not found clinical utility in patients with asthma, but it does offer an exciting future for more personalised medicine, especially with the increasing use of expensive products.

Recognition that 5–10% of patients with asthma have severe disease not adequately controlled with inhaled drugs means that the remainder of this review will be devoted to two new treatments being evaluated in chronic severe disease: anti-human IgE and anti-TNF biologics.

☐ IMMUNOGLOBULIN E AS A TARGET FOR TREATMENT IN PATIENTS WITH SEVERE CHRONIC ASTHMA

In 1921, Prausnitz and Küstner first identified 'reagin' – the circulating substance that could passively transfer immediate type allergic responses from one individual to another in the Prausnitz–Küstner (P–K) reaction. The molecular basis of reagin as the fifth immunoglobulin class IgE was recognised by Ishizaka and Johansson in 1968, and this provided a therapeutic target for intervention not only in asthma but also in other allergic diseases. Immunoglobulin E produced by B cells and plasma cells sensitises mast cells and basophils by binding with high affinity to the high-

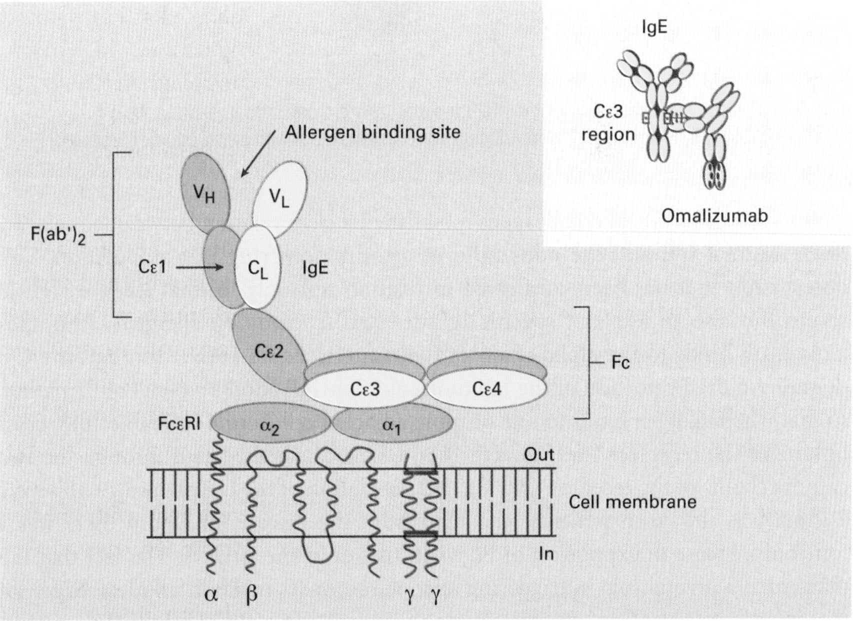

Fig 5 Immunoglobulin (Ig) E in a bent conformation when it binds to the high affinity IgE receptor. Cross linkage of two or more IgE molecules by allergen triggers mast cell activation via the two gamma chains. Top right: The humanised IgG anti-human IgE omalizumab binding to the Fc portion of IgE to block its binding to the high-affinity receptor.

affinity receptor ($Fc_{\varepsilon}R1$) (Fig 5). Cross linkage of cell-bound IgE then triggers release of preformed and newly generated mediators from mast cells and induces secretion of cytokines and chemokines. These mediators have direct effects on the airways, including smooth muscle contraction, microvascular leakage, stimulation of local and central neural reflexes, and increased secretion of mucus. They also lead to recruitment of inflammatory cells in the form of eosinophils and basophils and then T cells and monocytes, which, on migrating into the airways, become primed and activated to secrete their own mediators that contribute to the inflammatory milieu and an increase in disease expression (Fig 6).[21]

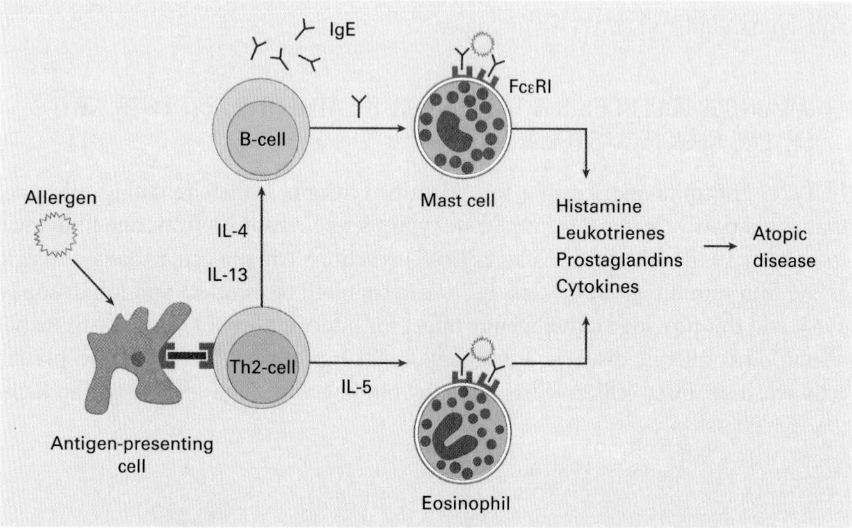

Fig 6 Schematic representation of the Th2-mediated allergic cascade in asthma. Ig = immunoglobulin; IL = interleukin. Reproduced from Holgate *et al* with permission of Elsevier.[21]

In 1989, Burrows and colleagues established a clear relation between circulating levels of total IgE and the odds ratio of asthma occurring in a population – an observation that has been confirmed in relation not only to total levels of IgE in serum but also to levels of specific IgE directed to common allergens. Immunoglobulin E binds to the alpha chain of the trimeric $Fc_{\varepsilon}R1$ ($\alpha\beta\gamma_2$) through the $C_{\varepsilon}3$ domain on the Fc portion of the IgE molecule. The IgE adopts a bent confirmation, so that when allergen binds to one or more adjacent cell-bound IgE molecules, cross linking of the receptors leads to activation of mast cells mediated through the two gamma chains of the receptor (Fig 5). The association of the IgE pathway with severe asthma was shown in patients who died from the disease, in whom there was a fourfold increase in expression of $Fc_{\varepsilon}R1$ in tissues in the airways. The fact that IgE plays such a pivotal role in triggering allergic responses makes it an ideal target for therapeutic intervention. The discovery that blockade of IgE with an IgG monoclonal antibody directed to the $C_{\varepsilon}3$ domain could attenuate allergen-induced early- and late-phase asthmatic responses led to this becoming a potential therapeutic target for patients with severe allergic asthma.[21]

The IgG2 monoclonal antibody omalizumab is humanised and contains <3% mouse peptide sequence in the antigen binding site. Omalizumab binds to IgE with high affinity, which results in the production of small trimeric and hexameric complexes that are rapidly eliminated by the reticuloendothelial system without activating complement. When administered by subcutaneous injection once or twice monthly to patients with moderate allergic asthma, omalizumab removes IgE immunoreactivity from the bronchial tissue in parallel with reduced expression of $Fc_{\varepsilon}R1$. This unusual response (that is, removal of IgE paralleled by loss of its receptor) is thought to be an important component of the therapeutic response (Fig 7).[22] The downstream consequence of interrupting the IgE signalling pathway is manifest as a reduction in eosinophil T-cell and B-cell infiltration of the wall of the airways and a reduction in sputum and airway mucosal eosinophilia.

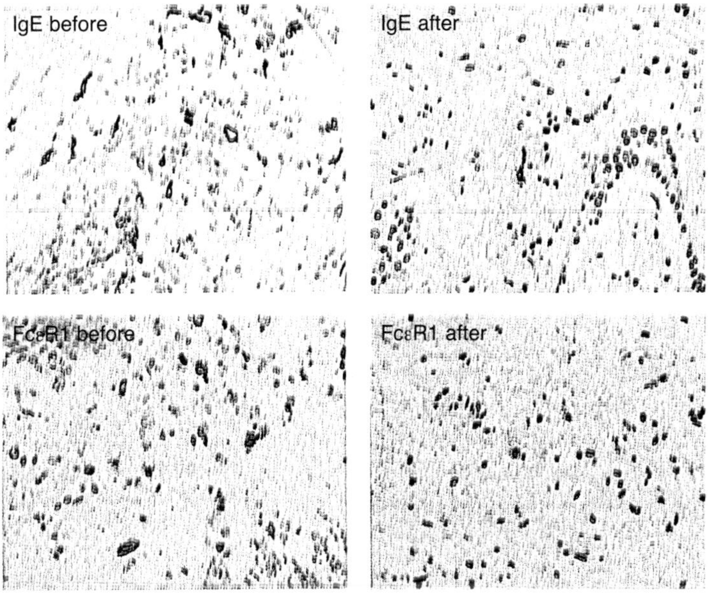

Fig 7 Sections of airway mucosa from patients with mild asthma immunostained for immunoglobulin (Ig) E (top) and the alpha chain of the high-affinity IgE receptor (bottom) before (left) and after (right) 12 weeks of treatment with omalizumab showing parallel loss of IgE and its receptor on mast cells and basophils. Reproduced from Djukanovic *et al* with permission of the American Thoracic Society.[22]

A series of seven clinical trials that involved 2,511 patients and 1,797 controls confirm the clinical efficacy of this drug in patients with severe allergic asthma, which was defined as baseline forced expiratory volume in one second (FEV_1) about 70% of predicted despite treatment with corticosteroids at a dose equivalent to up to 1500 μg of inhaled beclomethasone dipropionate (BDP) and, in 60% of patients, long-acting β_2 adrenoceptor agonists.[23] The annualised exacerbation rate across the treatment period was reduced by almost 40% with omalizumab, with even greater clinical impacts on hospital admissions, accident and emergency visits, and unscheduled doctor visits. The observations were confirmed in the subsequent investigation of omalizumab in severe asthma treatment (INNOVATE) study, which compared omalizumab with placebo in patients with even more severe asthma, which was defined as baseline FEV_1 61% predicted despite taking corticosteroids equivalent to an excess of 2300 μg BDP daily and, in all patients, a long-acting β_2 adrenoceptor agonist.[24] One fifth of this population was receiving regular oral corticosteroids, one third was taking xanthines, and one third was taking leukotriene receptor antagonists. This trial necessitated an adjustment of baseline prior to analysis because of a significant imbalance in the baseline values between the active and placebo arms of the study. At the end of the treatment, a significant 30% improvement in annual exacerbation rates was seen in the active group compared to the placebo group. This study also found a 40–50% reduction in severe exacerbations and total emergency visit rates, as well as an almost 50% increase in asthma-related quality of life (as measured on five domains of the Juniper questionnaire) with omalizumab.

The dose of omalizumab is calculated from an algorithm that involves total levels of IgE in serum and body weight. In effect, this means that treatment is restricted to those whose levels of IgE are >30 IU/ml but <700 IU/ml. In these studies, the only predictor of clinical response was the baseline level of total IgE in serum and the physicians' overall assessment of the clinical response taking into account symptom control, rescue treatment, and lung function.[25] The European licence for omalizumab states that treatment effectiveness must be assessed by the doctor 16 weeks after treatment is started in order for further injections to be administered, with the decision to continue treatment based on whether or not a marked improvement in overall asthma control is seen. With about 43,000 prescriptions in North America and an increasing number of patients using this treatment in the rest of the world, surprisingly little in the way of side-effects has been reported. A slight, but not significant, increase in the incidence of parasitic infections was reported in a study conducted in South America, and anaphylaxis has been reported occasionally.

Omalizumab undoubtedly is a step forward in the treatment of severe allergic asthma. Its true potential probably has not been realised, however, as it has been shown to have effects across a wide spectrum of allergic disorders, including rhinoconjunctivitis, sinusitis, and food allergy. It is becoming increasingly important to view asthma as part of a systemic allergic disorder and to develop new ways of measuring the effect of novel antiallergic treatments that extend beyond the lung.[26] The fact that the marked improvement in quality of life patients experience with omalizumab contrasts with the relatively small improvements in baseline lung function possibly reflects this drug's effects on aspects of asthma and allergic disease in organs that previously have not been the focus of attention.

Cost is the key issue that will influence whether or not omalizumab will become available for widespread use in the UK. At the time of writing, its cost effectiveness is being evaluated by the National Institute of Health and Clinical Excellence (NICE), and its use elsewhere in Europe is being monitored very carefully.

□ ANTI-TNF IN THE MANAGEMENT OF ASTHMA

Demonstration that epithelial injury and aberrant repair, in effect, create a chronic wound scenario that underpins severe refractory asthma has provided an opportunity to pursue further novel treatments. One feature of severe refractory asthma is the presence of neutrophils – alone or in addition to eosinophils – in sputum, fluid from bronchoalveolar lavage (BAL), and bronchial biopsies.[27] Neutrophilia is also a common feature of patients with asthma who smoke, whose response to corticosteroids is also impaired.[28] A study of bronchial biopsies in patients with severe asthma showed that airway neutrophilia occurs in parallel with increased epithelial injury and the secretion of the neutrophil chemokine IL-8. Other tissue-damaging immune diseases in which neutrophils dominate often involve the pleotropic cytokine TNF-α. Tumour necrosis factor is produced predominantly by macrophages, monocytes, Th1-type T cells, mast cells, epithelial cells, and eosinophils. Tumour necrosis factor α is a 17 kD type 2 membrane glycosylated protein that contains 157 amino acids; it is cleaved by ADAM17 (TNF-α cleaving enzyme (TACE)) to give an active soluble form of TNF-α that forms trimers. Soluble TNF-α acts via two receptors – p55 (CD120a) and p75 (CD120b) – and exerts a wide variety of effects on most cells in the lung, with the overall response being an increase in the expression of functions pertinent to that particular cell type. For example, TNF-α increases smooth muscle contractility, microvascular leakage, and secretion of mucus and augments secretion of mediators from most inflammatory cells.[27]

Patients who have died from asthma have increased immunostaining for TNF-α in their airways – an observation that was confirmed in bronchial biopsy studies in patients with severe asthma that required daily oral and high-dose inhaled corticosteroids and long-acting β adrenoceptor agonists.[29] In bronchial biopsies, TNF was predominantly localised to mast cells, eosinophils, and macrophages and was found in association with a 30-fold increase in mRNA for TNF-α when assessed by quantitative polymerase chain reaction (qPCR). Increased tissue expression of TNF-α, as well as increased levels in fluids from BAL and induced sputum, even in patients treated with oral and inhaled corticosteroids, suggest that this cytokine is not suppressed by conventional anti-inflammatory treatment.

A proof-of-concept clinical trial with etanercept (a soluble fusion protein of the p75 TNF receptor and the Fc region of human IgG) was investigated in 15 patients with chronic severe asthma who were taking regular oral corticosteroids, high-dose inhaled corticosteroids, salmeterol or theophylline, or their combination. Patients were given 25 mg etanercept by subcutaneous injection twice a week for 12 weeks, and efficacy was assessed as bronchial responsiveness to inhaled methacholine (a measure of non-specific bronchial hyper-responsiveness), symptoms of asthma, quality of life, and lung function. Although this was an open-label study, etanercept produced a marked reduction in symptoms and improvements in control of asthma in parallel with an overall 2.5-fold doubling dilution increase in provocation concentration producing a 20% fall from baseline FEV_1 (PC_{20}) for methacholine, which indicated a marked reduction in bronchial hyper-responsiveness beyond that achieved with corticosteroids (Fig 8[29]). In a subsequent double-blind, placebo-controlled, crossover study of etanercept in a similar group of patients with severe asthma, Berry and coworkers also found a marked improvement in asthma-related quality of life and symptoms, which was paralleled by a reduction in methacholine bronchial hyper-responsiveness (a 3.5-fold doubling dilution increase in PC_{20}) as well as improvements in baseline lung function (Fig 9).[30] This study also showed that patients with severe asthma had higher circulating mononuclear cell membrane-expression of TNF-α, ADAM17, and p55 and p75 receptors than patients with mild-to-moderate disease or normal controls, which suggests that these biomarkers are pathophysiologically relevant to this type of asthma. Of further interest was the fact that the clinical efficacy of anti-TNF treatment in patients with severe asthma was strongly predicted by the level of expression of membrane-associated TNF, which suggests that this might be a useful biomarker for differentiating treatment responders from non-responders. As with other chronic diseases such as rheumatoid arthritis, psoriasis, and inflammatory bowel disease, patients with asthma may be responders and non-responders to anti-TNF treatment. Thus, a method to identify patients with severe asthma most likely to respond to this type of treatment would be of great significance by enabling expensive treatments to be focused on those who would best benefit. Experience with anti-TNF antibodies in the treatment of asthma is limited; one recent study with infliximab is encouraging but emphasised the need for studies in patients with more severe disease.[31]

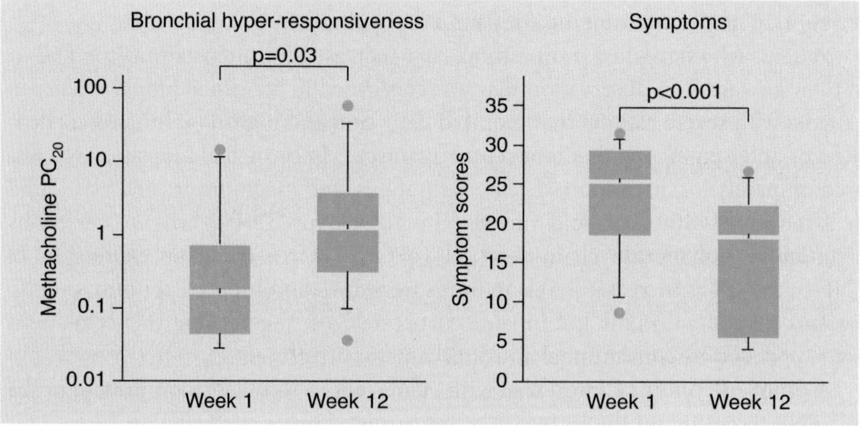

Fig 8 The effect of 10 weeks' treatment with etanercept on methacholine airway responsiveness (left) and asthma symptoms (right) in 15 symptomatic patients with severe asthma who were taking regular high-dose inhaled and oral corticosteroids. Reproduced from Howarth *et al* with permission of BMJ Publishing Group Ltd.[29]

In terms of possible mechanisms, TNF-α has many different effects on the airways, but the prominent mechanism seems to be its ability to increase hyper-responsiveness of the airways and contractility of smooth muscle by altering cellular calcium fluxes. Etanercept's marked effect on methacholine hyper-responsiveness despite the fact that patients were taking a wide variety of other asthma drugs including oral corticosteroids would support this as a mechanism. Other possible effects of anti-TNF treatment include a reduction in infiltration of inflammatory cells through inhibition of leukocyte recruitment and the priming of a large number of different inflammatory and structural cells within the airways. Large clinical trials are in progress to assess the clinical efficacy of anti-TNF, with a focus on chronic severe asthma as the target phenotype.

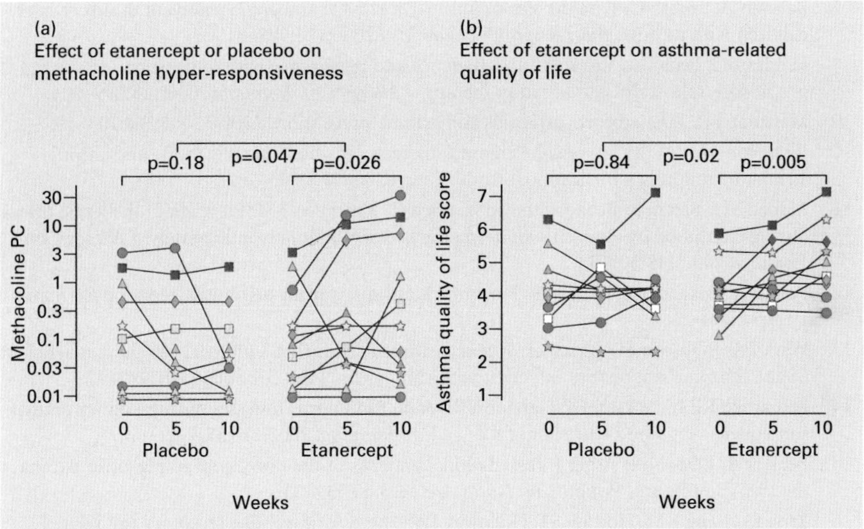

Fig 9 Effects of etanercept for 10 weeks on airway hyper-responsiveness and asthma-related quality of life in a crossover randomised controlled trial in 10 patients with severe corticosteroid-refractory asthma. Reproduced from Berry MA *et al* with permission of Massachusetts Medical Society.[30]

☐ CONCLUDING COMMENTS

Increased understanding of the cellular and molecular basis of chronic asthma is beginning to reveal novel therapeutic targets. Although attempts to manipulate the allergic cascade have shown benefits with the anti-IgE agent omalizumab, this biological agent is highly effective in only about half of the patients who receive it. Much still needs to be understood about the underlying basis of chronic severe asthma – not only with respect to the best interventions but also with respect to whether some phenotypes within the population of people with asthma will respond to specific types of therapy to a greater extent than others. The days when asthma was considered a homogenous disease are now passing, with renewed focus on subphenotypes and tailoring of specific treatments to the needs of individual patients.

REFERENCES

1 Holgate ST, Polosa R. The mechanisms, diagnosis, and management of severe asthma in adults. *Lancet* 2006;368:780–93.

2 Holgate ST, Holloway J, Wilson S *et al.* Understanding the pathophysiology of severe asthma to generate new therapeutic opportunities. *J Allergy Clin Immunol* 2006;117:496–506.

3 Janssen LJ, Killian K. Airway smooth muscle as a target of asthma therapy: history and new directions. *Respir Res* 2006;7:123.

4 Davies DE, Wicks J, Powell RM, Puddicombe SM, Holgate ST. Airway remodeling in asthma: new insights. *J Allergy Clin Immunol* 2003;111:215–25.

5 Wicks J, Haitchi HM, Holgate ST, Davies DE, Powell RM. Enhanced upregulation of smooth muscle related transcripts by TGF beta2 in asthmatic (myo) fibroblasts. *Thorax* 2006;61:313–9.

6 Holgate ST. Susceptibility genes in severe asthma. *Curr Allergy Asthma Rep* 2006;6:345–8.

7 Barbato A, Turato G, Baraldo S *et al.* Epithelial damage and angiogenesis in the airways of children with asthma. *Am J Respir Crit Care Med* 2006;174;975–81.
8 Bender BG, Pedan A, Varasteh LT. Adherence and persistence with fluticasone propionate/salmeterol combination therapy. *J Allergy Clin Immunol* 2006;118:899–904.
9 Martinez FD. Inhaled corticosteroids and asthma prevention. *Lancet* 2006;368:708–10.
10 Illi S, von Mutius S, Lau S *et al.* Perennial allergen sensitisation early in life and chronic asthma in children: a birth cohort study. *Lancet* 2006:368:763–70.
11 Arshad SH, Bateman B, Sadeghnejad A, Gant C, Matthews SM. Prevention of allergic disease during childhood by allergen avoidance: the Isle of Wight prevention study. *J Allergy Clin Immunol* 2007;119:307–13.
12 Pearce N, Pekkanen J, Beasley R. How much asthma is really attributable to atopy? *Thorax* 1999;54:268–72.
13 Wark PA, Johnston SL, Bucchieri F *et al.* Asthmatic bronchial epithelial cells have a deficient innate immune response to infection with rhinovirus. *J Exp Med* 2005;201;937–47.
14 Lemanske RF Jr, Jackson DJ, Gangnon RE *et al.* Rhinovirus illnesses during infancy predict subsequent childhood wheezing. *J Allergy Clin Immunol* 2005;116:571–7.
15 Beasley R, Ellwood P, Asher I. International patterns of the prevalence of pediatric asthma the ISAAC program. *Pediatr Clin North Am* 2003;50;539–53.
16 Yang IA, Fong KM, Holgate ST, Holloway JW. The role of toll-like receptors and related receptors of the innate immune system in asthma. *Curr Opin Allergy Clin Immunol* 2006; 6:23–8.
17 Liu YJ. Thymic stromal lymphopoeitin: master switch for allergic inflammation. *J Exp Med* 2006;203:269–73.
18 Holgate ST. The epithelium takes centre stage in asthma and atopic dermatitis. *Trends Immunol* 2007;28:248–51.
19 Dockrell M, Partridge MR, Valovirta E. The limitations of severe asthma: the results of a European survey. *Allergy* 2007;62:134–41.
20 Hall IP. Pharmacogenetics of asthma. *Chest* 2006;130:1873–8.
21 Holgate S, Casale T, Wenzel S *et al.* The anti-inflammatory effects of omalizumab confirm the central role of IgE in allergic inflammation. *J Allergy Clin Immunol* 2005;115:459–65.
22 Djukanovic R, Wilson SJ, Kraft M *et al.* Effects of treatment with anti-immunoglobulin E antibody omalizumab on airway inflammation in allergic asthma. *Am J Respir Crit Care Med* 2004;170:583–93.
23 D'Amato G. Role of anti-IgE monoclonal antibody (omalizumab) in the treatment of bronchial asthma and allergic respiratory diseases. *Eur J Pharmacol* 2006;533:302–7.
24 Humbert M, Beasley R, Ayres J *et al.* Benefits of omalizumab as add-on therapy in patients with severe persistent asthma who are inadequately controlled despite best available therapy (GINA 2002 step 4 treatment): INNOVATE. *Allergy* 2005;60:309–16.
25 Bousquet J, Rabe K, Humbert M *et al.* Predicting and evaluating response to omalizumab in patients with severe allergic asthma. *Respir Med* 2007;101:1483–92.
26 Price D, Holgate ST. Improving outcomes for asthma patients with allergic rhinitis: conclusions from the MetaForum conferences. *BMC Pulm Med* 2006;6(Suppl 1):S7.
27 Tomlinson JE, McMahon AD, Chaudhuri R *et al.* Efficacy of low and high dose inhaled corticosteroid in smokers versus non-smokers with mild asthma. *Thorax* 2005;60:282–7.
38 Russo C, Polosa R. TNF-alpha as a promising therapeutic target in chronic asthma: a lesson from rheumatoid arthritis. *Clin Sci (Lond)* 2005;109:135–42.
29 Howarth PH, Babu KS, Arshad HS *et al.* Tumour necrosis factor (TNF-alpha) as a novel therapeutic target in symptomatic corticosteroid dependant asthma. *Thorax* 2005;60:1012–8.
30 Berry MA, Hargadon B, Shelley M *et al.* Evidence of a role of tumor necrosis factor alpha in refractory asthma. *N Engl J Med* 2006;354:697–708.
31 Erin EM, Leaker BR, Nicholson GC *et al.* The effects of a monoclonal antibody directed against tumor necrosis factor-alpha in asthma. *Am J Respir Crit Care Med* 2006;174:753–62.

New developments in pleural disease

Najib M Rahman and Robert JO Davies

□ INTRODUCTION

Pleural effusion is a common problem in clinical practice, and although no high-quality epidemiological studies have addressed the incidence of the pleural effusion syndromes, there are estimated to be 250,000 new cases of malignant pleural effusion and 60,000 new cases of pleural infection per year in the United Kingdom and United States. This article will address recent advances in the diagnosis and management of the more common pleural fluid syndromes.

□ MALIGNANT PLEURAL EFFUSION – DIAGNOSTIC STRATEGIES

The incidence of malignant pleural effusion is estimated to be about 660 patients per million population per year. About 50% of patients referred to respiratory medicine for the investigation of pleural effusion are found to have malignancy, with more than 10% of cancers presenting de novo with pleural effusion. The most common causes of malignant pleural effusion are secondary spread from lung, breast, lymphoma, or ovarian primaries, with the primary remaining unknown in a substantial number of cases (often associated histologically with adenocarcinoma).[1] Malignant mesothelioma is the major primary pleural cancer, and an epidemic of deaths from mesothelioma over the next 20 years is predicted in association with high rates of asbestos importation in the 1960s and 1970s.

Diagnosis of malignant pleural effusion ultimately relies on histocytological confirmation of malignant cells within pleural fluid or tissue. The initial recommended investigation, therefore, is diagnostic thoracocentesis to establish the presence of a transudate or exudate (these are covered in detail elsewhere,[2] although it should be noted that up to 10% of unilateral transudative effusions are due to malignancy) and pleural infection and for cytological analysis. In the hands of an experienced pathologist, a single pleural aspiration will diagnose malignancy in around 60% of cases, and a second, although not a third, sample modestly increases diagnostic yield.[1]

Contrast-enhanced thoracic computed tomography (CT) is the next investigation of choice in the presence of negative cytology and has a high sensitivity for malignant pleural disease.[1] It shows the anatomy of the pleural surfaces and allows examination of the underlying lung (for intraparenchymal malignancy or major airway blockage) and mediastinal structures. Pleural thoracic CT is best performed before complete fluid drainage and with contrast enhancement during the late venous phase. This allows assessment of pleural nodularity and thickening, which have been shown to reliably predict malignant pleural disease (Fig 1).

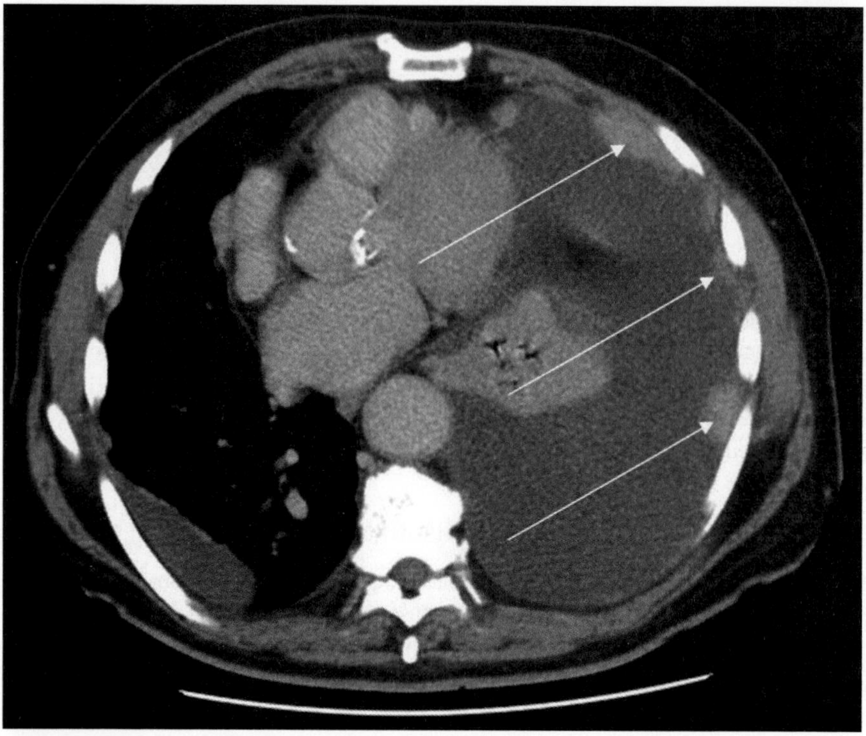

Fig 1 Contrast-enhanced thoracic computed tomography in the late venous phase, showing areas of pleural nodularity (arrows).

Although thoracic CT may suggest features of malignant pleural involvement, histological or cytological confirmation of diagnosis is required, as it will usually influence further treatment (in terms of chemotherapy, radiotherapy, and, specifically, tract site radiotherapy in mesothelioma), may permit compensation claims to be made, and is likely to inform prognosis. Traditionally, the next step in diagnosis was a closed or 'blind' pleural biopsy (eg Abram's biopsies), which increased yield by 7–27% above cytology alone in malignant pleural effusion, with lower diagnostic yields in mesothelioma.[1] The process of pleural malignancy often affects the pleura in a patchy way and preferentially in the basal pleural areas, so a 'blind' technique – usually that avoids the basal areas – is likely to have a low yield.

Recent evidence suggests that CT-guided pleural biopsy has a high diagnostic yield in malignant pleural effusion. Maskell *et al*[3] directly compared CT-guided pleural biopsy and Abram's pleural biopsy in a randomised trial in patients with cytologically negative pleural exudates. Fifty patients underwent thoracic CT and were then randomised to Abram's needle biopsy by an experienced operator or CT-guided biopsy. Thirty two patients, 19 of whom had mesothelioma, were randomised; the numbers of patients with minimal (<5 mm) pleural thickening on initial CT were equal in each group (n=17). Computed tomography-guided biopsy had a significantly higher diagnostic yield, with sensitivity of 47% for Abram's biopsy and 87% for CT-guided biopsy (p=0.02).[3] This translates to avoidance of repeat biopsy in 40% of cases when CT is used as the initial biopsy technique, and these results have led many centres to abandon the use of blind pleural biopsy for malignant pleural effusion.

Although CT-guided biopsy has a high diagnostic yield for malignant pleural effusion, patients may need subsequent invasive procedures to drain symptomatic pleural effusion and prevent recurrence. Physician-based local anaesthetic thoracoscopy (conducted under conscious sedation rather than general anaesthetic) is a valuable technique in this setting, permitting pleural biopsy of abnormal-looking tissue under direct vision, total drainage of the chest, and pleurodesis in a single procedure. The diagnostic rate of thoracoscopy is likely to be comparable to that of CT-guided biopsy, with retrospective series suggesting a sensitivity of more than 90% for malignant pleural disease.[4]

Given the higher diagnostic yield of other techniques, Abram's biopsy is not recommended in the diagnostic work up of potential malignant pleural effusion when facilities for other techniques are available.

□ TUBERCULOUS PLEURITIS – DIAGNOSTIC STRATEGY

Tuberculous pleuritis, which is a distinct clinical entity from tuberculous empyema, is a result of delayed hypersensitivity reaction to mycobacteria within the pleural space. The resulting pleural effusion is therefore relatively low in mycobacterial load, characteristically inflammatory according to biochemical criteria, and associated with a lymphocytic exudate. Pleural fluid thoracocentesis therefore is often negative for Ziehl–Nielsen stain and mycobacterial culture, and pleural histology (which shows a caseating granulomatous reaction) is usually needed to establish the diagnosis.

Tuberculous pleuritis affects the entire pleural surface in a diffuse uniform manner, and 'blind' pleural biopsy techniques therefore are associated with a high diagnostic yield. Most studies report a combined sensitivity for Abram's biopsy and culture of around 80%.[5] Abram's biopsy was recently compared directly with thoracoscopy in a trial of 51 patients in an area in which tuberculosis is endemic.[5] Thoracoscopy had a higher diagnostic yield for tuberculous pleuritis than closed pleural biopsy (sensitivity and specificity of 100% for thoracoscopy (for combined histology and culture) *v* sensitivity of 79% and specificity of 100% for closed pleural biopsy).[5] This results in a negative predictive value of 100% for thoracoscopy compared with 50% for Abram's biopsy. Thus, although the high diagnostic yield and ready availability of closed pleural biopsy make it a reasonable technique for suspected tuberculous pleuritis, thoracoscopy has been shown to have the highest diagnostic yield of any technique to date. It therefore is reasonable to use closed pleural biopsy as an initial investigation in patients with suspected tuberculous pleuritis unless local facilities for thoracoscopy exist.

□ PREVENTING RECURRENCE OF PLEURAL FLUID

Although most pleural effusions result from malignant disease, disabling and symptomatic recurrent effusions may occur in patients with cardiac, liver, and connective tissue diseases. Removal of pleural fluid by thoracocentesis or intercostal drainage alleviates symptoms, but it is painful as the chest wall and parietal pleura are heavily innervated by sensory nerves. Most malignant effusions recur after single drainage, with recurrence rates of up to 100% at one month. Definitive management is recommended in most patients with good performance status,[1] and pleurodesis achieves this by causing adherence of the visceral and parietal pleural surfaces through induction of irritant inflammation to ablate the pleural cavity.

A variety of agents have been investigated as potential pleurodesis agents; sterile talc (magnesium silicate) has been shown in trials to be the most effective, with efficacy of 88–100% at one month.[1] Pleurodesis with talc has been associated with a number of adverse effects, however; in an international survey of more than 800 respiratory physicians, more than half reported seeing cases of respiratory distress after talc pleurodesis either via chest drain (slurry) or during thoracoscopy (poudrage).[6] The literature contains 30 case reports of adult respiratory distress syndrome (ARDS) developing after the administration of talc (19 cases after slurry and 15 cases after poudrage), nine of which were fatal. Animal models of pleurodesis with talc have shown that talc particles are distributed widely throughout the tissues (including the abdominal cavity and brain),[7] and this is thought to be mediated by lymphatic pores within the parietal pleura (the pores of Wang), which have a fixed diameter of around 10 mm. Talc used in Europe was subsequently found to be 'graded' – ie sifted to exclude small particles (<15 mm) – whereas talc used in the United States does not undergo this process ('mixed' talc).[8] Most reported cases of ARDS occurred in areas with mixed talc that included small particles (<15 mm) rather than 'graded' talc, and toxicity was hypothesised to relate to the small particles escaping via the parietal pores.

A randomised trial to assess the systemic response to pleurodesis agents therefore was conducted. Maskell *et al* recruited patients who required pleurodesis for malignant pleural effusion and initially randomised them to receive tetracycline or talc pleurodesis.[8] Significantly higher levels of lung inflammation (measured by isotope scanning) and systemic inflammation (measured by levels of C-reactive protein (CRP)) were seen with talc than with tetracycline. Forty-eight patients were randomised to pleurodesis with mixed talc (n=24) and graded talc (n=24), and significantly larger effects on gas exchange and lung and systemic inflammation were seen in those who received pleurodesis with mixed talc. Graded talc resulted in a small change (0.7 kPA) in arterial oxygen after pleurodesis, whereas mixed talc caused a decrease of about 2 kPA; the difference was statistically significant (p=0.01). The systemic inflammatory response was higher in the graded talc group, as evidenced by a larger increase in levels of CRP in blood (100 µg/l *v* 150 µg/l, p=0.04)[8] (Fig 2). Taken together, these data suggest that the use of mixed talc is associated with increased systemic and pulmonary inflammatory responses, perhaps mediated by the mechanisms proposed above. Two large studies conducted recently enable indirect comparison of the talcs used in the United States (mixed) and Europe (graded). A large American study to assess the success rate of pleurodesis with thoracoscopy compared with the conventional tube method reported a rate of ARDS of around 4% in a population of 400 patients who received mixed talc.[9] In contrast, a large European cohort study prospectively analysed 500 cases in which graded talc was given at thoracoscopy and found not a single incidence of ARDS.[10]

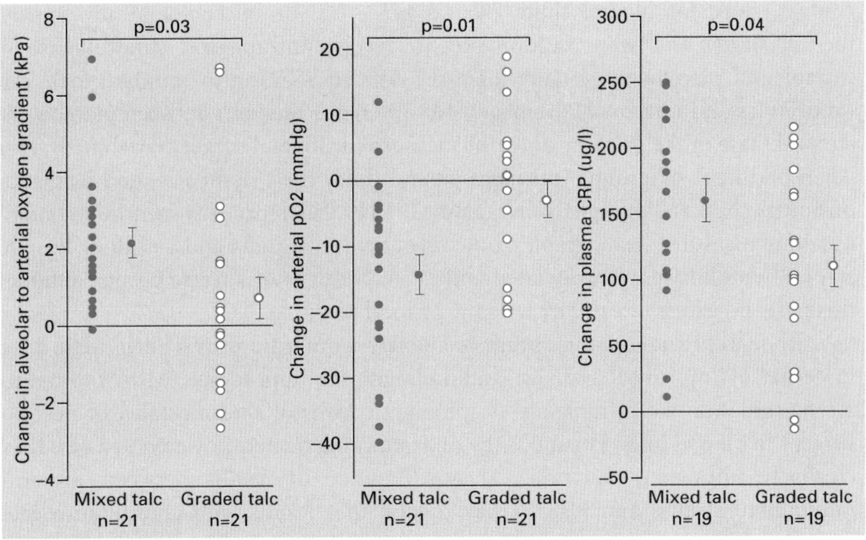

Fig 2 Changes in arterial oxygenation and levels of C-reactive protein (CRP) after pleurodesis with mixed and graded talc. Adapted from Maskell *et al* with permission of the American Thoracic Society.[8]

In summary, talc is the most effective pleurodesis agent for recurrent pleural effusion. Graded talc seems to be associated with fewer systemic side-effects, including ARDS.

☐ PLEURAL INFECTION: INTRAPLEURAL FIBRINOLYTIC TREATMENT

During the evolution of pleural infection, normal pleural physiology is altered in response to bacterial invasion. As proinflammatory cytokines are produced, tissue permeability increases, which results in the formation of a pleural exudate and downregulation of the normal fibrinolytic system. Fibrinous membranes and adhesions therefore form within the fluid, which results in a loculated pleural collection. Attempts to drain the collection with a single intercostal drain are likely to fail, so agents with the potential to lyse these septations (such as fibrinolytic drugs) have been investigated.[11]

A large number of case reports and case series have suggested benefit when fibrinolytic drugs are used to improve pleural drainage or reduce the size of radiographic collections. These reports led to five small randomised trials that included a total of 104 adults and showed benefit from the use of intrapleural streptokinase or urokinase over placebo in improving drainage and hospital stay in patients with pleural infection.[11] A meta-analysis, however, concluded that insufficient evidence existed to support the routine use of intrapleural fibrinolytic therapy in pleural infection.[12]

With this background, the first Multicentre Intrapleural Sepsis Trial (MIST1)[13] recruited 454 patients from 52 centres in the United Kingdom and was powered to assess whether intrapleural streptokinase changed the clinically meaningful endpoints of death or need for surgery, or both. Patients were recruited on the basis of established diagnostic criteria for pleural infection (that is, in the correct clinical context, purulent pleural fluid, pleural pH <7.2, or microbiologically positive pleural fluid) and were randomised to receive intrapleural streptokinase or intrapleural placebo twice daily for three days in addition to standard local care (antibiotics and intercostal drainage). No difference was seen between placebo and streptokinase in the primary outcome measure (death and surgery combined), even when pertinent subgroups (purulent pleural fluid, chest drain size, and loculation on initial chest radiograph) were analysed.[13] No difference was seen in secondary outcome measures (radiographic outcome at three months and length of hospital stay). Streptokinase was associated with a small excess of adverse events, although there was no excess of cases of systemic or local bleeding.

Although previous studies suggested benefit from intrapleural fibrinolytic drugs in terms of improved drainage and radiographic appearance, MIST1 provided strong evidence that intrapleural streptokinase does not alter mortality or need for surgery in pleural infection and is the only study adequately powered to assess these clinically important outcomes. The difference in results between previous randomised studies and MIST1 may suggest that results with clinical surrogates (such as radiographic change and length of hospital stay) do not necessarily translate to a benefit in terms of mortality or a decrease in the rate of surgery.

Although MIST1 suggested no benefit from the use of intrapleural streptokinase, other intrapleural agents are being investigated. Streptokinase may not be the optimal agent in the context of pleural infection, as it requires a minimum concentration of endogenous plasminogen to exert fibrinolytic effects. The level of endogenous plasminogen within the pleural space is likely to be low in patients with pleural infection, and direct plasminogen activators (which bypass the need for high levels of endogenous plasminogen) are therefore a potential candidate for lysing septations within an infected pleural space. In addition, a fibrinolytic drug alone may be inadequate for chest drainage because of the viscidity of intrapleural pus. Several in vitro studies suggest that fibrinolytic drugs do not decrease the viscidity of pus, which is thought to be due to the presence of uncoiled DNA strands, whereas enzymes capable of degrading DNA (for example, DNase) have significant effects on the viscidity of pus and have been shown to aid drainage of pus through a filter in vitro. The successful use of DNase after failed fibrinolytic treatment was reported in a case report[14] and DNase has been used successfully in three cases treated in our unit. The combination of a direct plasminogen activator and DNase is likely to be synergistic and is the subject of a randomised controlled trial (MIST2).

In summary, current evidence does not support the routine use of intrapleural fibrinolytic drugs in patients with pleural infection, as it does not alter clinically meaningful outcomes. It is perfectly reasonable, however, to use intrapleural fibrinolytic drugs when a large volume of loculated infected pleural fluid is producing respiratory embarrassment in order to aid decompression of the hemithorax.

☐ ADVANCES IN UNDERSTANDING – THE BACTERIOLOGY OF PLEURAL INFECTION

Studies that assessed the bacteriology of pleural infection have demonstrated varied patterns of microbiology but have consistently shown a difference between community-acquired disease and hospital-acquired disease (in a manner analogous to that with pneumonia) and consistently found that around 40% of cases remain bacteriologically obscure.[11] The high rate of 'culture-negative' empyema implies that empirical treatment will be needed for the duration of the treatment of a large number of cases. The microbiological pattern associated with pleural infection is increasingly recognised as distinct from that seen in pneumonia, which suggests that pneumonia may not be a necessary prerequisite for the development of pleural infection and perhaps suggests that the term 'parapneumonic effusion' is inaccurate in some cases.

The largest single series to address the bacteriology of pleural infection was published recently.[15] Samples from the cohort of patients enrolled to MIST1 (n=434) underwent detailed bacteriological analysis with standard methods (culture and Gram stain) and newer molecular techniques (bacterial DNA polymerase chain reaction (PCR)). Microbiological diagnosis was achieved with standard methods in 60% of cases, with a further 16% of cases diagnosed with bacterial PCR. The use of PCR decreased microbiologically obscure cases to 26% (from 42% using standard methods).[15] The importance of routine blood cultures in these patients is underlined by the finding in this cohort of 12% of patients with positive blood cultures but in whom all other microbiological tests were often negative.

This study showed that 36% of cases were due to a single aerobic organism, 9% were due to a single anaerobic organism, and 13% were polymicrobial infections.[15] Hospital- and community-acquired diseases were associated with distinct microbiological patterns, and the overall pattern of disease was quite different to that expected for pneumonia. The most common organisms seen in positive cultures from patients with community-acquired disease were from the *Streptococcus intermedius* group (around 30%, including *S. milleri*, *S. constellatus*, and *S. inonia*), *Streptococcus pneumoniae* (14%), and staphylococci (12%), with the remainder caused by a variety of other organisms, including Gram-negative organisms. Anaerobic infection was found – in isolation or in association with another organism – in 20% of cases. Multiresistant organisms were prevalent within the hospital-acquired subset – for example, staphylococci (50%) and Gram-negative organisms, including methicillin-resistant *Staphylococcus aureus* (MRSA, 28%), *Enterobacteriaceae* (20%), and enterococci (12%)[15] (Table 1).

The study also assessed whether survival was related to class of bacterial infection. Overall mortality for the study was 22%; patients with streptococcal disease had a relatively low mortality (17%) compared with those with Gram-negative infection (45%).[15] Streptococcal or anaerobic (including mixed anaerobic and aerobic) infection was associated with a substantially lower mortality than disease due to staphylococci, mixed aerobes, or *Enterobacteriaceae.* Although mortality was higher in patients with hospital-acquired infection, the difference in mortality according to bacterial class was independent of the source of infection. Organisms such as *Mycoplasma* and *Legionella* ('atypical' organisms) were rarely seen as a cause.

The bacteriological pattern seen in this study provides useful information to guide empirical antibiotic treatment by dividing cases according to the source of

Table 1 Results of positive bacteriology from the MIST1 cohort. Adapted from Maskell *et al* with permission of the American Thoracic Society.[15]

Organism	Positive isolates (%)
Community-acquired infection	
Streptococcus milleri group	32
Streptococcus pneumoniae	13
Other streptococci	7
Staphylococci*	11
Anaerobic organisms*	16
*Enterobacteriaceae**	7
Haemophilus influenzae	3
*Proteus**	3
Other	8
Hospital-acquired infection	
Methicillin-resistant *Staphylococcus aureus**	28
Staphylococci*	18
*Enterobacteriaceae**	16
Enterococci*	13
Anaerobic organisms*	5
Streptococcus milleri group	5
*Pseudomonas**	5
Other streptococci	5
Other	5

*Organism with resistance to 'standard' antibiotic therapy.

infection. In community-acquired pleural infection, 50% of organisms are resistant to penicillin and 20% have associated anaerobic infection that requires a combination of an anaerobic antibiotic and an agent such as penicillin plus a β-lactamase inhibitor. Most cases of hospital-acquired infection are associated with resistant organisms, with MRSA the cause in almost one third, so a combination of broad-spectrum antibiotic, antibiotic active against MRSA, and anaerobic cover is needed (for example, meropenem plus vancomycin).[11]

The implications of the different mortalities seen with different bacterial classes are uncertain. More aggressive treatment strategies for those with unfavourable bacteriology, perhaps including earlier surgical intervention, may be appropriate, although other factors that contribute to mortality in empyema have not been defined clearly, and further investigation is required.

REFERENCES

1 Antunes G, Neville E, Duffy J, Ali N. BTS guidelines for the management of malignant pleural effusions. *Thorax* 2003;58(Suppl 2):ii29–38.

2 Maskell NA, Butland RJ. BTS guidelines for the investigation of a unilateral pleural effusion in adults. *Thorax* 2003;58(Suppl 2):ii8–17.

3 Maskell NA, Gleeson FV, Davies RJ. Standard pleural biopsy versus CT-guided cutting-needle biopsy for diagnosis of malignant disease in pleural effusions: a randomised controlled trial. *Lancet* 2003;361:1326–30.

4 Blanc FX, Atassi K, Bignon J, Housset B. Diagnostic value of medical thoracoscopy in pleural disease: a 6-year retrospective study. *Chest* 2002;121:1677–83.

5 Diacon AH, Van de Wal BW, Wyser C *et al.* Diagnostic tools in tuberculous pleurisy: a direct comparative study. *Eur Respir J* 2003;22:589–91.

6 Lee YC, Baumann MH, Maskell NA *et al.* Pleurodesis practice for malignant pleural effusions in five English-speaking countries: survey of pulmonologists. *Chest* 2003;124:2229–38.

7 Werebe EC, Pazetti R, Milanez de Campos JR *et al.* Systemic distribution of talc after intrapleural administration in rats. *Chest* 1999;115:190–3.

8 Maskell NA, Lee YC, Gleeson FV *et al.* Randomized trials describing lung inflammation after pleurodesis with talc of varying particle size. *Am J Respir Crit Care Med* 2004;170:377–82.

9 Dresler CM, Olak J, Herndon JE *et al.* Phase III intergroup study of talc poudrage vs talc slurry sclerosis for malignant pleural effusion. *Chest* 2005;127:909–15.

10 Janssen JP, Collier G, Astoul P *et al.* Safety of pleurodesis with talc poudrage in malignant pleural effusion: a prospective cohort study. *Lancet* 2007;369:1535–9.

11 Davies CW, Gleeson FV, Davies RJ. BTS guidelines for the management of pleural infection. *Thorax* 2003;58(Suppl 2):ii18–28.

12 Cameron R, Davies HR. Intra-pleural fibrinolytic therapy versus conservative management in the treatment of parapneumonic effusions and empyema. *Cochrane Database Syst Rev* 2004;(1):CD002312.

13 Maskell NA, Davies CW, Nunn AJ *et al.* U.K. controlled trial of intrapleural streptokinase for pleural infection. *N Engl J Med* 2005;352:865–74.

14 Simpson G, Roomes D, Reeves B. Successful treatment of empyema thoracis with human recombinant deoxyribonuclease. *Thorax* 2003;58:365–6.

15 Maskell NA, Batt S, Hedley EL *et al.* The bacteriology of pleural infection by genetic and standard methods and its mortality significance. *Am J Respir Crit Care Med* 2006;174: 817–23.

Emphysema – lung volume reduction and beyond

Edward J Cetti and Duncan M Geddes

□ INTRODUCTION

Emphysema – from the Greek for 'to blow into' – is 'an increase beyond the normal in the size of the air spaces distal to the terminal bronchiole, accompanied by destruction of their walls'. It is one of the pathological lesions that characterises chronic obstructive pulmonary disease (COPD), with the others being large airway mucus gland hyperplasia and small airway fibrosis with inflammation. In the United Kingdom (UK), emphysema is estimated to affect about 3 million people and to kill 30,000 each year. The estimated prevalence of severe emphysema in the UK is 2%, and COPD is the only major chronic disease that continues to increase in prevalence and mortality.

The impact of severe emphysema on an individual's quality of life is profound, as is its effect on mortality. Severe emphysema, defined in terms of airflow obstruction as forced expiratory volume in one second (FEV_1) <35% predicted, has survival at five years of only 40%. When factors such as dyspnoea (measured by the Medical Research Council (MRC) dyspnoea scale) and exercise tolerance (measured by distance walked in six minutes) are added to FEV_1 to define severity, patients with the most severe disease (too breathless to leave the house and able to walk <150 m in six minutes) have survival at five years <20%.[1]

□ CURRENT TREATMENT OPTIONS

Standard treatment for severe emphysema currently comprises enrolment in a pulmonary rehabilitation programme, treatment with inhaled corticosteroids and long- or short-acting bronchodilators, and the addition of oxygen if the patient is hypoxic. Of these, only long-term oxygen treatment, in suitable patients, has definitively been shown to prolong life. Although standard drug treatment does improve quality of life, patients with severe emphysema tend to have significant disability despite optimum medical treatment. As emphysema is characterised by mechanical destruction at the alveolar level, it is perhaps not surprising that the benefits of current drug regimens are modest.

To date, surgical options for the treatment of severe emphysema have been limited to bullectomy, lung transplantation, and lung volume reduction surgery. Bullectomy is effective for patients with a 'giant bulla' (an air-filled space that occupies more than one third of a hemithorax) and produces benefits in terms of reduced dyspnoea and improved lung function that persist for up to five years postoperatively. This patient subset is very small, however, compared with the sum total of patients with severe emphysema. Severe emphysema (FEV_1 <35% predicted) is an accepted indication for lung transplantation, and, in fact, together with α1-antitrypsin deficiency, accounts for more than half of the single lung transplants in adults. The benefits of a single or double set of new lungs are obvious in terms of a dramatic improvement in symptoms and quality of life; however, donor shortage severely limits the number of possible transplants and very few patients older than 60 years will reach the transplant theatre. Apart from the perioperative mortality, chronic rejection continues to be a problem, and this still limits post-transplant survival to 50% at five years. Against this background, any new treatment that improves the mechanical properties of the lungs and so reduces breathlessness would be a major breakthrough.

□ UNDERLYING PHYSIOLOGY

The dyspnoea of emphysema reflects the underlying pathophysiology and is multifactorial. Patients with emphysema have destruction of lung parenchyma and of the attachments between the alveoli and the bronchioli. This uncouples the airways from the parenchyma, which causes a loss of elastic recoil and loss of traction support for the small airways,[2] leading to their collapse or expiration. This limits expiratory airflow (and reduces the FEV_1) and so causes air trapping and hyperinflation.

Patients with COPD exhibit resting hyperinflation (that is, their residual volume, functional residual capacity, and total lung capacity (TLC) are increased), but they also experience additional hyperinflation during exercise because the combination of flow limitation and increasing minute ventilation obliges them to shift, within the flow volume curve, towards TLC. This phenomenon, termed dynamic hyperinflation, is increasingly recognised as an important contributor to the generation of symptoms in patients with COPD,[3] and interventions that reduce resting and dynamic hyperinflation – for example, inhaled tiotropium – have proved value in this condition.

Hyperinflated areas of lung are poorly perfused because of the loss of alveolar capillaries along with the alveolar walls. This leads to ventilation–perfusion mismatch and a reduction in efficient gas exchange (and hence a reduced gas transfer factor).

Hyperinflation of the lungs compromises efficient contraction of the inspiratory muscles, principally the diaphragm, and also reduces the mechanical efficiency of the ribcage. Such hyperinflation causes flattening of the diaphragm, which reduces the curve of its normal 'domed' anatomical shape. This loss of curvature reduces the normal zone of apposition between the muscle and the chest wall and thereby reduces its capacity to generate intrathoracic pressure. Changes also occur within the muscle at a microscopic level – for example, a reduction in the passive tension of the muscle fibres when stretched.[4]

Another physiological change in emphysematous lungs – which is likely to be a beneficial adaptation to airflow obstruction – is the phenomenon of collateral ventilation. This may well prove to be an all-important factor in planning new treatments for emphysema. Collateral ventilation is defined as 'ventilation of alveolar structures through passages or channels that bypass the normal airways' – in other words, the development of new channels for airflow within the lungs. The existence of channels within the lungs through which such collateral flow could occur was recognised a century ago, but only with the recent advances in techniques aimed at producing lung volume reduction has the phenomenon attracted renewed interest.

In patients with emphysema, low-resistance channels exist at multiple levels because of the breakdown in the normal architecture of the lungs. If such channels allow airflow to bypass the airways with expiratory flow limitation, collateral ventilation might be of physiological benefit in patients with emphysema. Collateral ventilation has been measured in patients with emphysema and seems to be increased significantly compared with that in normal lungs, but it has not yet been measured in a large sample size or prospectively to assess its impact on the efficacy of new techniques for volume reduction.

□ LUNG VOLUME REDUCTION SURGERY

Attempts have been made to treat emphysema surgically since the 1950s. The rationale is that resection of hyperinflated regions of the lung will allow for improvement in the function of the less-affected areas and respiratory muscles. Interest in lung volume reduction surgery (LVRS) was reawakened in the 1990s, but concerns about associated morbidity and mortality led to a collection of trials, including the National Emphysema Treatment Trial (NETT) in the United States and a randomised controlled trial in the UK.[5,6] The results of these trials, as well as many uncontrolled series, now help define the use of LVRS. It is not surprising that it took randomised controlled trials to clarify the efficacy and safety of this approach, and these studies showed significantly higher rates of postoperative morbidity and mortality than earlier reports of uncontrolled case series.

In essence, the trials showed that LVRS works. In NETT, no overall difference in mortality at two years was seen between the surgical and medical arms, but cycle exercise tolerance increased in 15% of surgical patients compared with 3% of medically treated patients ($p<0.001$). Quality of life was also more likely to have improved in the surgical group than the medical group (33% *v* 9%, $p<0.001$). These results are broadly similar to those from other trials and are impressive considering the progressive deterioration in function normally seen in patients with emphysema; however, the overall mortality at 90 days was 8% in the surgical group – worryingly high for an operation that is not life saving. When 'high-risk patients' were excluded, postoperative morbidity was still significant.

An important part of NETT was a subgroup analysis that identified factors that predict which patients will benefit from LVRS and those for whom surgery is too risky. High-risk patients were those with severely reduced FEV_1 (<20% predicted) or gas transfer factor and those with non-upper lobe disease combined with high exercise capacity. The greatest benefit from surgery was found in those with disease predominant in the upper lobes and low exercise capacity. When the high-risk patients were excluded from analysis, mortality after surgery was 2% at 30 days and 5% at 90 days compared with 0.2% and 1.5%, respectively, in the medical arm.

Benefit from LVRS lasts two years on average, after which patients slip back to their baseline values in terms of exercise capacity and lung function. It is important, however, to compare these benefits with the outcomes in the control (medically treated) groups, in whom continued deterioration is the norm and measured parameters fall significantly below baseline by two years.

In summary, LVRS works with an acceptable surgical risk but only if patients are selected carefully. It is important to remember that LVRS is a major surgical procedure that involves a general anaesthetic and a postoperative stay in intensive care. It is irreversible and costs more than $60,000 (about £30,000) per patient when costs are assessed six months after surgery. Patient selection is paramount. Suitable patients are those with a heterogeneous pattern of emphysema, which is predominant in the upper lobes, severe disability but not FEV_1 or gas transfer <20% predicted, and no major comorbidities. The pool of suitable patients thus is not large, and in practice, at a typical centre, most suitable patients will already have undergone or declined LVRS. Lung volume reduction surgery, therefore, is not a common operation nowadays.

□ ENDOBRONCHIAL VALVES

Another strategy has been to induce atelectasis or collapse of the emphysematous lung by endobronchial obstruction with one-way valves. The rationale of this approach is that the distal lung will collapse and the pulmonary mechanics will improve if all segmental bronchi in the target lobe are occluded.

Emphasys Medical (Redwood City, CA) were the first company to develop a one-way endobronchial valve. Published case series[7,8] all involved the treatment of similar patients with severe heterogeneous emphysema – in other words, endobronchial valves were used as an alternative to LVRS. All groups initially used general anaesthesia but then moved to conscious sedation and local anaesthetic. The beneficial effects of valve insertion have been variable, including significant improvements in FEV_1, gas transfer, exercise capacity, and quality-of-life scores. None of the series involved controls, however, and the data must be prone to a significant placebo effect.

The latest generation endobronchial valve (Zephyr) is shown in Fig 1. The loading device is inserted through the working channel of the bronchoscope and deployed by squeezing a lever. The device consists of a frame of nickel–titanium alloy (Nitinol) around a one-way valve composed of silicone. The frame expands on deployment, lodging the valve in the segmental bronchus. The valves are easily removable with biopsy forceps. Fig 2 shows the valve in position after deployment.

Safety data from trials are similar. No problems with valve displacement or migration have been seen, and pneumonia in treated segments has not been a problem. Distal infection seems to have been avoided by the design of the valves, which allows drainage of secretions. Pneumothorax is the main risk. The rate of pneumothorax is about 10–20%, and it occurs at varying intervals after the procedure. Most cases occur ipsilaterally to the valves, but contralateral pneumothorax has occurred. Patients with severe emphysema are at risk of pneumothorax

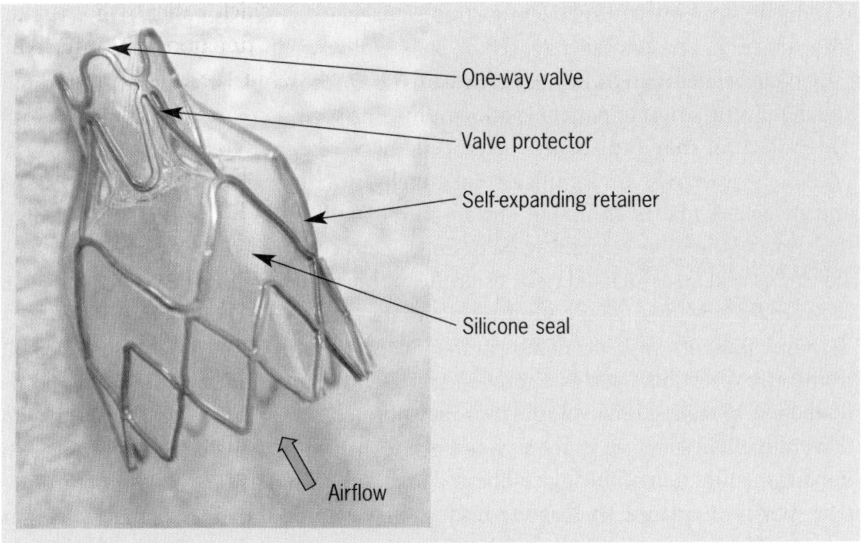

Fig 1 Endobronchial valve (Zephyr; Emphasys Medical, Redwood City, CA), with direction of airflow shown. Air flows on expiration out of the distal lung.

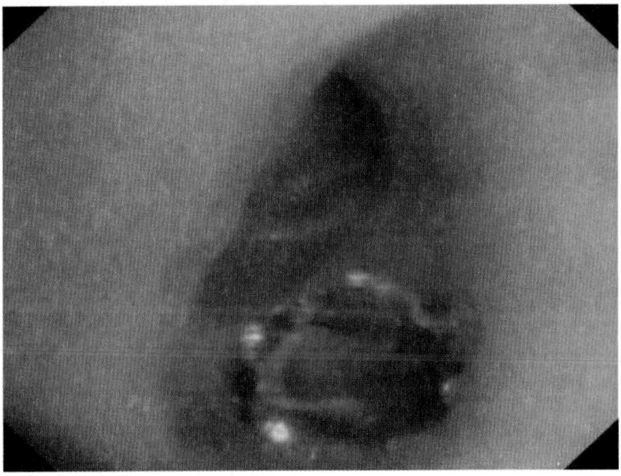

Fig 2 Endobronchial valve (Zephyr; Emphasys Medical, Redwood City, CA) in situ in a segmental airway.

because of pleural blebs and adhesions. The more effective and rapid the volume reduction, the greater the risk of pneumothorax. It may be that overeffective treatment is dangerous, and this has led to debate about the comparative benefits of unilateral and bilateral treatment.

Despite the risk of pneumothorax, a consistent feature of studies with endobronchial valves has been the frequent absence of atelectasis after insertion of the valve; rates of atelectasis have varied between 0% and 50%. Patients with demonstrable volume loss tend to be those with the greatest physiological improvements. In Hopkinson's series,[9] the one in four patients with atelectasis had greater improvements in exercise tolerance and lung function. The key question thus is 'Why do some patients get demonstrable atelectasis and its associated benefits and some do not?' The answer may well be collateral ventilation.

Collateral ventilation has been measured bronchoscopically, and the amount of collateral ventilation in patients with emphysema seems to vary from none to a lot.[10] This variation may explain the heterogeneity of response to valve insertion. If an occluded upper lobe has significant collateral ventilation, the valves will be bypassed and atelectasis may be minimal. The amount of collateral ventilation that is ideal for insertion of the valve remains to be defined. Zero collateral flow might lead to rapid atelectasis and an associated risk of significant pneumothorax, while substantial flow may negate valve insertion completely. Perhaps there is a happy medium?

Some patients with no demonstrable atelectasis still have physiological benefits from valve insertion, such as improved exercise tolerance and measured gas transfer. Reduction of resting lung volume thus may not necessarily be the only aim. It may be that differential changes in lobar volumes are crucial. If a hyperinflated upper lobe impairs the function of the lower lobe and loses volume after valve insertion, the lower lobe may well enlarge, so that the resting lung volume remains unchanged despite substantial physiological benefit. Dynamic hyperinflation may also be reduced, as suggested by a reduction in end-expiratory lung volume at peak exercise.[9]

Another endobronchial valve has been developed. The intrabronchial valve (Spiration, Redmond, WA) is shaped like an umbrella and consists of a polyurethane membrane on a self-expanding frame of nickel–titanium alloy (Nitinol). The 'umbrella' membrane acts as a one-way valve and thus allows distal air and secretions to drain. Pilot studies have shown encouraging results.

☐ AIRWAY BYPASS PROCEDURE

Broncus Technologies (Mountain View, CA) have developed a technique of bronchial fenestration to improve expiratory flow in patients with severe homogeneous emphysema, which takes advantage of collateral ventilation. The idea is to create small extra-anatomical communications between pulmonary parenchyma and the segmental airways. These cartilaginous airways do not collapse on expiration, and it is hoped that these new pathways would allow improved escape of air on expiration, bypassing the collapsed small airways and thus reducing resting and dynamic hyperinflation.

The concept was tested first in explanted emphysematous lungs from transplant recipients.[11] The lungs were placed in a sealed ventilation chamber, and communications were created between the parenchyma and segmental bronchi with a radiofrequency catheter (Broncus Technologies, Mountain View, CA). A stent was passed into each passage to keep the pathway open. With five stents in situ, the FEV_1 doubled.

A Doppler catheter probe was developed to reduce the risk of haemorrhage (Broncus Technologies). This radiofrequency probe is deployed through the working channel of the bronchoscope and placed against the bronchial wall. It can detect the presence or absence of peribronchial vessels through the wall and so identifies safe areas through which pathways can be created. The probe is then advanced through the bronchoscope to create a pathway before the stent is inserted. This Doppler probe allowed the technique of bronchial fenestration to undergo proof-of-concept testing in 10 patients at the time of lobectomy for cancer and in five patients undergoing transplantation.[12] A total of 29 passages were created in the patients who underwent lobectomy and 18 in the transplant recipients. Only two cases of minor bleeding developed, and these settled with suction and topical application of adrenaline.

As reported at the annual meeting of the American Association of Thoracic Surgeons in 2006, 29 patients were treated in a feasibility study with a current version of the system, in which the radiofrequency probe is replaced by a combination needle and dilation balloon device (Broncus Technologies) for the creation of passages and a drug-eluting stent (Broncus Technologies) is included to prolong patency of the stented extra-anatomical passages. Fig 3 shows one of these passages in situ viewed via the bronchoscope. Preliminary results from this pilot study, in which 242 stents were placed, showed that the procedure reduced hyperinflation and dyspnoea in selected patients. One death occurred after intraoperative bleeding due to a stent being placed away from the area identified by the Doppler probe. Thorough investigation of this event resulted in several modifications to the procedure. The duration of benefit from airway bypass seems to correlate with the degree of hyperinflation before treatment. Complete results for this feasibility study have been submitted for publication.

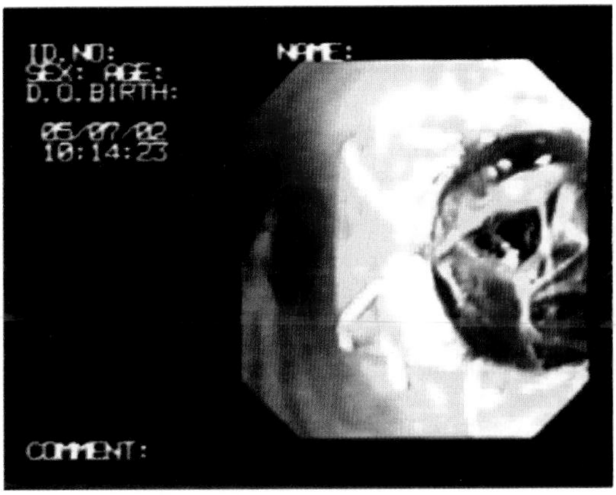

Fig 3 Airway stent (Exhale; Broncus Technologies, Mountain View, CA) in situ across the wall of a segmental airway; emphysematous lung parenchyma is visible through the stent.

Problems with the stents blocking or the holes healing occurred in earlier studies, and the drug-eluting design is a response to this. Longevity of effect is as yet unknown, and the technique has been taken forward to a worldwide randomised controlled study. The Exhale Airway Stents for Emphysema (EASE) trial started in late 2006 and will recruit participants for up to two years, including at the Royal Brompton Hospital.

Airway bypass is suited to patients with a homogenous pattern of emphysema and so is a promising treatment for a different group of patients than those treated with valves. In contrast with valves, collateral ventilation will likely play an important role in the effectiveness of airway bypass. If trapped air is 'drained' by the insertion of one of these stents, the treated area of lung will be increased if collateral interconnections exist to a great degree.

□ CONCLUSIONS

The field of interventional treatment for emphysema is likely to be fast changing over the next few years. Large-scale randomised trials of the new techniques are needed. These trials will not fixate on resting 'volume reduction' as the outcome measure but will include dynamic hyperinflation, exercise data, and quality of life. The Emphasys valve is currently the subject of a large multicentre randomised controlled trial – the Endobronchial Valve for Emphysema PalliatioN Trial (VENT); results are expected in 2007. The future use of endobronchial valves is likely to be defined by this trial. Spiration is also starting a randomised trial this year. Collateral ventilation is likely to be important, and it may be that measurement of the amount of collateral ventilation before valve insertion will predict the response to treatment. The airway bypass procedure is also the subject of a large randomised controlled trial. In this area, patient selection is likely to be paramount, and this will be clarified by the trials.

We can envisage a future in which some patients with heterogeneous emphysema are more suitable for conventional LVRS, while others, with little collateral ventilation, will be more suitable for endobronchial valves, and patients with homogeneous disease perhaps will be suitable for airway bypass stents. It is even possible to see a future where a single patient is treated with more than one technique. This approach may well offer new therapeutic options in this group of very disabled patients in whom medical treatment has limited efficacy and current surgical options, including transplantation and surgical volume reduction, carry significant risks.

REFERENCES

1 Celli BR, Cote CG, Marin JM *et al.* The body-mass index, airflow obstruction, dyspnea, and exercise capacity index in chronic obstructive pulmonary disease. *N Engl J Med* 2004;350: 1005–12.

2 Gibson J, Geddes D, Costabel U, Sterk P, Corrin B, eds. *Respiratory medicine.* Philadelphia, PA: WB Saunders, 2002.

3 O'Donnell DE, Revill SM, Webb KA. Dynamic hyperinflation and exercise intolerance in chronic obstructive pulmonary disease. *Am J Respir Crit Care Med* 2001;164:770–7.

4 Moore AJ, Stubbings A, Swallow EB *et al.* Passive properties of the diaphragm in COPD. *J Appl Physiol* 2006;101:1400–5.

5 Fishman A, Martinez F, Naunheim K *et al.* A randomized trial comparing lung-volume-reduction surgery with medical therapy for severe emphysema. *N Engl J Med* 2003;348: 2059–73.

6 Geddes D, Davies M, Koyama H *et al.* Effect of lung-volume-reduction surgery in patients with severe emphysema. *N Engl J Med* 2000;343:239–45.

7 Snell GI, Holsworth L, Borrill ZL *et al.* The potential for bronchoscopic lung volume reduction using bronchial prostheses: a pilot study. *Chest* 2003;124:1073–80.

8 Toma TP, Hopkinson NS, Hillier J *et al.* Bronchoscopic volume reduction with valve implants in patients with severe emphysema. *Lancet* 2003;361:931–3.

9 Hopkinson NS, Toma TP, Hansell DM *et al.* Effect of bronchoscopic lung volume reduction on dynamic hyperinflation and exercise in emphysema. *Am J Respir Crit Care Med* 2005;171:453–60.

10 Morrell NW, Wignall BK, Biggs T, Seed WA. Collateral ventilation and gas exchange in emphysema. *Am J Respir Crit Care Med* 1994;150:635–41.

11 Lausberg HF, Chino K, Patterson GA *et al.* Bronchial fenestration improves expiratory flow in emphysematous human lungs. *Ann Thorac Surg* 2003;75:393–7.

12 Rendina EA, De Giacomo T, Venuta F *et al.* Feasibility and safety of the airway bypass procedure for patients with emphysema. *J Thorac Cardiovasc Surg* 2003;125:1294–9.

☐ RESPIRATORY MEDICINE SELF-ASSESSMENT QUESTIONS

New treatments for severe asthma in relation to pathophsyiology

1 Cytokines associated with T helper (Th) 2 T lymphocyte-driven, allergic-type inflammation in asthma include:
(a) Interleukin (IL)-7
(b) Thymic stromal lymphopoeitin (TSLP)
(c) IL-13
(d) IL-9
(e) Epidermal growth factor (EGF)

2 Neutralisation of immunoglobulin (Ig) E with the anti-IgE monoclonal antibody omalizumab results in:
(a) The formation of immune complexes
(b) Greater improvements in lung function than in asthma-related quality of life
(c) Reduced levels of eosinophils in the airways
(d) Increased levels of T lymphocytes in the airways
(e) Protection against anaphylaxis

3 In patients with asthma, tumour necrosis factor alpha is a dominant cytokine associated with:
(a) Mild corticosteroid-sensitive asthma
(b) Increased airway responsiveness to non-specific stimuli
(c) Mast cells
(d) Reduced microvascular permeability
(e) Influx of neutrophils into the airway

4 Chronic severe symptomatic asthma frequently is accompanied by:
(a) Thickening of the airway wall
(b) Refractoriness to corticosteroids
(c) Preferential influx of basophils into the airways
(d) A greater occurrence of atopy than mild asthma
(e) An association with tobacco smoking

New developments in pleural disease

1 Concerning malignant pleural effusion:
(a) It is most commonly due to mesothelioma
(b) The diagnosis is excluded by negative cytological tests on pleural fluid
(c) Pleural fluid recurs in most cases after thoracocentesis
(d) Computed tomography is best performed after full drainage of fluid
(e) Abram's pleural biopsy has a sensitivity of >80%

2 Concerning pleurodesis for malignant pleural effusion:
(a) Talc has an efficacy of 40% at one month

(b) Talc pleurodesis results in adult respiratory distress syndrome (ARDS) in 50% of patients
(c) Death due to talc pleurodesis has been reported
(d) Larger particles within talc are associated with systemic distribution and side effects

3 Pleural infection:
(a) Is associated with positive standard microbiology in 60% of cases
(b) Is most commonly due to *Staphylococcus aureus* in patients with community acquired disease
(c) Should be treated routinely with intrapleural tissue plasminogen activator
(d) Is always due to underlying pneumonia
(e) Has a higher mortality with mixed aerobic infection

Emphysema – lung volume reduction and beyond

1 In severe emphysema:
(a) Lung volume reduction surgery (LVRS) prolongs survival
(b) Airflow across lung fissures is uncommon
(c) Survival at five years is around 40%
(d) LVRS is indicated only for patients with disease predominant in the upper lobe

2 Endobronchial valves:
(a) Must be inserted under general anaesthetic
(b) Have been approved for use by the National Institute for Clinical Excellence
(c) Cause collapse of the distal lung in most patients
(d) When used, rely on little collateral ventilation
(e) Are associated with a risk of pneumothorax

3 The airway bypass procedure:
(a) Uses drug-eluting stents
(b) Is indicated in patients with severe disease predominant in the upper lobe
(c) Is associated with a risk of haemorrhage
(d) Leads to an improvement in expiratory airflow
(e) Relies on the absence of collateral ventilation

Multi-system disease

Systemic amyloidosis

Philip N Hawkins

□ INTRODUCTION

Amyloidosis is caused by extracellular deposition of insoluble abnormal fibrils that are derived from the aggregation of misfolded normally soluble proteins. Some 20 different unrelated proteins are known to form amyloid fibrils in vivo, which share a pathognomonic ultrastructure. Systemic amyloidosis – in which amyloid deposits are present in the viscera, walls of the blood vessels, and connective tissues – is usually fatal and is the cause of about one per 1,000 deaths in developed countries. In various localised forms of amyloidosis, the deposits are confined to specific foci or a particular organ or tissue. These may be clinically silent or trivial or they may be associated with serious disease, such as haemorrhage in patients with AL amyloidosis local to the respiratory or urogenital tract. In addition, local deposition of amyloid fibrils can be associated with important diseases in which the pathogenetic role of the amyloid remains unclear; these notably include Alzheimer's disease, prion disorders, and type 2 diabetes mellitus.

In addition to fibrils, amyloid deposits always contain the normal plasma protein serum amyloid P component (SAP), which binds specifically to a ligand expressed on all amyloid fibrils. Radiolabelled SAP has been developed as a specific, quantitative tracer for scintigraphic imaging of amyloid deposits.[1] Treatment of amyloidosis involves measures to support impaired organ function, including dialysis and transplantation, along with vigorous efforts to control underlying conditions responsible for the production of fibril precursors. Serial scintigraphy with SAP has shown that reducing the supply of precursor proteins leads to regression of amyloid deposits in many cases.

□ PATHOGENESIS OF AMYLOIDOSIS

Amyloidogenesis involves substantial refolding of the native structures, and sometimes cleavage of the various amyloid precursor proteins, which enables them to autoaggregate in a highly ordered manner to form fibrils with a characteristic β_2-sheet structure. Wild-type transthyretin (TTR) is inherently amyloidogenic and forms amyloid fibrils in almost all people older than 80 years to some extent and in some in amounts sufficient to cause senile cardiac amyloidosis. The other amyloidogenic wild-type proteins – serum amyloid A protein (SAA) and β_2-microglobulin (β_2M) – form amyloid fibrils only when they have been present at grossly supraphysiological concentrations for prolonged periods. Aberrant proteins with enhanced amyloidogenicity can be acquired (as is the case with the monoclonal immunoglobulin light chains responsible for AL amyloidosis) or inherited (as is the case in patients with familial amyloidosis). A lag period, often of many years, exists between first appearance of a potentially amyloidogenic protein and the deposition of clinically significant amyloid, but accumulation of amyloid can occur very rapidly once the process has begun. Amyloidosis is exceptionally rare in children and young adults, but it can occur.

All amyloid deposits contain abundant proteoglycans and glycosaminoglycan chains, which contribute to amyloid fibrillogenesis or stabilisation of the fibril's structure. In addition, SAP undergoes avid, specific, calcium-dependent binding to amyloid fibrils of all types, which leads to its remarkably specific concentration in amyloid deposits; SAP also contributes to amyloidogenesis.

The mechanisms by which amyloid deposits damage tissues and compromise organ function are incompletely understood. Massive deposits, quite plainly, are structurally disruptive and incompatible with normal function, as are strategically located small deposits – for example, in the glomeruli or nerves. The relation between quantity of amyloid and organ dysfunction is inconsistent, however, and the rate of deposition of new amyloid also may be a factor in progressive organ failure. In vitro studies, and some clinical studies, also have suggested that certain amyloid proteins may have cytotoxic properties.

□ CLINICAL AMYLOIDOSIS

Acquired systemic amyloidosis

Acquired systemic amyloidosis is the cause of death in about one in 1000 people in the United Kingdom (UK) and is probably much underdiagnosed in the elderly population. Systemic AL amyloidosis is the most commonly diagnosed and most serious form, with the number of referrals to the National Health Service (NHS) National Amyloidosis Centre in the UK outnumbering those of AA amyloidosis fourfold.

Systemic AA amyloidosis, formerly known as secondary amyloidosis, is a complication of chronic inflammatory disorders characterised by sustained increased production of the acute-phase reactant SAA. Up to about 5% of people with rheumatoid arthritis, other inflammatory arthritides, Crohn's disease, and an endless list of rarer inflammatory disorders (including hereditary periodic fever syndromes) eventually develop AA amyloidosis.

More than 95% of patients with AA amyloidosis present with non-selective proteinuria or renal failure. End-stage chronic renal failure is the most common cause of death. Hepatosplenomegaly and occasionally thyroid goitre occur in some cases, but clinically significant involvement of the heart is rare, as is liver failure. A variety of lower gastrointestinal symptoms can occur in patients with advanced disease.

The median duration of inflammatory disorders associated with AA amyloidosis is 17 years, but the duration can be as little as just one year. Prognosis is related closely to the degree of renal dysfunction, the effectiveness of anti-inflammatory treatment, and the availability of renal replacement therapy.

Systemic AL amyloidosis, previously known as primary amyloidosis, is the most common form of clinical amyloid disease in developed countries. The AL fibrils are derived from monoclonal immunoglobulin light chains, and almost any clonal B-cell dyscrasia (including myeloma, lymphomas, and macroglobulinaemia) may be complicated by AL amyloidosis. More than 80% of cases, however, are associated with subtle and otherwise 'benign' monoclonal gammopathies. A monoclonal paraprotein or free light chain can be detected by conventional electrophoresis and immunofixation in the serum or urine of only about 80–90% of patients with AL amyloidosis, but high-sensitivity assays of free light chains in serum can confirm monoclonal gammopathy in most of the remaining cases.

Systemic AL amyloidosis occurs equally in men and women, usually in those older than 50 years but as early as the third decade. The clinical manifestations are protean, as virtually any tissue other than the brain may be involved directly.[2] Renal presentation is most frequent, although the heart is affected in more than 50% of cases, and peripheral and autonomic neuropathies, liver involvement, gastrointestinal disturbances, skin deposits, and bruising all are common. Systemic AL amyloidosis also may affect the joints and lungs and can cause acquired bleeding diatheses. Uraemia, heart failure, and other effects of the amyloid usually cause death within 1–2 years unless the underlying B-cell clone is suppressed.

Hereditary systemic amyloidosis

Just a decade ago, hereditary systemic amyloidosis was thought to be extraordinarily rare. It since has been recognised often to be poorly penetrant and to have a late onset, so the expected autosomal dominant family history often is absent.[3] Indeed, the introduction of routine DNA analysis at the NHS National Amyloidosis Centre has shown that more than 10% of patients who present with non-AA amyloidosis have hereditary non-AL forms of the disease. The proteins implicated in amyloid fibrils in patients with hereditary systemic amyloidosis are transthyretin, apolipoproteins AI and AII, fibrinogen A α-chain, gelsolin, and lysozyme.

Severe and ultimately fatal peripheral and autonomic neuropathies are the major features of hereditary TTR amyloidosis (familial amyloid polyneuropathy). Apolipoprotein AI (ApoAI) amyloidosis sometimes causes neuropathy, but this is not a feature of the other hereditary types, which typically involve the viscera. Age of onset, distribution of amyloid deposits, and clinical presentation can vary widely within and between families – even those with the same mutation. All amyloidogenic mutations are dominant, but they are variably penetrant and there may be no family history. Although AA amyloidosis can be diagnosed reliably through immunohistochemistry, such diagnosis often is not possible in patients with the AL form of the disease, and the assumption that non-AA amyloidosis in a patient with a monoclonal gammopathy is AL amyloidosis therefore can be erroneous. It thus is absolutely mandatory that the type of amyloid fibrils is identified positively in all patients with systemic amyloidosis and/or that comprehensive testing for all known amyloidogenic mutations is undertaken to exclude the hereditary forms.

Familial amyloidotic polyneuropathy (FAP), which is caused by more than 100 point mutations in the gene for the plasma protein TTR, is an autosomal dominant syndrome with variable penetrance. Symptoms typically present between the third and seventh decades, and the condition is characterised by progressive and disabling peripheral and autonomic neuropathy and varying degrees of visceral amyloid involvement. Severe cardiac amyloidosis is common. Deposits within the vitreous of the eye can occur and are very characteristic.

Hereditary lysosyme amyloidosis usually presents in middle age with proteinuria and very slowly progressive renal impairment. Marked hepatosplenomegaly is common, and virtually all patients have substantial amyloid deposits in the upper gastrointestinal tract, which can cause serious bleeding and perforation.

Hereditary ApoAI amyloidosis is associated with about a dozen amyloidogenic variants that can present quite diversely with renal disease, hepatic involvement, predominant cardiomyopathy, hoarseness, and even an FAP-like syndrome.

Hereditary fibrinogen A alpha chain amyloidosis is the most common cause of hereditary renal amyloidosis in the UK. Several amyloidogenic fibrinogen A alpha chain variants have been identified, but Val526 is by far the most common. This has very low penetrance in most families, and most patients present in middle age with proteinuria or hypertension and progress to end-stage renal failure within 5–10 years. Other organs are rarely involved clinically.

□ DIAGNOSIS OF AMYLOIDOSIS

Until recently, amyloidosis was diagnosed exclusively through histology, and green birefringence of deposits stained with Congo red when viewed in cross-polarised light remains the gold-standard test. The stain is unstable, however, and must be freshly prepared at least every two months. Sections with a thickness of 5–10 μm and inclusion of a positive control tissue containing modest amounts of amyloid in every staining run are critical. Immunohistochemical staining of amyloid-containing tissue is the simplest method for identifying the type of amyloid fibril, and commercially available antibodies to SAA and β_2M generally yield definitive results, but AL deposits stain with standard antisera to κ or λ light chains in only about half of fixed biopsies. Immunohistochemical staining of amyloid fibrils may require pretreatment of sections with formic acid or alkaline guanidine or deglycosylation. Electron microscopy shows the typical fibrillar ultrastructure of tissue amyloid deposits, but fibrils cannot always be identified convincingly, and electron microscopy alone is not sufficient to confirm the diagnosis of amyloidosis.

'Screening' biopsies of rectal or abdominal fat are positive for amyloid fibrils in about 50–80% of patients with systemic amyloidosis, while biopsies of affected target organs such as the kidney are diagnostic in >95% of cases. It is important, however, to appreciate that biopsies provide small samples that cannot provide information on the extent, localisation, progression, or regression of amyloid deposits – aspects in which histology is complemented by whole-body scintigraphy with radiolabelled SAP (see below). In addition, biopsies, especially those of the liver, carry a higher risk of bleeding in patients with amyloidosis.

Non-histological investigations

Echocardiographs that show small concentrically thickened ventricles, diastolic dysfunction, dilated atria, and homogeneously echogenic valves are characteristic of patients with cardiac amyloidosis. Measurements of levels of B-natriuretic peptide (BNP) and troponin in the serum and magnetic resonance imaging of the heart are being evaluated in patients with cardiac amyloidosis, and all seem very promising.

In cases of known or suspected hereditary amyloidosis, or indeed any case of presumed AL amyloidosis, DNA studies must be performed, but corroboration of DNA findings through confirmation, one way or another, that the respective variant protein is indeed the main constituent of the amyloid fibrils remains essential.

Immunoassays of free light chains in serum

A high-sensitivity immunoassay that can quantify circulating levels of free immunoglobulin light chains with remarkable sensitivity was developed recently.[4] The detection limits of this assay compare with the typical detection limits of 150–500 mg/l for immunofixation and 500–2000 mg/l for electrophoresis. In a series of 262 patients who were undergoing assessment at the NHS National Amyloidosis Centre,[5] a monoclonal immunoglobulin could not be detected by electrophoresis or immunofixation in the serum or urine of 21% of patients at presentation. In a further 26% of patients, monoclonal light chains could be detected only qualitatively by immunofixation. In contrast, the immunoassay for free light chains in serum showed monoclonal free immunoglobulin light chains in 98% of patients. Serial assays for free light chains enable much more rational administration and monitoring of chemotherapy in patients with AL amyloidosis than previously.

Scintigraphy with SAP

Serum amyloid P component is a normal plasma protein that binds specifically to all amyloid fibrils and radiolabelled SAP enables amyloid deposits in solid organs to be imaged and quantified,[6] which provides information on the diagnosis, distribution, and extent of amyloid deposits throughout the body. Serial scans with radiolabelled SAP monitor progress and response to treatment and have unequivocally shown regression of many types of amyloid fibril when the supply of the respective precursor proteins is reduced by treatment. This technique is not available commercially but is used routinely in the NHS National Amyloidosis Centre in the UK.

□ MANAGEMENT OF AMYLOIDOSIS

Although no treatments that specifically promote mobilisation of amyloid fibrils are available yet, measures to support failing organ function while attempts are made to reduce the supply of the precursor proteins can be very effective. Although scintigraphy with SAP in more than 2,000 patients showed that suppression of the primary disease process often results in regression of existing deposits, the process is slow and recovery of organ function is often much delayed. Production of the precursor proteins should be monitored to help guide the need for and intensity of treatment for the underlying primary condition. This involves frequent estimation of the level of SAA in plasma in patients with AA amyloidosis[7] and monitoring of the levels of free light chains in serum[5] or other markers of the underlying monoclonal plasma cell dyscrasia in those with AL amyloidosis.

Treatment of AA amyloidosis ranges from anti-inflammatory and immunosuppressive drugs in patients with rheumatoid arthritis to lifelong prophylactic colchicine in familial Mediterranean fever and surgery in conditions such as refractory osteomyelitis and Castleman's disease.[7] Biologic anti-TNF and interleukin 1 antagonists can induce rapid and complete remission in patients with inflammatory arthritis and some inherited periodic fever syndromes.

Treatment of AL amyloidosis is derived from the approaches used in myeloma. In more than 50% of patients, cyclic chemotherapy regimens that include melphalan and dexamethasone and thalidomide-based regimens are associated with haematological responses, along with manageable toxicity.[5] Slightly higher response rates with autologous stem cell transplantation are offset by substantial procedural mortality in people with amyloid involvement of multiple organs.[8]

Hepatic transplantation can be effective in patients with familial amyloid polyneuropathy associated with transthyretin gene mutations, as the variant amyloidogenic protein is produced mainly in the liver. Outcome is best among younger patients with the methionine 30 variant, although peripheral neuropathy usually only stabilises even in this group.[9] Unfortunately, paradoxical worsening of cardiac amyloidosis with wild-type transthyretin has occurred in many older patients. On a similar basis, hepatic transplantation lately has also been undertaken successfully in selected patients with hereditary fibrinogen A α-chain[10] and ApoAI amyloidosis.

Supportive management remains critical, as it has the potential to delay target organ failure, maintain quality of life, and prolong survival while the underlying process is treated. Rigorous control of hypertension is vital in patients with renal amyloidosis. Surgical resection of amyloidotic tissue occasionally is beneficial, but, in general, a conservative approach to surgery, anaesthesia, and other invasive procedures is advisable. Amyloidotic tissues may heal poorly and are liable to bleed. Diuretics and vasoactive drugs should be used cautiously in patients with cardiac amyloidosis, because they can reduce cardiac output substantially. Replacement of vital organ function, notably through dialysis, may be necessary, and cardiac, renal, and liver transplant procedures have a role in selected cases.

Finally, a number of different treatments aimed specifically at inhibiting the formation of amyloid fibrils or promoting regression of fibrils are under development, and some are already being evaluated clinically. The latter include approaches directed at production of precursor proteins, glycosaminoglycans,[11] and SAP;[12] prevention of aberrant protein folding; and various kinds of immunotherapy, and this offers the hope that amyloidosis may become more readily treatable.

□ ACKNOWLEDGMENTS

The work of the Centre for Amyloidosis and Acute Phase Proteins is supported by Medical Research Council Programme Grant G79/00051 to MB Pepys and PN Hawkins, the Wolfson Foundation, and NHS research and development funds. The NHS National Amyloidosis Centre is funded entirely by the Department of Health in the UK.

REFERENCES

1 Hawkins PN. Serum amyloid P component scintigraphy for diagnosis and monitoring amyloidosis. *Curr Opin Nephrol Hypertens* 2002;11:649–55.

2 K.yle RA, Gertz MA. Primary systemic amyloidosis: clinical and laboratory features in 474 cases. *Semin Hematol* 1995;32:45–59

3 Lachmann HJ, Booth DR, Booth SE *et al.* Misdiagnosis of hereditary amyloidosis as AL (primary) amyloidosis. *N Engl J Med* 2002;346:1786–91.

4 Bradwell AR, Carr-Smith HD, Mead GP *et al.* Highly sensitive, automated immunoassay for immunoglobulin free light chains in serum and urine. *Clin Chem* 2001;47:673–80.

5 Lachmann HJ, Gallimore R, Gillmore JD *et al.* Outcome in systemic AL amyloidosis in relation to changes in concentration of circulating free immunoglobulin light chains following chemotherapy. *Br J Haematol* 2003;122:78–84.

6 Hawkins PN, Lavender JP, Pepys MB. Evaluation of systemic amyloidosis by scintigraphy with 123I-labeled serum amyloid P component. *N Engl J Med* 1990;323:508–13.

7 Gillmore JD, Lovat LB, Persey MR, Pepys MB, Hawkins PN. Amyloid load and clinical outcome in AA amyloidosis in relation to circulating concentration of serum amyloid A protein. *Lancet* 2001;358:24–9.

8 Comenzo RL, Gertz MA. Autologous stem cell transplantation for primary systemic amyloidosis. *Blood* 2002;99:4276–82.

9 Herlenius G, Wilczek HE, Larsson M, Ericzon BG. Ten years of international experience with liver transplantation for familial amyloidotic polyneuropathy: results from the Familial Amyloidotic Polyneuropathy World Transplant Registry. *Transplantation* 2004;77:64–71.

10 Gillmore JD, Booth DR, Rela M *et al.* Curative hepatorenal transplantation in systemic amyloidosis caused by the Glu526Val fibrinogen a-chain variant in an English family. *QJ Med* 2000;93:269–75.

11 Kisilevsky R, Lemieux LJ, Fraser PE *et al.* Arresting amyloidosis in vivo using small molecule anionic sulphonates or sulphates: implications for Alzheimer's disease. *Nature Med* 1995;1:143–8.

12 Pepys MB, Herbert J, Hutchinson WL *et al.* Targeted pharmacological depletion of serum amyloid P component for treatment of human amyloidosis. *Nature* 2002;417:254–9.

The porphyrias

Timothy M Cox

☐ INTRODUCTION

Porphyrias are caused by disturbances in the multistep pathway that leads to the formation of an essential iron-containing pigment, ferroprotohaem, known more familiarly as 'haem' (Fig 1). The ancient biosynthetic enzymes of haem biosynthesis have been strongly conserved in evolution: they contribute to the generation of other pigments essential for life, including the magnesium-containing chlorophyll molecule and the corrins – of which the unique cobalt-containing vitamin B12, is the sole representative in humans.[1] Inherited and acquired defects in seven of the eight enzymes that bring about the formation of haem cause the human porphyrias (Table 1).[2–4] Porphyria may cause dramatic episodes of neurovisceral disease with or without photosensitivity and characteristic cutaneous manifestations that are the province of general and specialist physicians, as well as doctors in numerous other fields of clinical practice.

Biosynthesis of haem is regulated tightly and subject to complex mechanisms that ensure negative feedback control by its end product. This means that acquired or inherited defects of any of the component reactions lead to the overproduction of unwanted toxic precursor molecules.

Porphyrias with neurovisceral manifestations

The neurovisceral aspects of the porphyrias are perhaps the most challenging for doctors and hitherto have remained a largely unfathomable mystery in the canon of human pathophysiology. Profound and severe neurological manifestations are associated with histological abnormalities in peripheral autonomic nerves, signs of muscle denervation, and hypothalamic malfunction with sympathomimetic overactivity. Increased levels of ALA itself, and possibly other precursors, are now widely believed to be responsible for these neurotoxic manifestations as part of the disturbed biosynthetic metabolism associated with acute porphyric attacks.[2–5]

Overproduction of the first committed porphyrin precursor of haem, δ- (or 5-) aminolaevulinic acid (ALA), is associated with the acute neurovisceral manifestations of human porphyria. Under these circumstances, induction of ALA synthase type 1 (ALAS-1) – the primary isoenzyme that leads to formation of ALA in the liver – seems to be responsible.[2,3]

Porphyrias with cutaneous manifestations (photosensitivity)

The four-ringed macrocyclic porphyrins (tetrapyrroles) that arise before chelation of the iron atom by protoporphyrin IX are highly photoactive – a property attributable

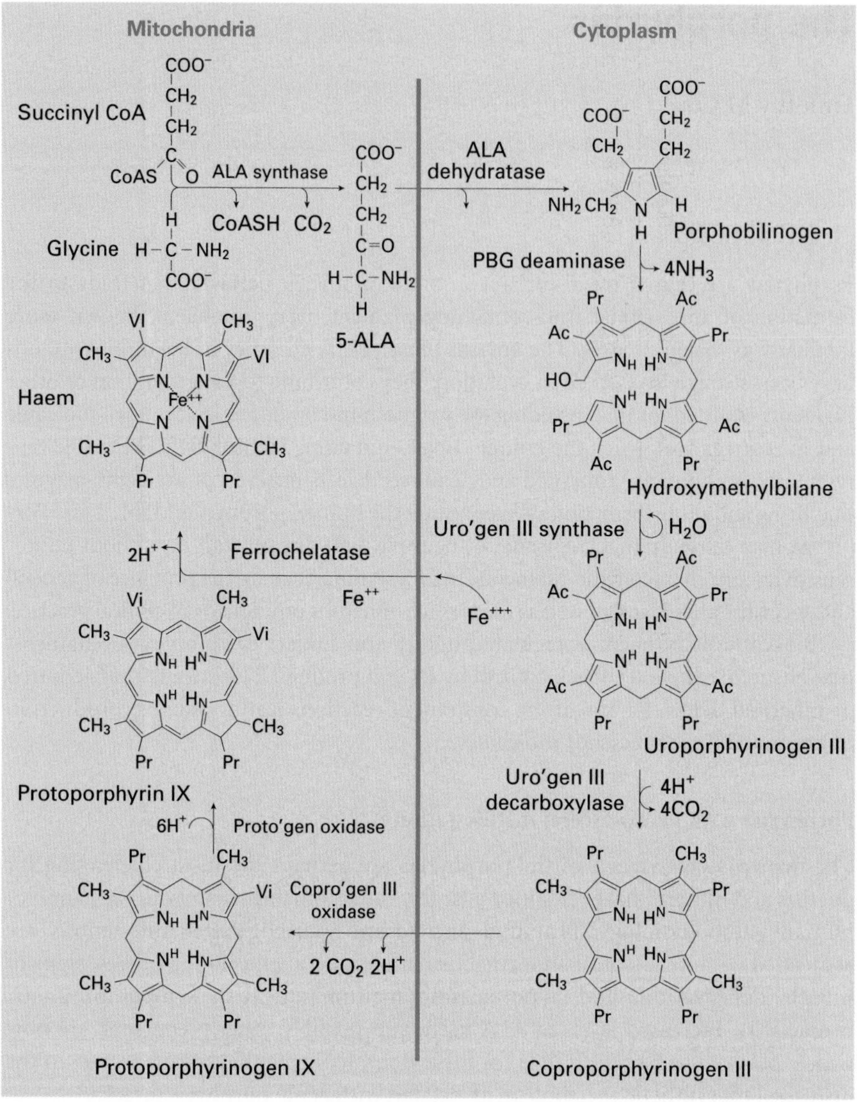

Fig 1 Biosynthesis of haem in eukaryotic cells. PGB = porphobilinogen. Note that the first and last three steps occur in the mitochondria.

to their extensive double-bond resonance structure. Absorbance of light energy occurs principally in the Soret region (400–420 nm, violet) and in the green-to-yellow range (530–595 nm). The oxidised macrocyclic porphyrins that are precursors of haem are fluorescent molecules, and after excitation at these wavelengths they emit light in the *visible* range. Emission of fluorescence and internal energy conversion are physical processes that enable the excited-state molecules to return to their ground state without alterations in chemical structure. These processes lead to the characteristic photosensitivity of several of the porphyrias – the so-called *photodynamic effect* that is dependent principally on the presence of ambient tissue oxygen.[6]

Table 1 The human inherited porphyrias. Adapted and reproduced from Kauppinen with kind permission from Elsevier.[4]

Porphyria	Enzyme	Inheritance	Gene	Source	Manifestations
ALA dehydratase deficiency 'Doss'	Aminolaevulinate dehydratase	Autosomal recessive	*ALAD* 9q34 (<10 mutations)	Hepatic	Acute attacks* Neuropathy
Acute intermittent	Porphobilinogen deaminase	Autosomal dominant	*PBDG* 11q23.3 (~230 mutations)	Hepatic	Acute attacks*
Congenital erythropoietic	Uroporphyrinogen III cosynthase	Autosomal recessive	*UROS* 10q25.2q26.3 (35 mutations)	Erythroid	Photosensitivity Haemolysis
Cutanea tarda	Uroporphyrinogen III decarboxylase	Autosomal dominant (also bigenic and 'acquired')	*UROD* 1p34 (60 mutations)	Hepatic	Photosensitivity (associated liver injury)
Coproporphyria	Coproporphyrinogen III oxidase	Autosomal dominant	*CPOX* 3q12 (<40 mutations)	Hepatic	Acute attacks* Photosensitivity
Variegate	Protoporphyrinogen IX oxidase	Autosomal dominant	*PPOX* 1q22 (~120 mutations)	Hepatic	Acute attacks* Photosensitivity
Protoporphyria	Ferrochelatase	Autosomal dominant/ recessive (bigenic)	*FECH* 18q21.3 (~75 mutations)	Erythroid	Photosensitivity Cholestatic liver disease

*Porphyrias associated with acute neurovisceral attacks.

Cholestasis in porphyria

Another manifestation of the porphyrias is cholestasis, which is caused by the poor aqueous solubility of the late porphyrin precursor protoporphyrin IX. Protoporphyrin IX is associated with formation of gallstones, as well as microscopic paracrystalline masses within biliary canaliculi and hepatocytes.

□ HEREDITARY AND ENVIRONMENTAL FACTORS IN PORPHYRIAS

Most human porphyria syndromes are caused by inherited deficiencies of single enzymes in the haem biosynthetic pathway. Certain toxins and xenobiotic metabolites, including several hydrocarbons, influence the pathway, however, and exacerbate porphyria in susceptible individuals. Metals such as mercury and lead, as well as arsenic and iron, may disturb porphyrin metabolism in humans.[3,7] The mechanisms by which the metabolism of ingested compounds, including alcohol (and many therapeutic drugs), as well as endogenous molecules, including steroid hormones, disrupt the tightly regulated equilibrium and provoke porphyria remain largely unexplained.

Such gene–environment interactions in apparently healthy people may be associated with sporadic attacks of porphyria. Examples of this include the outbreak of severe cutaneous porphyria resembling porphyria cutanea tarda that occurred as a result of consumption of hexachlorobenzene (HCB) intended as a fungicide for seed corn delivered compassionately to impoverished regions of Turkey in the 1950s;[8] toxic porphyria still persists in those exposed to HCB as a legacy of this tragic but highly instructive biological accident.

□ BIOSYNTHESIS OF HAEM

The main site of haem biosynthesis is the erythropoietic bone marrow (erythron). About 300 mg of haem per day is formed constitutively in the erythron (as determined by isotopic studies with nitrogen, carbon, or iron labelling), and this compensates for the physiological destruction of effete red cells. Hepatic biosynthesis accounts for about 50 mg of the haem produced each day, but this can be induced rapidly and can increase severalfold. Formation of haem at peripheral sites accounts for only about 1% of the total. It is worth noting that the breakdown of haem and haem proteins does not lead to the production of porphyrins, rather it is the means of generating bile pigments. Biosynthesis of haem in the liver undergoes rapid oscillations and represents the principal component of the so-called early-labelled peak of bilirubin. This component is derived from the rapid turnover of haem proteins in the liver, largely those in the endoplasmic reticulum that belong to the vast family of cytochrome P450 molecules, whose turnover rate is disproportionately high.

Formation of the metal-chelating tetrapyrrole ring system in the eight enzymatic steps of haem biosynthesis represents an astonishing feat of biological economy (see Fig 1). Generation of 5'-aminolaevulinate in the mitochondrion is the first committed reaction of haem biosynthesis. The activity and abundance of ALA synthase found in the liver – ALAS-1 – is subject to rapid fluctuations and regulation; in the bone marrow, a separate enzyme, ALAS-2, which is encoded by a gene located on the X chromosome, is separately responsible for the formation of ALA in erythroid cells. Both isozymes of ALA synthase require pyridoxal-5-phosphate, derived from vitamin B6, as a cofactor.

Biosynthesis of haem is orchestrated in distinct cellular compartments: after initiation in the mitochondrion, intermediate reactions take place in the cytosol; but the final steps again take place in the mitochondrion. Once 5'-aminolaevulinic acid is formed, it is converted to the tetrapyrrole macrocycle through three reactions: first, two molecules are condensed to form the basic pyrrolic constituent porphobilinogen; polymerisation of four molecules of porphobilinogen follows to generate an unstable tetrapyrrolic chain structure (hydroxymethylbilane or preuroporphyrinogen); finally, cyclisation of preuroporphyrinogen, with a specific rearrangement of one of the rings, yields the universal intermediate uroporphyrinogen III. This is the conserved precursor from which all haem molecules and the other formed porphyrins, corrins, and chlorophylls found in living organisms are derived. Uroporphyrinogen III is successively oxidised by decarboxylation: first to coproporphyrinogen III, then to protoporphyrinogen IX and finally to protoporphyrin IX. An iron atom is inserted into protoporphyrin IX by ferrochelatase (the last enzyme of the pathway in the mitochondrion) to bring about formation of the metalloporphyrin ferroprotohaem (haem).

The three-dimensional crystal structures of all mammalian and many plant, bacterial, and yeast haem biosynthetic enzymes have been determined; at the same time, the detailed molecular mechanisms of the often complex reactions they catalyse have been worked out.

□ THE PORPHYRIA SYNDROMES

An operational conspectus of the porphyrias is provided in Table 1, together with a summary of their genetics and principal manifestations. Highly efficient reactions in the finely regulated haem pathway minimise the production of excess toxic intermediates. Photoactive macrocyclic porphyrins (tetrapyrroles), or the neurotoxic 5-aminolaevulinic acid precursor, account for the principal clinical manifestations of porphyria.[2–6]

Cutaneous porphyrias

Photosensitivity

Photosensitive reactions associated with the porphyrias are a consequence of the unique double bond-containing structure of the tetrapyrrolic nucleus of the formed porphyrins that serve as metabolic intermediates in the formation of haem. Each individual molecule has a structure that determines its particular electronic energy states and absorption spectrum for photons. Absorption of photon energy increases the electronic state of tetrapyrroles to discrete quantised molecular energy levels. Under these circumstances, when the energy value of an integral electronic state is reached, the molecule is raised to an excited state and is able to participate in photochemical reactions. After excitation, the electronic states of the porphyrins are termed singlet or triplet; this reflects distinct spin assignments of those outer electrons that possess the greatest energies.

Once the energy of the photon has been absorbed to generate an excited singlet state molecule, the distribution of electrons is altered and the whole molecule acquires more total energy, which is distributed into various components. In this state, several processes may result: the emission of light at a lower wavelength than the exciting wavelength (fluorescence); formation of a photochemical product; interconversion between singlet and triplet states; and internal conversion in which the energy of the excited state is lost as heat and the molecule returns to its ground state. Intersystem crossing, by which a singlet excited-state molecule is converted to a triplet excited-state molecule, is the source of important photochemical reactions in biological systems and a relatively slow photophysical process. Triplet excited-state molecules have lifetimes prolonged to several hundred milliseconds, particularly in the presence of ambient oxygen. Under these circumstances, energy is transferred to ground state oxygen, thereby terminating the life of the triplet state molecule, which leads to the photodynamic effect. Singlet oxygen is a highly reactive species that interacts with many biological molecules, including proteins, lipids, and DNA. Singlet oxygen also forms hydroperoxides, which may be quenched by several biological molecules.

In summary, many of the photodynamic effects of porphyrins seem to involve excitation to the triplet state, with energy transfer to molecular oxygen. This induces formation of singlet oxygen and other highly reactive oxygen species that lead to tissue injury. If the porphyrin is relatively soluble in biological membranes – for example, protoporphyrin – the presence of dissolved oxygen induces local injury to biological membranes and lipids. Light-induced formation of reactive oxygen species causes inflammation, with complement-mediated injury affecting blood vessels: oedema results because of increased permeability in light-exposed tissues, especially where local concentrations of porphyrins are high and oxygen is present.

Porphyria cutanea tarda

Porphyria cutanea tarda (PCT) is by far the most common porphyria.[9] It is never associated with life-threatening neurovisceral attacks provoked by drugs or other factors and is not usually inherited with a simple pattern of Mendelian transmission. Most cases of PCT occur in susceptible individuals in whom toxins – such as alcohol, steroid hormones (particularly oestrogens), and iron – seem to be environmental cofactors in disease expression. Certain viruses, particularly hepatitis C and HIV, provoke expression of PCT. It is associated with skin fragility, formation of milia, blistering, and pigmentary changes, as well as scarring and hypertrichosis. The condition responds very well to two treatments: iron depletion by phlebotomy or low-dose chloroquine, which seems to solubilise excess hexacarboxylic porphyrins in the liver and promote their biliary excretion as a complex. Rare forms of PCT occur in families in which mutations in the gene for uroporphyrinogen decarboxylase have been identified. Toxic porphyria cutanea tarda may follow exposure to halogenated aromatic hydrocarbons – as in the outbreak in Turkey. Other hydrocarbons, including derivatives of dioxin, have similar effects; dioxin has been implicated in a recent political poisoning in the Ukraine. Porphyria cutanea tarda is important for general physicians, because it is associated with iron overload and liver disease, and it is encountered in the general clinic and dialysis unit; in the latter, it is associated with inadvertently excessive iron supplementation given to compensate for perceived chronic blood loss.

Many patients with sporadic or familial PCT possess at least one copy of the C282Y allele of the *HFE* gene, which predisposes to adult haemochromatosis. Where homozygosity for this mutation is present, a more florid clinical presentation with PCT occurs at an earlier age. Other factors that cause an excess of iron, including untoward dietary intake and consumption of alcoholic drinks, are cofactors in the expression of PCT. Minor abnormalities of serum aminotransferase activities are found in many patients, including those who drink alcohol to excess or have pre-existing iron overload. Even when patients who harbour the hepatitis C virus are excluded, however, PCT is associated with cirrhosis of the liver and carries an appreciable independent risk of hepatocellular carcinoma – a complication that has occurred in the absence of cirrhosis. Patients with PCT thus should be investigated for hepatocellular carcinoma at diagnosis and ideally should be monitored by ultrasound of the liver combined with measurement of α-fetoprotein and vitamin B12 in serum.

The treatment usually recommended for patients with iron overload involves phlebotomy of one unit of blood removed at weekly or fortnightly intervals until the patient has mild anaemia and the level of ferritin in serum is <20–40 mg/l. Levels of porphyrin in urine and plasma almost invariably return to normal. In patients unable to withstand phlebotomy, parenteral administration of desferrioxamine may achieve remission; in adults, chloroquine at a dose of 125 mg twice weekly produces clinical improvements over several months and should be continued until the pathological excess of uroporphyrin excretion has been corrected.

Protoporphyria

Erythropoietic protoporphyria is caused by inherited deficiency of ferrochelatase, the last enzyme in the haem biosynthetic pathway. It is probably the second most frequent porphyria and is characterised by an unusual syndrome of photosensitivity in infancy or childhood.[2,3,6] Unlike in patients with PCT, variegate porphyria, and coproporphyria (the other porphyrias associated with photosensitivity), light-exposed skin that contains an excess of protoporphyrin does not develop blisters; instead, exposure to light in patients with protoporphyria induces burning pain followed by erythema, oedema, and occasional scarring.

Protoporphyria has a complex pattern of inheritance. About 10% of patients inherit the condition from an affected parent. This is an example of pseudodominant transmission, in which a widely distributed allele that leads to deficiency of functional messenger RNA for ferrocheletase occurs at high frequency in the population at large. Co-inheritance of an individual private mutation in the other parental ferrochelatase allele leads to the expression of disease as a result of greatly decreased ferrochelatase activity.

In patients with protoporphyria, the acute effects of exposure to light are associated with itching, burning, and cutaneous oedema with erythema. More severe exposure leads to purpura and excoriation. In the chronic phase, thickening and hyperkeratosis occurs in sun-exposed skin. The skin may have a waxy or leathery texture, particularly over the interphalangeal joints, with a lichenoid and papular appearance. Pseudoragades (shallow elliptical or linear scars) may be seen on the malar regions of patients or as linear perioral furrows. Milia and nail changes are absent. Patients with protoporphyria occasionally develop generalised pigmentation as a result of the deposition of melanin.

Protoporphyrin hepatopathy

Very rarely, patients with protoporphyria (<5%) may develop an unusual hepatopathy associated with extreme photosensitivity, cholestatic features (including itching and excoriation), jaundice, and increasing pigmentation.[2,6,10] There is a high frequency protoporphyrin gallstones (Fig 2).

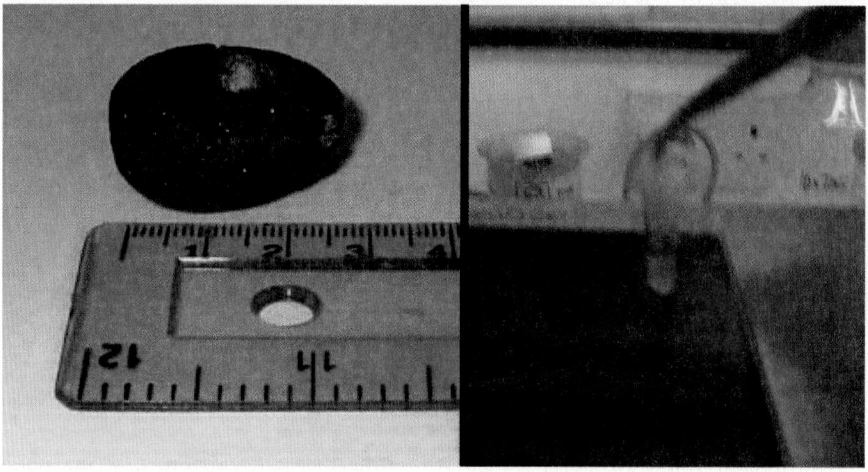

Fig 2 Gallbladder calculus from a patient with protoporphyria. The fluorescent porphyrin was extracted into organic solvent (right-hand panel).

It is now clear that protoporphyria has a rare association with cirrhosis, which is accompanied by cholestatic features as described above. Once established, these progress rapidly as a result of a vicious cycle of increasing cholestasis, haemolysis, and extreme photosensitivity. Deteriorating hepatic disease is heralded by generalised upper abdominal pain, tender splenomegaly, and signs of haemolyis with jaundice. Under these circumstances, hepatic transplantation is effective, but it presents a formidable technical challenge because of the danger that operative lights may cause enhanced tissue injury, so special filters may be needed to reduce phototoxicity. Reducing the protoporphyrin excess by exchange transfusion and hypertransfusion, as well as the use of bile acid treatment and charcoal, enhances disposal of protoporphyrin and decreases its production in the erythropoietic marrow.

Protoporphyria can be diagnosed easily on the basis of the history and examination of a wet blood film under ultraviolet light; this shows highly fluorescent red cells and reticulocytes in the circulation. The diagnosis can be confirmed by spectroscopy of plasma porphyrins and red cell porphyrins, as well as examination of the stool for evidence of excess excretion of protoporphyrin IX.

Treatment of protoporphyria

Treatment includes local measures such as cold compresses, corticosteroids, and analgesia for the acute cutaneous manifestations; exposure to light should be minimised. Reflectant sunscreen preparations and oral ingestion of the potential light-quenching agent β-carotene also may be beneficial. Early reports suggest that narrow-band ultraviolet phototherapy combined with a psoralen may be beneficial. Referral to a liver centre is recommended in patients with established hepatic disease. Measures to reduce levels of protoporphyrin by transfusion, light avoidance, and splenectomy may be beneficial in combination with methods to promote the secretion of protoporphyrin by bile acid therapy and the use of bile sequestrants and charcoal to interrupt the enterohepatic circulation. Hepatic transplantation is often successful for some years; but consideration might be given in the future to bone marrow transplantation in patients in the early stages of protoporphyrin hepatopathy. Marrow transplantation addresses the primary source of the toxic protoporphyrin that is responsible for the liver disease and acceleration of light sensitivity with haemolysis that characterises the fulminant stages of protoporphyria.[10]

Other porphyrias with photosensitivity

The porphyrias associated with photosensitivity include variegate porphyria and hereditary coproporphyria, as well as the extremely rare congenital erythropoietic porphyria. The latter disorder, an autosomal recessive disease, is not associated with acute neurovisceral attacks but causes extreme photosensitivity and photodestruction of skin in exposed areas, with hypertrichosis, porphyrin staining of the teeth, persistent haemolysis, and splenomegaly: referral to a specialist centre is recommended. Blistering lesions and formation of bullae characterise the photosensitive reactions of the other acute porphyrias, variegate porphyria, and coproporphyria, in which formed macrocyclic porphyrins contribute to the clinical manifestations.

□ THE ACUTE PORPHYRIAS[2,3,11]

Knowledge of the acute porphyrias is of key importance to general physicians and those who have responsibility for patients who present with an acute illness in the emergent situation, including surgeons and anaesthetists. During the prolonged period needed for recovery from an acute episode of porphyria, the assistance of many personnel as part of multidisciplinary teams may be needed to promote satisfactory rehabilitation. Neurologists and physiotherapists are often consulted – but all physicians need to be aware of the precipitating factors and principal features of these potentially fatal disorders.

Acute neurovisceral attacks occur in four of the porphyrias, as indicated in Table 1. In all but one – the so-called Doss porphyria (in which there is a deficiency of aminolaevulinate dehydratase) – the inheritance pattern is that of an autosomal dominant disease with variable penetrance; such features are typical of inborn errors that affect structural proteins or components of highly regulated pathways.

Clinical expression is marked by acute life-threatening attacks of neuropathy. Table 2 sets out the frequency of the main clinical manifestations of acute porphyria from three large published series.[12–14] Of note, abdominal pain, psychiatric symptoms, and signs of sympathetic and hypothalamic autonomic overactivity with severe hyponatraemia occur, sometimes accompanied by life-threatening seizures and motor defects. Unlike depictions in the media, porphyria is *not* frequently associated with long-term madness, but patients with acute attacks may seem hysterical and certainly are often very perturbed; when unwell, they may become violent and exhibit psychotic behaviour. Sympathetic overactivity causes anxiety, tremor, and marked tachycardia with arterial hypertension. Progressive neurological disease is characterised by generalised seizures, bulbar paresis, ventilatory failure, and profound limb weakness due to an axonal motor neuropathy, which often resembles an ascending paralysis of the Landry type. Once established, these neurological sequelae lead to persistent disability and the need for prolonged periods of mental, as well physical, rehabilitation and support.

Acute attacks of porphyria are precipitated when formation of haem in the liver is stimulated by induction of ALAS-1. This characteristically occurs when drugs that

Table 2 Principal clinical manifestations of acute porphyria.

	Prevalence of manifestation (%)		
Symptoms/signs	**Waldenström (1957)[12] (n=321)**	**Goldberg (1959)[13] (n=50)**	**Stein and Tschudy (1970)[14] (n=46)**
Abdominal pain	85	94	95
Vomiting	59	88	43
Constipation	48	84	48
Diarrhoea	9	12	5
Muscle weakness	42	68	60
Sensory loss	9	38	26
Convulsions	10	16	20
Respiratory paralysis	14	10	9
Mental symptoms	55	58	40
Hypertension	40	54	36
Tachycardia	28	64	80
Fever	37	14	9

are metabolised by the hepatic cytochrome P450 system are given. Despite the emergence of a convincing model of human acute intermittent porphyria in a genetically modified strain of mice, the pathogenesis of the acute attack remains mysterious, and axonal degeneration and central neuronal chromatolysis involving the anterior horn and hypothalamic and periventricular nuclei have been observed in fatal cases. Electrophysiological studies often show denervation associated with severe primary axonal degeneration of peripheral nerves, which in severe attacks leads to disabling paralysis.

Recent studies in a few patients treated for recurrent attacks by liver transplantation provide mounting evidence that ALA (or its metabolic derivatives) is the toxin responsible for the acute neurovisceral manifestations of porphyria. In support of this hypothesis, overproduction of ALA is associated with lead poisoning, which has many features in common with acute porphyria; overproduction of ALA also occurs in hereditary tyrosinaemia type 1, the rare inherited disorder with acute neurovisceral features, in which acquired deficiency of aminolaevulinate dehydratase results from inhibition by the tyrosine metabolite succinylacetone (dioxoheptanoic acid). Finally, neuronopathic effects of acute porphyria are seen in patients with ALA dehydratase deficiency – a recessive disease that presents solely with neurovisceral attacks; interestingly, individuals heterozygous for ALA dehydratase deficiency seem to be unusually susceptible to environmental lead poisoning.

Precipitating factors in acute porphyria

Acute attacks that are associated with induction of ALAS-1 in the liver are induced by nutritional, endocrine, and xenobiotic factors. Overall, it seems that 80–90% of patients heterozygous for mutations responsible for acute porphyria syndromes remain asymptomatic.

Endocrine factors

Acute attacks are very rare before puberty; after puberty, they are more common in women in the reproductive age group, in whom they often show periodicity – indeed, the attacks almost invariably decrease in frequency and severity after the menopause. Other precipitating factors include starvation, intercurrent illness, sepsis, and surgical procedures (often those associated with barbiturates used as short-acting anaesthetics or premedication agents).

Drugs

Barbiturates, many anticonvulsants, sulphonamides, numerous analgesics (including diclofenac and other non-steroidal anti-inflammatory drugs (NSAIDs)), antihypertensive drugs, cough medicines, and sex steroids (particularly progestogens) are all implicated in acute porphyrias. Alcohol and heavy metals also are implicated, and those such as lead and arsenic found in moonshine whisky have been reported to precipitate attacks.

Lead poisoning is, in effect, an acquired porphyria: the sulphydryl-rich enzymes ALA dehydratase and ferrochelatase seem to be particularly sensitive to lead, and acute lead poisoning is associated with abdominal pain ('lead colic') and neuropathy that resembles the manifestations of acute porphyrias (see below); excess ALA appears in the urine. At the same time, chronic exposure to lead, for example in long-term industrial poisoning, leads to hypochromic anaemia and inhibition of ferrochelatase, as well as other enzymes in the late steps of haem biosynthesis; under these circumstances, levels of erythrocyte protoporphyrins are increased and the urinary excretion of other formed porphyrins is increased. These metabolites are used to monitor exposure to lead in industrial workers and other individuals with suspected lead poisoning.

In relation to xenobiotic factors other than pharmaceutical agents, there is a strong suspicion (as yet unproved) that tobacco smoking is an aggravating factor in frequency and severity of acute porphyric crises in those patients with an established pattern of attacks.

Although the mechanism by which acute attacks of porphyria are induced is unknown, recent studies have identified an inducible gene transcription coactivator – the peroxisome proliferator-activated receptor-gene coactivator PGC-1α.[15] This molecule interacts with transcription factors involved in the regulation of energy metabolism, including adaptive thermogenesis and metabolism of glucose and fatty acids, and the gene product seems to have a role in the development of the heart. Mice that lack the gene that encodes for PGC-1α do not induce ALAS-1 in the liver, and mice with double mutations that lack porphobilinogen deaminase and are at risk from acute porphyria induced by starvation who also lack this transcription coactivator fail to develop porphyria under conditions of nutritional stress. These animals remain susceptible to acute porphyric disturbances when challenged with porphyrinogenic drugs such as barbiturates. Although PGC-1α seems to be a promising avenue of research, other components with inducible transcriptional gene coactivators are likely to be implicated in acute attacks of porphyria in affected individuals.

The most common acute porphyria is acute intermittent porphyria, which is caused by deficiency of porphobilinogen deaminase and inherited as a dominant disorder with variable penetrance and expressivity – as with the other two most familiar acute porphyrias, variegate and hereditary coproporphyria. The very rare ALA dehydratase deficiency is, in contrast, inherited as an autosomal recessive trait. Molecular heterogeneity is considerable, and hundreds of mutations have been described in people with this acute intermittent porphyria, as well as the other genes implicated in the acute porphyrias. Individuals who harbour genes that predispose to acute porphyria are estimated to have a frequency of about one in 10,000–12,000 of the population.

Laboratory abnormalities in an acute attack

In an acute attack, concentrations of early haem precursors (such as aminolaevulinate and porphobilinogen) in the urine and body fluids are markedly increased;[2–4] formed porphyrins may arise as a result of non-enzymatic cyclisation, but their appearance is not diagnostic of an acute attack. Useful screening tests include the Watson–Schwartz test or the Hoesch test, which is based on the use of Erhlich's reagent (2% dimethylbenzaldehyde in 2M hydrochloric acid) to detect porphobilinogen. Occasionally, overnight exposure of the urine to light may show the presence of excess porphobilinogen and other pyrrolic adducts in colours ranging from a little recognised mud-grey through tea-coloured or oxidised dilute Burgundy wine to frank crimson – and sometimes a wine-dark colour that resembles strong solutions of potassium permanganate. Quantitative tests that use simple chromatographic separation of ALA and porphobilinogen in the urine (such as the Mauzerall–Granick test) are to be recommended. Molecular analysis of the cognate gene is indicated for first-degree relatives with suspected or latent porphyria; in family studies, such investigations provide definitive information that can usefully allay anxiety or inform prescription of drugs. This service is provided in the UK with a high level of responsiveness, reliability, and professional assistance by Dr Michael Badminton and his colleagues of the Porphyria Service of the Department of Medical Biochemistry at the University Hospital of Wales in Cardiff.

Treatment of the acute attack

The most important aspect of treatment is to suspect porphyria in patients with unexplained abdominal and/or neurological symptoms. Diagnosis is of critical importance, and it is far better to set about the somewhat obsessive task of collecting and sending appropriate samples for this purpose and find them normal in an acutely ill patient (thus rejecting the diagnosis of an acute porphyric attack) than to vainly reject the rare diagnostic possibility on clinical grounds alone.

In patients with an acute attack, it is prudent to increase oral intake of carbohydrates, but the use of high-calorie infusion fluids, such as laevulose or high concentrations of dextrose, is no longer recommended as intravenous glucose preparations may compound the devastating effects of rapid hyponatraemia that characterise the acute attack and may lead to catastrophic consequences, including death from cerebral oedema. All precipitating drugs should be removed with a scrupulous review of the treatment chart and all drugs. Any attack severe enough to warrant hospital admission should be treated with intravenous haematin (available in the United States) or haem arginate (available in Europe and the United Kingdom). Pain should be treated with narcotic analgesics that are safe in porphyria, such as morphine or pethidine; anxiety often responds to tranquillisers such as chlorpromazine or haloperidol. Tachycardia, hypertension, and agitation also respond well to β-blocker drugs such as propranolol and labetalol.

The porphyric attack should be treated as an acute medical emergency and all precipitating factors should be identified as quickly as possible.[11] As a general rule, no drug, including non-prescription and proprietary medications, should ever be administered to a patient with an acute attack of porphyria without explicit and meticulous consultation of an approved pharmaceutical list. Respiratory function and blood pressure should be monitored. In acutely ill patients, it is mandatory to determine levels of sodium in plasma during the acute phases of an attack; I recommend that levels of sodium are determined on a daily basis. Levels of sodium in plasma decrease rapidly during acute porphyria, and hyponatraemia may be severe enough to induce seizures. The causes of hyponatraemia are multifactorial in patients with porphyria, but the syndrome of inappropriate release of antidiuretic hormone is pre-eminent in my experience. Patients with acute porphyria require regular checks for neurological paralysis and respiratory failure due to impaired ventilation as a result of motor dysfunction.

Specific treatment with haem arginate

This treatment is predicated on the concept of negative feedback control of the induced synthetic pathway based on the end-product in the liver at the level of activity of ALAS-1. Parenteral administration of haem arginate induces rapid clinical improvement, with a shortened duration of abdominal pain and hospital stay compared with those patients admitted to hospital and treated by general measures before the introduction of this specific therapy. The drug induces a rapid decrease in the excretion of the urinary precursors ALA and porphobilinogen over 2–3 days without major side effects.

Haem arginate (Normosang) is provided in ampoules containing 25 mg/ml. These need to be diluted immediately before use at a dose of 3 mg/kg body weight and infused into a large vein; the solutions are irritant but not as irritant as the haematin preparations available only in the United States. Haem arginate is infused over at least 30 minutes immediately after *prior* dilution in 100 ml of physiological saline for injection. A maximum dose of 250 mg daily is administered for four days. The clinical and biochemical response, with special reference to urinary porphyrin precursors, should be monitored closely.

Haem arginate is supplied as Normosang by Orphan Europe (Henley-on-Thames, UK). A review by the Centre for Porphyrin Research in Paris by Dr Yves Nordmann provides strong evidence for the benefit of haem arginate in acute attacks of porphyria. Although not explicitly sanctioned for use in pregnancy, haem arginate has been used to treat attacks of acute porphyria in pregnant women – apparently without ill effect.

Management after the acute porphyric attack

After an acute attack of porphyria, it is important to discuss the diagnosis with the patient and to offer, through them, family screening for potentially affected first-degree relatives. Advice about all drugs should be considered; this includes contraception, as progestogens are best avoided. The British National Formulary supplies an up-to-date list of drugs that are *unsafe* for use in patients with acute or latent acute porphyria; invaluable information is also provided by the Welsh Medicines Information Centre at the University Hospital of Wales in Cardiff (telephone: 029 2074 2979). Valuable information can be also obtained from the European Porphyria Initiative's website (www.porphyria-europe.com). Patients with porphyria are strongly advised to seek membership and advice of the appropriate disease association, such as the British Porphyria Association (BPA) in the UK (helpline: 01474 369231; website: www.porphyria.org.uk). This body can provide invaluable support for affected patients, key information about the diseases, a comprehensive drug list, and contact addresses for other members of the relevant porphyria 'community'. We recommend that patients wear warning jewellery that states the diagnosis and provides ready access to, and contact details for, key clinical information – for example, the bracelet, medallion, or brooch provided by the MedicAlert Foundation in London.

Some special problems in acute porphyria

Hyponatraemia

Hyponatraemia in patients with porphyria is associated with seizures and potentially fatal sequelae. Seizures may develop in the absence of hyponatraemia; they may be caused by hypertensive encephalopathy or, as part of the toxic state, may be associated with the ill-understood general 'nervous excitability' that characterises the acute porphyric attack.

Many acute attacks of porphyria are complicated by hyponatraemia, and an excess of antidiuretic hormone seems to be a major component, although overzealous replacement of fluids with hypotonic (dextrose-containing) fluids and excessive loss of salts caused by vomiting and diarrhoea may contribute. Hyponatraemia, however, cannot be explained by these mechanisms in every instance.

Management challenges: recurrent acute neurovisceral attacks

The author's experience is that recurrent attacks of acute porphyria almost invariably occur in young women and that many are related closely to the time of ovulation or menstruation, or both (that is, the progestogenic phases of the cycle). Periodic attacks can be extremely debilitating, and they are associated not only with abdominal and limb pain distinct from those that accompany menstruation but also with overt motor neuropathy and paralysis that are aggravated by each episode. The attacks characteristically last 8–15 days when untreated and occur periodically – usually immediately after ovulation or during the 1–2 days that precede the onset of menstruation. In the author's experience and in anecdotal reports in the literature, prophylactic infusions of haem arginate (one or two infusions of 250 mg on a daily basis) may reduce the severity of attacks or, when given in anticipation of a regular attack, effectively prevent these attacks. Difficulties frequently arise in young women with inconspicuous peripheral veins, so that venous access by means of indwelling infusion cannulae, such as portacath devices, is needed for the facile regular administration of haem arginate and other, unstable preparations of haem. The use of high-dose gonadotrophin analogues such as goserelin or buserelin in severely affected patients with recalcitrant disease has been reported. By acting as luteinising hormone-releasing hormone (LHRH) agonists to inhibit ovulation, these drugs induce functional hypogonadism and thereby arrest the cyclical hormonal changes that are associated with the porphyric attacks. In the author's experience, although this draconian intervention may have useful immediate effects, it rarely has been successful in the long term, and at least one patient continues to have attacks with comparable periodicity while receiving the drug at the standard depot dose; another patient with acute porphyria has conceived a second pregnancy while receiving buserelin by depot injection. Further investigations are to be welcomed to determine the most appropriate application of LHRH agonists: in the author's view, prescription of agents that cause profound physical and psychological effects due to hypogonadism but that are not guaranteed to prevent porphyric attacks in young women in the prime of life should not be undertaken other than as a desperate measure to assist those with frequent life-threatening episodes of disease.

The mechanism for the periodic attacks in young women is unknown, but previous research had suggested abnormalities of steroid hormone metabolism and progestogens. One can only hope that an improved mechanistic understanding of these influences will emerge from deepening research into the mechanism of ALAS-1 induction, especially in relation to transcriptional coactivator proteins such as PGC-1α and its potential molecular partners. Several transcriptional coactivators are known to interact with drugs that induce peroxisomal proliferation, and a number of such agents are approved for other indications in the pharmacopoeia. It thus seems probable that agents will be available to modify the induction mechanisms for ALAS-1 and will lead to better control of the devastating acute attacks of porphyria.

Although recurrent severe acute attacks of porphyria affect a very small number of patients nationally, a full understanding of the disease clearly will have broad implications for the outcome of porphyria in other more general circumstances. Indeed, a few patients have been so severely afflicted that heterotopic liver transplantation has been undertaken. In at least one reported case, this heroic procedure corrected the biochemical abnormality and abrogated the acute attacks of porphyria in a young woman. In most cases, however, liver transplantation would not be the preferred option of treatment, since, in the main, once recognised, porphyric attacks can be satisfactorily avoided by adjustment of lifestyle factors. Generally, with informed assistance and improved self education about porphyria for patients and those who provide care for them, future severe attacks in susceptible individuals can be avoided. Liver transplantation is not a generally attractive option for porphyria and should be considered as a matter of last resort;[5] indeed, it is chastening to note that the young woman who underwent successful liver transplantation for control of acute porphyria subsequently died of the complications of the transplant within a few years of the procedure.

REFERENCES

1 Ajioka RS, Phillips JD, Kushner JP. Biosynthesis of heme in mammals. *Biochim Biophys Acta* 2006;1763:723–36.

2 Schmid R, ed. The porphyrias. *Semin Liver Dis* 1998;18:1–101.

3 Anderson KE, Sassa S, Bishop DF, Desnick RJ. Disorders of heme biosynthesis: X-linked sideroblastic anemia and the porphyrias. In: Scriver CR, Beaudet AL, Sly WS, Valle D, eds. *The metabolic and molecular bases of inherited disease*, 8th edition, volume II. New York: McGraw-Hill, 2001:2991–3062.

4 Kauppinen R. Porphyrias. *Lancet* 2005;365:241–52.

5 Soonawalla ZF, Orug T, Badminton MN *et al.* Liver transplantation as a cure for acute intermittent porphyria. *Lancet* 2004;363:705–6.

6 Cox TM. Protoporphyria. In: Kadish KM, Smith KM, Guilard R, eds. *The porphyrin handbook, volume 14: medical aspects of porphyrins.* San Diego, CA: Academic Press, 2003: 121–49.

7 Cox TM, Jack N, Lofthouse S *et al.* King George III and porphyria: an elemental hypothesis and investigation. *Lancet* 2005;366:332–5.

8 Schmid R. Cutaneous porphyria in Turkey. *N Engl J Med* 1960;263:397–8.

9 Elder GH. Porphyria cutanea tarda. *Semin Liver Dis* 1998;18:67–75.

10 Wahlin S, Aschan J, Björnstedt M, Broomé U, Harper P. Curative bone marrow transplantation in erythropoietic protoporphyria after reversal of severe cholestasis. *J Hepatol* 2007;46:174–9.

11 Anderson KE, Bloomer JR, Bonkovsky HL *et al.* Recommendations for the diagnosis and treatment of the acute porphyrias. *Ann Intern Med* 2005;142:439–50.

12 Waldenström J. The porphyrias as inborn errors of metabolism. *Am J Med* 1957;22:758–73.

13 Goldberg A. Acute intermittent porphyria. A study of 50 cases. *Q J Med* 1959;28:183–209.

14 Stein JA, Tschudy DP. Acute intermittent porphyria: a clinical study of 46 patients. *Medicine (Baltimore)* 1970;41:1–16.

15 Handschin C, Lin J, Rhee J *et al.* Nutritional regulation of hepatic heme biosynthesis and porphyria through PGC-1alpha. *Cell* 2005;122:505–15.

The eye in multi-system disease: intravitreal use of systemic drugs in ocular infection, inflammation, and retinal vascular disease

Richard Andrews

Ophthalmologists are increasingly injecting drugs directly into the vitreous cavity to treat a growing number of ocular diseases. So-called 'intravitreal injections' have an established role in the management of infective and inflammatory eye disease. Over the past 12 months, the intravitreal injection of agents that inhibit vascular endothelial growth factor (VEGF) has radically altered the treatment of 'wet' age-related macular degeneration. These agents also offer a potential benefit in other common retinal vascular disorders such as diabetic retinopathy.

□ OCULAR INFECTION

Bacterial

The first established use of intravitreal injections was for the treatment of bacterial infections in the eye. Any focus of bacterial infection can spread to the eye, and this should be considered in any patient with a concurrent or recent infection who complains of ocular pain, reduced vision, or redness in one eye. All suspected cases should be seen urgently the same day by an ophthalmologist, as bacterial endophthalmitis typically progresses rapidly over several hours rather than days with even apparently appropriate systemic antibiotics. This manifests with an increasingly profound reduction in vision accompanied by reduction or loss of the red reflex and the formation of a hypopyon (Fig 1).

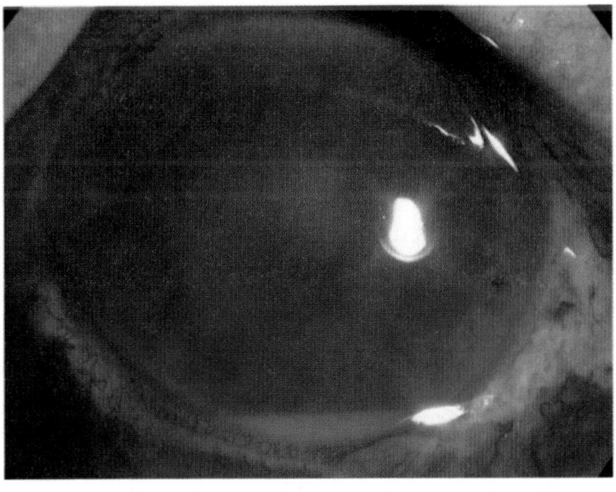

Fig 1 Bacterial endophthalmitis.

Why does bacterial infection in the eye progress so rapidly despite systemic antibiotics? Figure 2 uses gentamicin and vancomycin as representative examples to show why. When intravitreal levels of antibiotic are measured after oral or intravenous administration, levels of the drug within the eye are substantially lower than in the serum and well below the minimum inhibitory concentration for most pathogens. Penetration is limited by the blood–retina barrier, which is analogous to the blood–brain barrier and is formed by the tight junctions between cells of the retinal capillary endothelium and those of the retinal pigment epithelium. The only way to bypass this barrier and achieve adequate intravitreal concentrations of antibiotic is to inject them directly into the eye. In practice, patients are treated empirically with a combination of 2 mg/0.1 ml vancomycin and 0.4 mg/0.1 ml amikacin. This can be repeated after 48 hours if required.

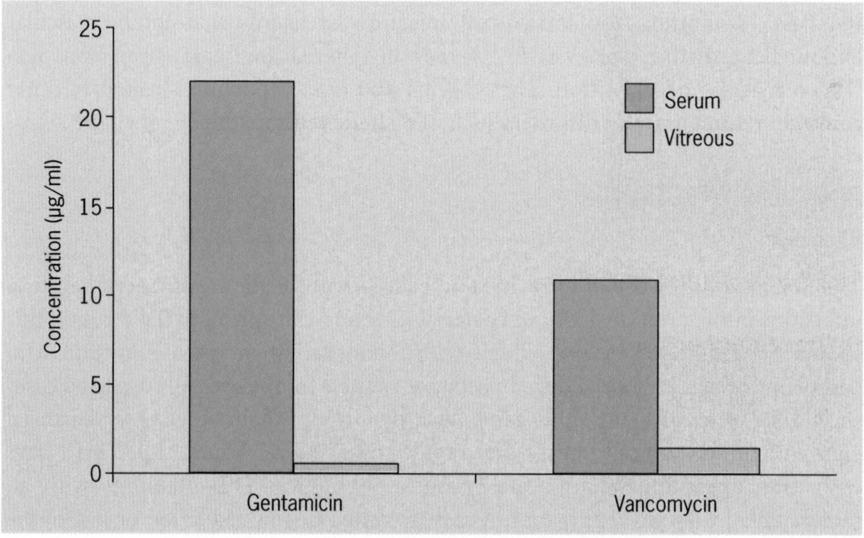

Fig 2 Serum and vitreous levels of antibiotic following systemic administration.

Fungal

Endogenous fungal endophthalmitis is less common than bacterial endophthalmitis. *Candida* species are the most common cause, with *Aspergillus*, *Fusarium* and others seen relatively rarely. Ocular infection occurs via the blood or direct from the sinuses, and traditionally is seen in intravenous drug abusers and people who have had a recent septic or other hospital episode in which intravenous lines were used.

In common with antibiotics, antifungals have poor or limited penetration into the eye. Treatment is therefore determined by the site of the lesion. Candidal foci confined to the choroid, which appear as yellow or yellowish-white areas deep to the retina, lie outside the blood–retina barrier and can be treated successfully with oral fluconazole. Extension of infection into and beyond the retina gives rise to characteristic floating white 'cotton-ball' colonies within the vitreous (Fig 3). Management at this stage requires surgical removal of the vitreous plus 5–10 µg intravitreal amphotericin in combination with treatment for systemic infection. Infection with *Aspergillus* is less common but may produce a panophthalmitis manifest by fullness of the lids and marked conjunctival chemosis (Fig 4). Treatment similarly requires a combination of systemic therapy together with vitrectomy and intravitreal amphotericin.

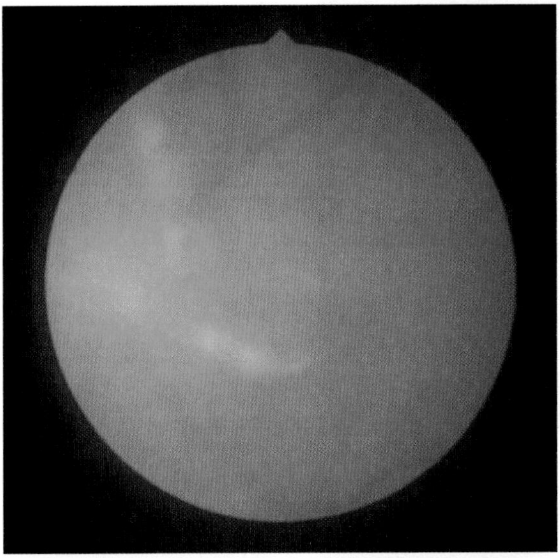

Fig 3 'String of pearl' appearance of Candida within the vitreous.

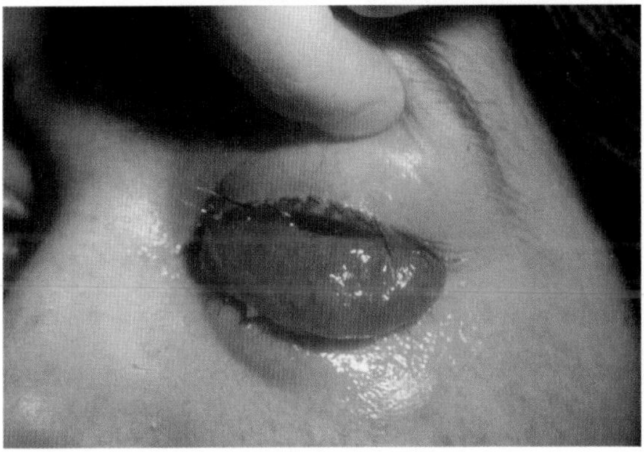

Fig 4 Panophthalmitis associated with *Aspergillus* infection.

Viral

Cytomegalovirus is the most common cause of viral retinitis, although the incidence has decreased dramatically since the introduction of highly active antiretroviral therapy (HAART). The infection appears first as dense white areas of retinitis in a perivascular distribution. This gradually spreads and is associated with haemorrhage that produces a so-called 'pizza-top' appearance (Fig 5). Without treatment, blindness ensues. Intravitreal injection of ganciclovir is effective at inducing remission of the retinitis but needs to be given twice weekly, which clearly has practical implications as a method of long-term maintenance treatment. Ganciclovir implants circumvent this through slow sustained release of the drug over a period of about 6–8 months (Fig 6). If treatment is required beyond the active life of the implant, it is simply replaced.

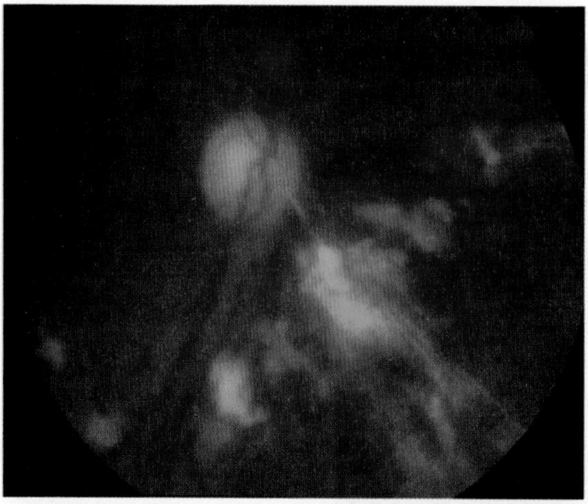

Fig 5 Fulminating CMV retinitis.

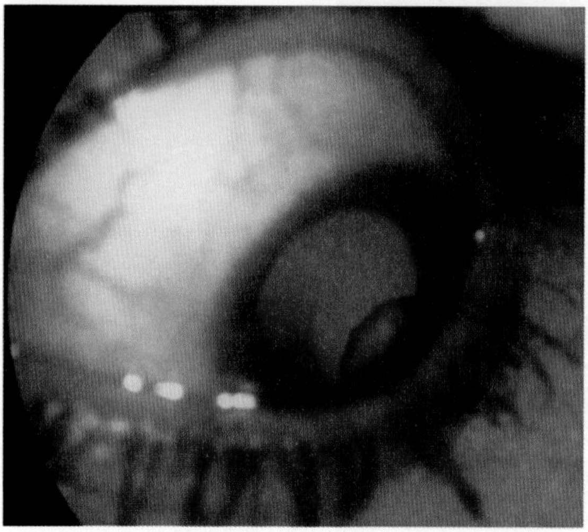

Fig 6 Slow-release ganciclovir implant visible through dilated pupil.

□ OCULAR INFLAMMATION

Beyond intraocular infection, intravitreal injections also have an established role in the management of patients with intraocular inflammation primarily centred at the back of the eye – so-called intermediate and posterior uveitis. In many patients, the inflammatory disease is limited to the eye, but in others it is part of a much broader multi-system disease such as sarcoidosis or Behçet's disease. In some patients, ocular and systemic disease activity may mirror each other, but in others visual loss or threat may occur when the extraocular disease is essentially quiescent.

In contrast with antibiotics, oral steroids penetrate readily into the eye. They are the only treatment choice when vision is imminently threatened. In many patients, vision is compromised more insidiously, with the most common cause being the accumulation of fluid in the retina – so-called macular oedema. In such instances, the benefits of oral treatment need to be weighed against the systemic side-effects. Every effort is made by ophthalmologists to administer steroids locally where possible.

A variety of local treatment options are available. Drops, although safe, convenient, and easy to use, unfortunately do not penetrate to the back of the eye. Orbital injection of depomedrone around the eye, performed by passing a needle through the lower lid and along the floor of the orbit below the eye, can be effective in some patients. In others, the disease remains refractory despite up to three injections given six weeks apart. In these circumstances, intravitreal injection of 4 mg/0.1 ml of triamcinolone offers the potential to control the inflammation, resolve macular oedema, and potentially restore vision. The effects of triamcinolone last for up to 3–4 months. Repeat injections may be given to those in whom macular oedema subsequently recurs. Sustained-release intravitreal steroid implants are now becoming available. Posurdex is a micro-sized intraocular drug delivery system in which the active drug, dexamethasone, is released slowly from a biodegradable polymer matrix over approximately six months.

☐ AGENTS THAT INHIBIT VASCULAR ENDOTHELIAL GROWTH FACTOR

Agents that inhibit vascular endothelial growth factor (VEGF) are the current hot topic in ophthalmology, with pegaptanib sodium injection (Macugen), ranibizumab injection (Lucentis) and bevacizumab (Avastin) even making it to the front pages of the national press. The ophthalmic use of these drugs at the present time is restricted largely to the treatment of choroidal neovascularisation in patients with 'wet' age-related macular degeneration. Anti-VEGF agents, however, may prove to have more widespread applications in the treatment of a variety of other retinal vascular diseases, including diabetic retinopathy and retinal vein occlusions, as well as end-stage complications such as rubeotic glaucoma.

Vascular endothelial growth factor regulates angiogenesis and vascular permeability – both important features of diabetic retinopathy. Levels of VEGF are increased in experimental models of diabetes, and increased levels are found in the eyes of people with proliferative diabetic retinopathy. Injection of VEGF into the eyes of primates induces changes in the retinal vasculature similar to those seen in the eyes of people with diabetes. The obvious question is whether anti-VEGF agents are of value in the treatment of diabetic retinopathy above and beyond conventional laser treatment. Phase III trial data is lacking, but results of preliminary trials and published case series suggest they may have a number of benefits, including regression of retinal neovascularisation, improvements in the retinopathy severity score, involution of microaneurysms, and a beneficial anatomical effect. In patients with severe ischaemic eye disease, neovascularisation may extend onto the iris and encroach into the trabecular meshwork. The resulting obstruction of aqueous outflow and increase in intraocular pressure can be difficult to treat, with some patients developing intractable ocular pain. Anti-VEGF agents can induce regression of the iris' new vessels and, alone or in combination with existing treatments, can lower the intraocular pressure and alleviate pain.

□ SUMMARY

The number of intravitreal injections of drugs is likely to increase rapidly over the next couple of years. Some patients undoubtedly will be cared for jointly by ophthalmologists and physicians. For patients with endogenous infection, intravitreal injection allows the blood–retina barrier to be bypassed so that therapeutic levels of antibiotics and antifungals can be achieved. The use of such injections in patients with inflammatory eye disease limits the need for systemic corticosteroids. The intravitreal role of anti-VEGF agents beyond macular degeneration is not yet defined clearly, but preliminary studies suggest they may have a broader role in selected patients with common retinal vascular disorders.

☐ MULTI-SYSTEM DISEASE SELF-ASSESSMENT QUESTIONS

Systemic amyloidosis

1 In amyloid A (AA) amyloidosis:
  (a) Patients may have no clear history of chronic inflammatory disease
  (b) Clinically significant cardiac involvement is very rare
  (c) Kidney involvement predominates the clinical picture and outcome
  (d) The prognosis is generally much better than in AL amyloidosis
  (e) Proteinuria is present in almost all cases at diagnosis

2 AL amyloidosis:
  (a) Can be localised to a single anatomical site
  (b) Is always associated with underlying multiple myeloma
  (c) Often responds to systemic chemotherapy
  (d) Can be hereditary
  (e) May occur in patients with no evidence of monoclonal gammopathy

3 Hereditary amyloidosis
  (a) Can be inherited recessively or dominantly
  (b) In some cases can be treated effectively by liver transplantation
  (c) May occur in patients who have monoclonal gammopathy
  (d) Occurs in many patients in the absence of any family history
  (e) Most commonly has a predominately neuropathic or renal phenotype

The porphyrias

1 Regarding acute porphyria:
  (a) It is always associated with haematuria
  (b) It is frequently associated with haematuria
  (c) The porphyrins excreted in excess may give positive stick test results for altered blood in the urine
  (d) The appearance of discoloured urine is an indication that the patient will be photosensitive
  (e) Acute attacks are always associated with abnormal excretion of porphyrin precursors in the urine

2 Acute porphyric attacks:
  (a) Are associated with marked hypokalaemia
  (b) Are associated with marked hyponatraemia
  (c) Are best treated with large volumes of intravenous solutions of 5% weight by volume D-glucose
  (d) Are aggravated by the inappropriate use of pethidine or morphine
  (e) Occur in most patients who inherit a single copy of the mutant allele responsible for porphyria in their family

3 Regarding porphyria cutanea tarda:
(a) It is usually transmitted as an autosomal dominant trait
(b) It does not blister or injure the skin
(c) It is frequently associated with excess iron in the liver
(d) Starvation and/or barbiturate anaesthetics should be avoided
(e) Abdominal symptoms respond well to infusions of haem arginate

Haematology

The modern management of chronic myeloid leukaemia

Puja Mehta, Brian Huntly and Jane F Apperley

☐ INTRODUCTION

Chronic myeloid leukaemia (CML) is a triphasic myeloproliferative disorder characterised by a consistent chromosomal translocation – the Philadephia (Ph) chromosome. The *BCR* gene from chromosome 22 becomes juxtaposed to the *ABL* gene, which is normally resident on chromosome 9, and this results in the formation of the hybrid gene *BCR-ABL* and consequently the fusion protein Bcr-Abl – a dysregulated tyrosine kinase. Uncontrolled expression of Bcr-Abl leads to the defining characteristics of leukaemic cells – enhanced proliferation, resistance to apoptosis, and altered adhesion.[1]

The management and prognosis of CML were revolutionised very recently by the introduction of the targeted tyrosine kinase inhibitors (TKIs) into clinical practice. Before this, the management options were allogeneic stem-cell transplantation (alloSCT), interferon-based treatment, and simple cytoreduction with hydroxyurea. All eligible patients of appropriate age and with human leucocyte antigen (HLA)-matched donors proceeded to alloSCT, which even today is the only curative treatment. All other patients received α-interferon, which, when tolerated in the long term, achieved a median survival of 6.5–7 years by prolonging the chronic phase (CP). Progression to the more advanced phases of disease – 'acceleration' and 'blast transformation' – was not amenable to available treatment.

Imatinib (Glivec) was the first TKI to be introduced into clinical practice in 1998. It competitively occupies the adenosine triphosphate (ATP)-binding pocket of Abl kinase, thus preventing a conformational change to the active form of the molecule and resulting in death of target cells. Imatinib initially was used for patients with suboptimal response to α-interferon or those in the accelerated or blastic phases. Phase II studies showed complete haematological remission (CHR) in 95%, 53%, 15%, and 19% of those in CP, accelerated phase, myeloid blast crisis, and lymphoid blast crisis, respectively, and impressive complete cytogenetic responses (CCyR) in 41%, 17%, 7%, and 17%, respectively.[2–4] These results led to a pivotal phase III randomised trial of imatinib versus α-interferon plus cytosine arabinoside (IFN-ara-C) (the IRIS study).[5] Overall, CHR and CCyR were achieved in 95% and 94%, respectively, of those on imatinib and in 55% and 8.5%, respectively, of those on IFN-ara-C. Progression-free survival (PFS) at 18 months was achieved in 96.7% of those on imatinib and 91.5% of those on IFN-ara-C; a significant difference despite a high rate of crossover from the IFN-ara-C arm to the imatinib arm. After five years, 70% of patients in the imatinib-only group remained on treatment, and the probabilities of attaining CHR and CCyR on treatment were 98% and 87%, respectively.[6] Imatinib gained accelerated regulatory approval for all disease phases and became first-line treatment for all newly diagnosed patients. Some 20% of patients do not achieve CCyR, however, and a small but significant proportion of good responders will subsequently lose their response. Furthermore, leukaemic cells remain detectable by sensitive reverse transcriptase polymerase chain reaction (RT-PCR) even in most patients with CCyR, which suggests that the disease is well controlled but not eradicated permanently. This has led to an intensive pursuit of the mechanisms of imatinib resistance, with the aim of identifying alternative effective therapeutic interventions.

□ RESPONSE AND RESISTANCE

Response to treatment is defined in three distinct stages. The initial aim of treatment is achievement of normal peripheral blood counts and <5% of bone marrow blasts (CHR) ideally within four weeks of starting treatment and certainly by the twelfth week of treatment. Complete cytogenetic remission is defined as the absence of the Ph chromosome by conventional cytogenetic analysis of bone marrow metaphases and ideally should be obtained within 18 months of initiation of imatinib. Once a patient has achieved CCyR, further monitoring of disease response requires the measurement of *BCR-ABL* transcripts by RT-PCR (sensitivity of 10^5) or fluorescence in situ hybridisation (FISH; (sensitivity of 10^{-3}; false positive rate of 2–5%). Once an individual has achieved a 3-log reduction in their disease burden (only calculable through RT-PCR), they are deemed to be in 'major molecular response' (MMolR). About 5% of patients who have achieved CCyR become negative on RT-PCR ('molecular negativity'), which means that that leukaemic load has decreased to below the level detectable by the test. In most cases, RT-PCR levels decrease until they eventually plateau at an individual-specific level.

The definition of 'lack of response' has proved controversial (Table 1) as it has been unclear how long treatment should continue before a patient can be defined as 'failing' on imatinib; timeframes are not absolute and should not dictate discontinuation of imatinib without an effective alternative treatment. Loss of CHR and CCyR are easy to identify. Loss of molecular response is more difficult to define precisely, partly because RT-PCR assays are not yet standardised,[7] so individual results should be monitored to identify definite trends.

'Primary resistance' (or 'refractoriness') is defined as failure to elicit a response to imatinib. 'Acquired resistance' is the loss of previously established response: haematological, cytogenetic, or molecular.

□ MECHANISMS OF 'RESISTANCE'

The mechanisms of primary resistance are yet to be elucidated fully and are thought to be due to mechanisms independent of the *BCR-ABL* gene. Mechanisms of secondary resistance are better understood and are due to mutations in the Abl

Table 1 Suggested thresholds to define failure, suboptimal response, and optimal response. Reproduced from Mauro and Deininger with permission of the American Society of Hematology.[14]

	Month			
Outcome	**3**	**6**	**12**	**18**
Failure	No haematological response	>95% Ph+	>35% Ph+	>0% Ph+
Suboptimal response	No complete haematological response	35–95% Ph+	1–35% Ph+	0% Ph+ <3 log decrease in *BCR-ABL* transcripts
Optimal response	1–2 log decrease in *BCR-ABL* transcripts	<35% Ph+	0% Ph+ >3 log decrease in *BCR-ABL* transcripts	0% Ph+ >3 log decrease in *BCR-ABL* transcripts

Ph+ = positive for Philadelphia chromosome.

kinase domain in 50–90% of cases.[8] Amplification of *BCR-ABL* may also contribute to resistance, most commonly via genomic amplification or the acquisition of additional Ph chromosomes.[9]

Mutations in the Abl kinase domain

Fifty different mutations have been associated with clinical resistance to imatinib; they generally cluster into four categories: T315 mutants; activation loop (A loop) (particularly H396 mutants); ATP-binding loop (P loop) (particularly Y253 and E255 mutants); and M351 mutants. Mutations may interrupt critical drug–protein contact points, although most induce a conformational change in the Abl kinase that decreases or precludes binding of the drug. Dose escalation recaptures response in some patients, albeit modest or lacking in durability, therefore some mutations are thought to confer only partial resistance.

Fifteen amino acid substitutions account for more than 85% of the mutations, and, interestingly, mutations at only seven sites (G250, Y253, E255, T315, M351, F359, and H396) are responsible for about two thirds of the reported cases. Substitutions can occur at the same residue and may confer different sensitivities to imatinib. Whether certain mutations induce disease progression or simply signify genetic instability associated with acceleration is unclear.

Imatinib critically recognises and binds the inactive conformation of Abl when the activation (A) loop – the major regulatory element of the kinase domain – blocks the catalytic centre. Mutations within the A loop (Abl residues 381–402) are likely to prevent the kinase adopting the inactive conformation. Binding of the A loop to imatinib causes the P loop (Abl residues 244–255) to fold over the drug. P loop mutations have been associated with more rapid progression to advanced phase disease and poorer prognosis than mutations in other regions of the molecule.[10]

Mutations can antedate treatment with imatinib and commonly are described in patients who receive imatinib in the advanced phases. This suggests that the mutation occurs in a proliferating stem cell early in the disease and that the mutation offers no survival advantage until the patient is exposed to imatinib. In patients with mutations, imatinib may exert an in-vivo selection pressure for the resistant clone. The implications of mutations are uncertain. The development of mutations in patients with stable disease may not alter immediate treatment response; however, in patients who lose their response or have progressed to advanced disease, cells from mutated clones are likely to increase and predominate.

Increased expression of Bcr-Abl

The most frequent cause of resistance to imatinib in cell lines that have been engineered to develop resistance is overexpression of Bcr-Abl. Surprisingly, this is not a frequent observation in patients with acquired resistance, although it has been described in clinical practice. Amplification of the *BCR-ABL* gene was seen in 3/11 patients studied with acquired resistance, and in one individual it coexisted with the presence of a point mutation in the Abl kinase domain.[9] Others have since confirmed this latter phenomenon.

Cell lines that express high amounts of Bcr-Abl are less sensitive to imatinib and take a substantially shorter time to produce resistant subclones. As the numbers of *BCR-ABL* transcripts correlate with disease phase, it is possible that the relatively high levels of oncoprotein in advanced-phase disease may underlie the observed rapid development of resistance.

Clonal evolution

Disease progression is associated with the acquisition of additional chromosomal aberrations in the Ph-positive population – 'clonal evolution'. In some classification systems, clonal evolution satisfies the criteria for disease acceleration. Clonal evolution has been shown to correspond with decreased response to imatinib in terms of achievement of cytogenetic response, loss of haematological response, and overall survival.

Quiescent stem cells

Despite optimal response to treatment and the absence of point mutations, imatinib fails to completely remove all leukaemic cells, and patients continue to have molecularly detectable disease. These 'quiescent' or 'dormant' cells are thought to then form a reservoir of disease with the capacity to develop resistance.

□ NOVEL TREATMENT TO ADDRESS IMATINIB-RESISTANT DISEASE

Due to the heterogeneity of resistance mechanisms, a single strategy to combat imatinib-resistant CML is unlikely to be uniformly successful. The most promising approach involves the development of novel TKIs such as dasatinib (Sprycel, BMS-354835) and nilotinib (Tasigna, AMN-107), which are designed to target resistant clones. Nilotinib was developed from imatinib and modified to bind the Abl kinase with higher affinity and less stringent bonding requirements. Dasatinib was developed as a Src kinase inhibitor but was found to inhibit Bcr-Abl in the active and inactive conformations. Both compounds inhibit Abl and all known mutant Abl kinases in vitro, except for mutations at the 'gatekeeper position' T315I.

In 2004, nilotinib entered a dose-escalating phase I study (n=119), with CHR obtained in 39%, 74%, and 92% of imatinib-resistant patients in blast crisis, acceleration phase, and CP, respectively. Major cytogenetic response (MCyR) was seen in 5/33 patients in blast crisis, 15/56 in the accelerated phase, and 6/17 in CP.[11] Dasatinib entered phase I trials in 2003 initially with patients in resistant CP (n=84), but the study was extended to other disease phases after efficacy was shown. In patients in CP, the accelerated phase, myeloid blast crisis, and lymphoblastic crisis/leukaemia, the rates of CHR were 92%, 45%, 45%, and 27%, respectively, and the rates of MCyR were 35%, 35%, 70%, and 80%, respectively.[12]

Dasatinib (15–240 mg/day) did not exhibit dose-limiting toxicity, but nilotinib 600 mg twice daily was associated with hepatic and pancreatic enzyme derangement. Treatment-induced pleural effusions occurred in 18% of patients treated with dasatinib. Nilotinib was associated with prolongation of the QT interval by 5–15 msec without clinical cardiotoxicity. Myelosuppression was more marked with both drugs compared with imatinib, particularly with dasatinib; however, failure or intolerance of imatinib may be confounded by other consequences of longer disease duration.

In phase I, both drugs elicited responses in patients with advanced CML and Ph-positive acute lymphoblastic leukaemia (ALL). Overall, 70% of patients treated with dasatinib and 41% treated with nilotinib had Abl kinase mutations before treatment. Patients with and without mutations generally responded to both agents; however, T315I mutant clones prohibited a response and commonly were detected at the time of treatment failure.

The phase II results for both drugs in patients in CP are encouraging (Table 2); most attained CHR, about half attained MCyR, and one-third attained CCyR. The phase II studies of dasatinib in all phases of CML and Ph-positive ALL supported the granting of its licence in December 2006.

□ MANAGEMENT OF IMATINIB RESISTANCE

The management of patients with suboptimal or failing responses to imatinib is complex (Fig 1). It is important to look for a cause for the resistance, as the approach to treatment may differ in the presence of clonal evolution, gene amplification, or point mutations, or their combination. Unless the mutated clone is present to a significant degree, however, the likelihood of detection will be low as the sensitivity of most techniques is relatively low.

The choices available at the time of imatinib failure essentially include increasing the imatinib dose; changing to a new TKI; alloSCT; returning to conventional treatment with hydroxyurea or interferon, or both; or entry into a trial of a novel therapeutic agent. Ideally, all patients who fail on imatinib should be entered into a clinical trial of one or other therapeutic approach, as little evidence at the present

Table 2 Phase II results for nilotinib and dasatinib across all phases of chronic myeloid leukaemia (CML). Adapted and reproduced from Mauro and Deininger with permission of the American Society of Hematology.[14]

Iminitab-refractory or -intolerant disease	No of patients	No of patients with response (%)						Median follow up (months)
		Haemato-logical	Complete haematological	Cytogenetic				
				Any	Minor	Major	Complete	
Nilotinib								
CML								
Chronic phase	81	NR	69	68	11	46	32	6
Accelerated phase	25	40	16	56	8	28	16	5.5
Myeloid blast crisis	13	8	NR	NR	NR	16	8	2.5
Lymphoid blast crisis	6	NR	17	NR	NR	50	33	2.5
Ph+ ALL	15	27*	NR	NR	NR	NR	NR	2.3
Dasatinib								
CML								
Chronic phase	387	NR	90	NR	NR	51	40	8
Accelerated phase	174	59	34	39	5	34	25	7
Myeloid blast crisis	109	49	25	44	13	31	25	3.5
Lymphoid blast crisis	48	39	29	NR	NR	44	38	2.3
Ph+ ALL	46	48	33	NR	NR	46	44	2.7

ALL = acute lymphoblastic leukemia; NR = not reported; Ph+ = positive for Philadelphia chromosome.
*Response to nilotinib in patients with ALL positive for Philadelphia chromosome was recorded as 'complete response' (haematological recovery and <5% marrow blasts).

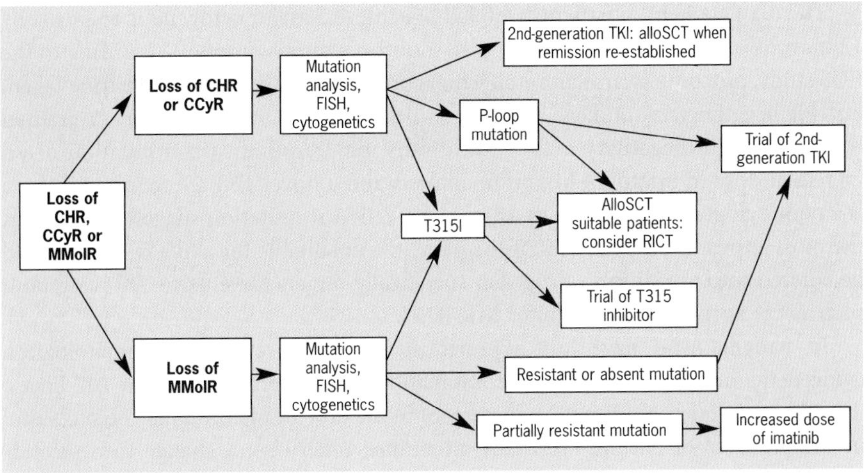

Fig 1 Management of lack of complete haematological response (CHR) or complete cytogenetic response (CCyR). AlloSCT = allogeneic stem-cell transplantation; FISH = fluorescence in situ hybridisation; Ph = Philadelphia chromosome; RICT = reduced-intensity conditioning; TKI = tyrosine kinase inhibitor.

time can guide these decisions. The rationale for increasing the dose of imatinib to 600 or 800 mg a day is based on three factors. Firstly, studies of higher doses in newly diagnosed patients show that responses (CHR, CCyR, and MMolR) are obtained more rapidly, but it is unclear whether they are achieved in a higher proportion of patients in the long term. Secondly, some point mutations show only partial resistance to imatinib in vitro. Finally, some groups have shown that the mutation is not always the cause of resistance, as the disease remains stable and the level of the mutated clone is unchanged in the presence of ongoing treatment with imatinib. In a recent study that compared dasatinib with imatinib 800 mg a day in patients who were deemed to have failed imatinib 600 mg a day, dasatinib showed a higher rate of response with respect to CHR and CCyR than imatinib.[13]

The role and timing of alloSCT is controversial. Despite a significant procedural-related risk of mortality, alloSCT usually eradicates leukaemic cells according to sensitive RT-PCR. The graft-versus-leukaemia effect may serve as consolidation after salvage with a second-generation TKI or as an alternative with high relapse or risk of progression.

In patients who tolerate imatinib but fail to achieve CHR by three months, early alternative treatment is needed. Mutation analysis rarely is helpful. Allogeneic stem-cell transplantation should be considered in patients of a suitable age. Those ineligible for transplant may benefit from a trial of an alternative TKI.

Intolerance to the dose of imatinib may require corticosteroids and supportive measures (granulocyte colony-stimulating factor (G-CSF), erythropoietin, and platelet transfusions). Perseverance usually allows continuation of imatinib and withdrawal of supportive treatment. Failing this, alloSCT or conventional chemotherapy should be offered rather than nilotinib and dasatinib, which are more myelotoxic than imatinib.

The management of patients who fail to achieve a major cytogenetic response by 12 months or a complete response by 18 months is more complex. According to the IRIS study, outcome is similar for all who achieve CCyR regardless of the time taken, but Ph negativity is unlikely if MCyR is not achieved by 18 months. A gradual reduction in Ph negativity before 18 months may respond to continuation or an increased dose of imatinib. Mutation analysis and a novel TKI are required if there is a poor cytogenetic response by 18 months. A T315I mutation suggests alloSCT as the most appropriate treatment; if the patient is unsuitable for alloSCT, they should be entered into a trial for a drug that specifically targets the elusive T315I mutant, such as the aurora kinase inhibitor MK-0457.

In patients who have lost a previously obtained response (haematological, cytogenetic, or molecular, or their combination), point mutations in the Abl kinase domain are frequent findings. An increment in the dose of imatinib may be successful in the presence of partially resistant mutations; otherwise, a change to a second-generation TKI is indicated. Loss of cytogenetic and haematological responses suggests a higher tumour burden. A trial of a second-generation TKI may recapture response. Preliminary results with nilotinib and dasatinib suggest that responses are obtained early, and all suitable patients should proceed to alloSCT if they are absent.

Progression to acceleration or blast crisis while a patient is taking imatinib warrants prompt alloSCT in suitable patients after a second chronic phase has been established – either by the use of a second-generation TKI or conventional acute myelogenous leukaemia (AML)-like therapy. If alloSCT is not possible, a second-generation TKI, conventional chemotherapy, or autologous transplant should be considered.

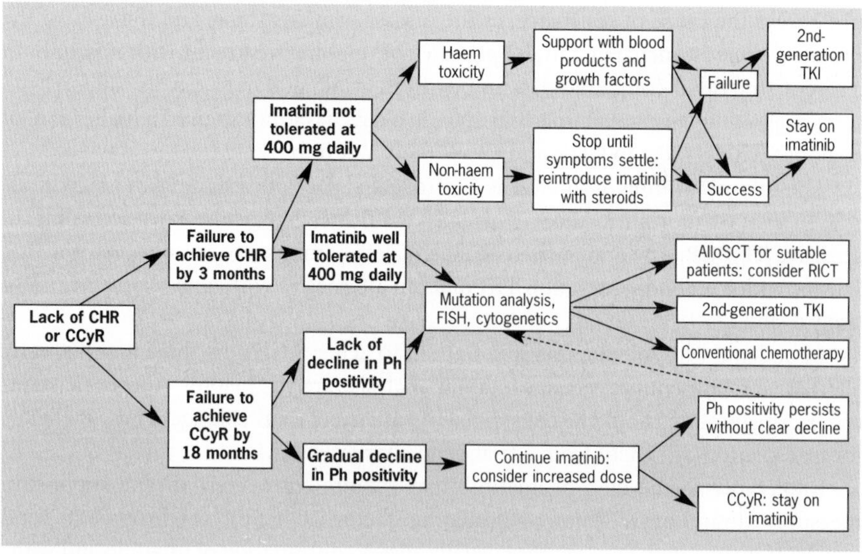

Fig 2 Management of loss of response. AlloSCT = allogeneic stem-cell transplantation; CCyR = complete cytogenetic response; CHR = complete haematological response; FISH = fluorescence in situ hybridisation; RICT = reduced-intensity conditioning; MMolR = major molecular response; TKI = tyrosine kinase inhibitor.

☐ SUMMARY

The TKIs have dramatically altered the management of CML. Most patients respond excellently to imatinib for many years, but the drug does not eradicate all leukaemic cells. Dasatinib and nilotinib represent important advances for challenging resistant disease. New treatments undoubtedly must be developed for patients with T315I mutants. Emerging data will enable better understanding of the significance of Abl kinase mutations and novel targeted therapies and will contribute to individualised management strategies.

REFERENCES

1. Goldman JM, Melo JV. Chronic myeloid leukaemia – advances in biology and new approaches to treatment. *N Engl J Med* 2003;349:1451–64.
2. Kantarjian H, Sawyers C, Hochhaus A *et al.* Hematologic and cytogenetic responses to imatinib mesylate in chronic myelogenous leukemia. *N Engl J Med* 2002;346:645–52.
3. Talpaz M, Silver RT, Druker BJ *et al.* Imatinib induces durable hematologic and cytogenetic responses in patients with accelerated phase chronic myeloid leukemia: results of a phase 2 study. *Blood* 2002;99:1928–37.
4. Sawyers CL, Hochhaus A, Feldman E *et al.* Imatinib induces hematologic and cytogenetic responses in patients with chronic myelogenous leukemia in myeloid blast crisis: results of a phase II study. *Blood* 2002;99:3530–9.
5. O'Brien SG, Guilhot F, Larson RA *et al.* Imatinib compared with interferon and low-dose cytarabine for newly diagnosed chronic-phase chronic myeloid leukemia. *N Engl J Med* 2003;348:994–1004.
6. Druker BJ, Guilhot F, O'Brien SG *et al.* Five-year follow-up of patients receiving imatinib for chronic myeloid leukemia. *N Engl J Med* 2006;355:2408–17.
7. Hughes T, Deininger M, Hochhaus A *et al.* Monitoring CML patients responding to treatment with tyrosine kinase inhibitors: review and recommendations for harmonizing current methodology for detecting BCR-ABL transcripts and kinase domain mutations and for expressing results. *Blood* 2006;108:28–37.
8. Shah NP. Loss of response to imatinib: mechanisms and management. *Hematology Am Soc Hematol Educ Program* 2005:183–7.
9. Gorre ME, Mohammed M, Ellwood K *et al.* Clinical resistance to STI-571 cancer therapy caused by BCR-ABL gene mutation or amplification. *Science* 2001;293:876–80.
10. Branford S, Rudzki Z, Walsh S *et al.* Detection of BCR-ABL mutations in patients with CML treated with imatinib is virtually always accompanied by clinical resistance, and mutations in the ATP phosphate-binding loop (P-loop) are associated with a poor prognosis. *Blood* 2003;102:276–83.
11. Kantarjian H, Giles F, Wunderle L *et al.* Nilotinib in imatinib-resistant CML and Philadelphia chromosome-positive ALL. *N Engl J Med* 2006;354:2542–51.
12. Talpaz M, Shah NP, Kantarjian H *et al.* Dasatinib in imatinib-resistant Philadelphia chromosome-positive leukemias. *N Engl J Med* 2006;354:2531–41.
13. Kantarjian H, Pasquini R, Hamerschlak N *et al.* Dasatinib or high-dose imatinib for chronic-phase chronic myeloid leukemia after failure of first-line imatinib: a randomized phase 2 trial. *Blood* 2007;109:5143–50.
14. Mauro MJ, Deininger MW. Chronic myeloid leukemia in 2006: a perspective. *Haematologica* 2006;91:152.

The myeloproliferative disorders: management and molecular pathogenesis

Anthony R Green

The past two years have seen major advances in our understanding of both the pathogenesis and the management of myeloproliferative disorders (MPDs). First, the two largest randomised clinical trials in myeloproliferative disorders have been published[1,2] – one in polycythaemia vera (PV) and one in essential thrombocythaemia (ET). Second, the discovery of the *JAK2* V617F mutation[3–7] promises to redefine the diagnostic work-up, classification, and management of these disorders.

☐ MANAGEMENT

Polycythaemia vera

The Collaboration on Low-Dose Aspirin in Polycythemia Vera (ECLAP) trial included a randomised comparison of aspirin and placebo in patients with newly or previously diagnosed PV.[2] In addition to aspirin or placebo, all patients had cytoreduction or phlebotomy to control haematocrit, platelet count managed according to their local haematologists' preferences, or both. Patients who had a clear indication for aspirin (that is, those at high risk) were excluded from the randomisation; these represented a larger number of patients (n=742) than those actually randomised (n=518), which indicates that the ECLAP trial represented the approximately 40% of patients with PV who are at lowest risk of thrombosis. The mean age of randomised patients thus was about 61 years compared with 65 years for the full cohort, and fewer than 5% had had a previous arterial thrombosis in the aspirin trial compared with 28.7% in the overall study.[2,8]

The key finding of the randomised trial was a significantly reduced risk of the combined primary endpoint of non-fatal myocardial infarction, non-fatal stroke, pulmonary embolism, major venous thrombosis, or death from cardiovascular causes in patients randomised to receive aspirin.[2] Subgroup analyses showed that the benefits of aspirin were homogeneous across groups stratified by duration of disease, cytoreductive therapy, and platelet counts and haematocrit at trial entry. The benefits of aspirin came with no increased risk of major haemorrhage and a minimal (if any) increase in minor bleeding (relative risk 1.83; p=0.10).[2]

Essential thrombocythaemia

The Medical Research Council (MRC)'s primary thombocythemia-1 (PT-1) trial randomised high-risk patients (those with prior thrombosis, age >60 years, or platelets $>1000\times10^9/l$) to receive hydroxyurea plus aspirin or anagrelide plus aspirin.[1] With more than 800 patients randomised and with central clinical and histological review of endpoints, the PT-1 trial is the largest and most comprehensive study of ET performed to date. The results show several major differences between the two arms. Compared with hydroxyurea plus aspirin, treatment with anagrelide plus aspirin was associated with increased rates of arterial thrombosis, major haemorrhage, myelofibrotic transformation, and treatment withdrawal but a decreased rate of venous thromboembolism.

The difference in the rates of thrombosis in the two arms of the PT-1 trial is intriguing given the equivalent long-term control of the platelet count. These data imply that, in addition to lowering the platelet count, hydroxyurea and anagrelide may modulate thrombosis by other mechanisms (for example, altered white cell count or function or altered endothelial function). The unexpected increase in major haemorrhage seen in patients who received anagrelide plus aspirin may reflect an ability of anagrelide to interfere with platelet function in a way that synergises with low-dose aspirin. Although most assays of platelet function are normal in patients with ET who receive anagrelide, some subtle effects on platelet function have been reported. The results from the PT-1 study suggest that a decision to use concurrent aspirin when anagrelide is used should depend on the relative risk of arterial thrombosis and hemorrhage in each individual patient.

Patients who received anagrelide plus aspirin had a higher rate of transformation to myelofibrosis than patients who received hydroxyurea plus aspirin. It is important to emphasise that a diagnosis of myelofibrotic transformation required not only a trephine biopsy showing grade 3 fibrosis or higher but also the development of other clinical or laboratory evidence of transformation. The incidence of myelofibrosis in patients with untreated ET is unknown, so it is not clear whether the observed differences reflect a protective effect of hydroxyurea or an acceleration of myelofibrosis by anagrelide. Hydroxyurea has been reported to reduce reticulin fibrosis in a variety of myeloproliferative disorders, including ET. On the other hand, anagrelide blocks megakaryocyte differentiation, and the resultant relative increase in immature forms could conceivably result in altered production of profibrotic cytokines.

□ MOLECULAR PATHOGENESIS

The human myeloproliferative disorders represent a spectrum of clonal haematological malignancies with three main members: PV, ET, and idiopathic myelofibrosis (IMF). For more than a quarter of a century, these diseases have been realised to reflect transformation of a multipotent haematopoietic stem cell, but the identity of underlying target gene(s) has remained elusive.

In 2005, we and others showed that a single acquired point mutation in the *JAK2* gene is present in virtually all patients with PV and in about half those with ET or

IMF.[3–6] In our cohort, a single point mutation (V617F) was identified in the *JAK2* gene in 71 (97%) of 73 patients with PV, 29 (57%) of 51 patients with ET, and eight (50%) of 16 patients with IMF. The mutation is acquired, is present in a variable proportion of granulocytes, alters a highly conserved valine present in the negative regulatory JH2 domain, and is predicted to dysregulate kinase activity. It was heterozygous in most patients, was homozygous in a subset as a result of mitotic recombination, and arose in a multipotent progenitor capable of giving rise to erythroid and myeloid cells. The mutation was present in all erythropoietin-independent erythroid colonies, which demonstrates a link with growth factor hypersensitivity – a key biological feature of these disorders. The V617F mutation in *JAK2* was not detected in 418 cancer cell lines that represented more than 30 different tumour types, and it was seen in only 5% of patients with myelodysplasia or acute myeloid leukemia (AML). The mutation also increases kinase activity and confers cytokine independence in vitro together with erythrocytosis in vivo.

Identification of the mutation in *JAK2* has made it possible to address a number of outstanding issues concerning the pathogenesis of the myeloproliferative disorders. Analysis of individual haematopoietic colonies and flow-sorted progenitor populations showed that the mutation arises in the haematopoietic stem cell compartment.[3] It is possible to detect progenitors homozygous for the mutation in *JAK2* in the vast majority of patients with PV but not in those with ET.[9] The latter observation suggests that homozygous progenitors have a particular selective advantage in patients with PV (possibly because of low serum erythropoietin levels) or that mitotic recombination occurs more frequently in patients with PV. We have also been able to investigate four patients with a *JAK2* V617F-positive myeloproliferative disorder who subsequently developed AML. Unexpectedly, in three of the four patients, the AML blasts lacked the mutation in *JAK2*, which shows that mutant *JAK2* is not necessary for leukaemic transformation.[10]

In an example of scientific serendipity, these results coincided with our publication of the results of the MRC's PT-1 trial,[1] the largest randomised study of any myeloproliferative disorder yet performed. Analysis of prospective data from 776 patients with ET in this study showed that *JAK2* mutation status defines two biologically distinct subtypes of ET, with differences in presentation, outcome, and response to treatment.[7] Patients negative for the mutation in *JAK2* do not become *JAK2* positive, which suggests that JAK mutation status defines two distinct diseases rather than separate stages of the same disorder. Mutation-positive patients displayed multiple features that resembled PV – an observation also noted in patients with IMF.[11] Moreover, compared with mutation-negative patients, patients with ET positive for the V617F mutation in *JAK2* were more sensitive to treatment with hydroxyurea but not anagrelide. These results suggest that mutation-positive ET and PV form a continuum, with the degree of erythrocytosis determined by physiological or genetic modifiers, and that mutation-negative ET represents a distinct disorder. Similar arguments may explain interindividual differences in platelet count and reticulin fibrosis.

Taken together, these data lay the foundation for new approaches to the diagnosis, classification, and treatment of the myeloproliferative disorders.

REFERENCES

1 Harrison CN, Campbell PJ, Buck G *et al.* Hydroxyurea compared with anagrelide in high-risk essential thrombocythemia. *N Engl J Med* 2005;353:33–45.

2 Landolfi R, Marchioli R, Kutti J *et al.* Efficacy and safety of low-dose aspirin in polycythemia vera. *N Engl J Med* 2004;350:114–24.

3 Baxter EJ, Scott LM, Campbell PJ *et al.* Acquired mutation of the tyrosine kinase JAK2 in human myeloproliferative disorders. *Lancet* 2005;365:1054–61.

4 James C, Ugo V, Le Couedic JP *et al.* A unique clonal JAK2 mutation leading to constitutive signalling causes polycythaemia vera. *Nature* 2005;434:1144–8.

5 Levine RL, Wadleigh M, Cools J *et al.* Activating mutation in the tyrosine kinase JAK2 in polycythemia vera, essential thrombocythemia, and myeloid metaplasia with myelofibrosis. *Cancer Cell* 2005:7:387–97.

6 Kralovics R, Passamonti F, Buser AS *et al.* A gain-of-function mutation in JAK2 in myeloproliferative disorders. *N Engl J Med* 2005;352:1779–90.

7 Campbell PJ, Scott LM, Buck G *et al.* Definition of subtypes of essential thrombocythaemia and relation to polycythaemia vera based on JAK2 V617F mutation status: a prospective study. *Lancet* 2005;366:1945–53.

8 Marchioli R, Finazzi G, Landolfi R *et al.* Vascular and neoplastic risk in a large cohort of patients with polycythemia vera. *J Clin Oncol* 2005;23:2224–32.

9 Scott LM, Scott MA, Campbell PJ, Green AR. Progenitors homozygous for the V617F mutation occur in most patients with polycythemia vera, but not essential thrombocythemia. *Blood* 2006;108:2435–7.

10 Campbell PJ, Baxter EJ, Beer PA *et al.* Mutation of JAK2 in the myeloproliferative disorders: timing, clonality studies, cytogenetic associations, and role in leukemic transformation. *Blood* 2006;108:3548–55.

11 Campbell PJ, Griesshammer M, Dohner K *et al.* V617F mutation in JAK2 is associated with poorer survival in idiopathic myelofibrosis. *Blood* 2005:107:2098–100.

☐ HAEMATOLOGY SELF-ASSESSMENT QUESTIONS

The modern management of chronic myeloid leukaemia

1 Levels of which of the following are often increased in patients with chronic myeloid leukaemia (CML)?
(a) Vitamin B1
(b) Leucocyte alkaline phosphatase
(c) Vitamin B12
(d) Magnesium
(e) Urate

2 The Philadelphia chromosome – the hallmark of CML – may also be found in patients with the following conditions:
(a) Waldenström's macroglobulinaemia
(b) Myelodysplasia
(c) Acute lymphocytic leukaemia
(d) Chronic lymphocytic leukaemia
(e) Acute myeloid leukaemia

3 The following features indicate a poor prognosis for patients with CML:
(a) Positivity for Philadelphia chromosome
(b) Myelofibrosis
(c) Family history of CML
(d) Size of the spleen
(e) Older age

4 In the treatment of CML:
(a) Imatinib is recommended as first-line treatment for all patients with CML
(b) Imatinib induces durable cytogenetic responses in >90% of patients
(c) The most frequent cause of imatinib resistance in newly diagnosed patients is mutations in the kinase domain
(d) The most frequent side effect of imatinib is skin rash
(e) The best treatment after failure of imatinib because of a T315I mutant is dasatinib

5 Imatinib has been successfully used to treatment other conditions, in addition to CML, including:
(a) Ovarian carcinoma
(b) Malignant pleural mesothelioma
(c) Gastrointestinal stromal tumour (GIST)
(d) Carcinoma of the nasopharynx
(e) Hypereosinophilic leukaemia

The myeloproliferative disorders: management and molecular pathogenesis

1 The JAK2 V617 mutation is found in:
  (a) More than 90% of patients with polycythaemia vera
  (b) More than 90% of patients with essential thrombocythemia
  (c) About 50% of patients with sarcomas
  (d) About 50% of patients with myelofibrosis
  (e) About 50% of patients with acute myeloid leukaemia

2 For patients with essential thrombocythaemia at high risk of vascular events:
  (a) Hydroxyurea plus aspirin represents first-line treatment
  (b) Anagrelide plus aspirin represents first-line treatment
  (c) Anagrelide is associated with more side effects than hydroxyurea
  (d) Anagrelide is associated with more myelofibrosis than hydroxyurea
  (e) Anagrelide is associated with more arterial thrombosis than hydroxyurea

3 Compared to patients with essential thrombocythaemia who are negative for JAK2 V617F, those who are positive for JAK2 V617F:
  (a) Have a higher mean level of haemoglobin
  (b) Develop more venous thrombosis
  (c) Develop more arterial thrombosis
  (d) Transform to polycythaemia vera more frequently
  (e) Transform to acute myeloid leukaemia more frequently

Skin and bones

Drug allergies

Peter S Friedmann

□ INTRODUCTION

Adverse drug reactions (ADRs) are responsible for about 5% of all hospital admissions, and between 10–20% of hospital inpatients develop ADRs.[1] They can have many manifestations, and it is important to understand their classification (see below) in order to approach diagnosis and identification of the culprit drug. Most ADRs result from augmented effects of the normal pharmacological effects of drugs, but allergic hypersensitivity reactions generally are unrelated to a drug's pharmacological properties.

Classification of adverse drug reactions

Adverse drug reactions can be classified into five types. Type A (augmented) ADRs are the most common. They are predictable from the primary and secondary pharmacology of the drug and are dose related. Type B (bizarre or idiosyncratic) ADRs are not predictable from the known pharmacology of the drug. The term reflects patient individuality rather than mechanism. The dose relation is less obvious. Type C (chemical) ADRs are predictable from the structure of the drug or its metabolites. Examples include reactions to paracetamol (which is bioactivated in the liver to a toxic quinone imine that is hepatotoxic) and azathioprine (which is metabolised to 6-mercaptopurine, which is myelotoxic and must be further converted by the enzyme thiopurine methyltransferase (TPMT)). Type D (delayed) ADRs are late effects that include teratogenicity and carcinogenicity. Type E (end of dose) ADRs are withdrawal reactions that follow discontinuation of the drug – for example, seizures after the discontinuation of benzodiazepines.

Interpretation of the clinical patterns of immune-mediated drug hypersensitivities is facilitated by reference to the classification of immune hypersensitivity mechanisms defined by Gell and Coombs (Table 1).[2]

Factors that determine susceptibility to type B reactions

Drug disposition

Most drugs are chemical entities of low molecular weight (<1000 Da). In order for small molecules to be recognised by the T-cell receptor, they must act as so-called haptens, binding to proteins that act as carriers. The hapten-conjugated protein is complexed with major histocompatibility complex (MHC) molecules, and the

Table 1 Types of hypersensitivity and the underlying immune effector mechanisms. Adapted from Coombs with permission of Blackwell Science.[2]

Type of hypersensitivity	Effector mechanisms
Type I Immediate or anaphylactic	• Immunoglobulin E (IgE) bound to surface of mast cells or basophils • Antigen binding causes mast-cell degranulation and release of histamine and other mediators
Type II Cytotoxic	• Antigenic determinants on cell surfaces are the target of antibodies, which may be IgG or IgM • Antibodies damage cells or tissues by activating complement or activating cytotoxic killing – for example, K cells, by binding to cells through Fc? receptors
Type III Immune complex	• Circulating immune complexes are deposited in vascular beds or on tissue surfaces • Complement is activated, neutrophils are attracted, and their products damage tissues
Type IV Delayed	• Effector T lymphocytes are activated after recognition of the 'antigen' for which they are specific • CD4+ T cells are activated via major histocompatibility complex (MHC) class 2 and CD8+ T cells via MHC class 1 • T cells (mainly CD8+ but also CD4+) can act as cytotoxic cells, inflicting tissue damage

whole complex is recognised by the T-cell receptor. Many drug molecules are not intrinsically reactive, but protein-reactive intermediate metabolites can be generated during metabolic detoxication of the drug. Normal detoxication of foreign chemicals generally comprises two phases. In phase 1, cytochrome P450 enzymes perform oxygen-addition reactions. The intermediates produced may be highly toxic or reactive and so must be rapidly detoxified by phase 2 metabolism (Fig 1). Phase 2 enzymes may 'neutralise' reactive epoxides by hydrolysis (epoxide hydrolase) or attach groups such as acetate (acetyl transferases) or glutathione (glutathione S transferase), which renders the target water soluble and capable of excretion. One hypothesis to explain the differences in individuals who develop ADRs (at least of types B and C) suggests that phase 2 detoxication processes are deficient and thus allow persistence of higher levels of toxic or immunogenic metabolites.[3,4] So far, however, this general hypothesis has not been supported clearly by identification of specific failure of detoxication.

Immune recognition and response

In order to activate an immune response, drugs must act as haptens and bind to proteins; however, what the proteins are or whether the protein carriers are different in people who generate immune hypersensitivities is not known. A currently arising hypothesis is that differences in control of the immune system mean that people who develop immune hypersensitivity to a drug have somehow failed to generate immunological tolerance – perhaps mediated by suppressive 'regulatory T cells'.[5]

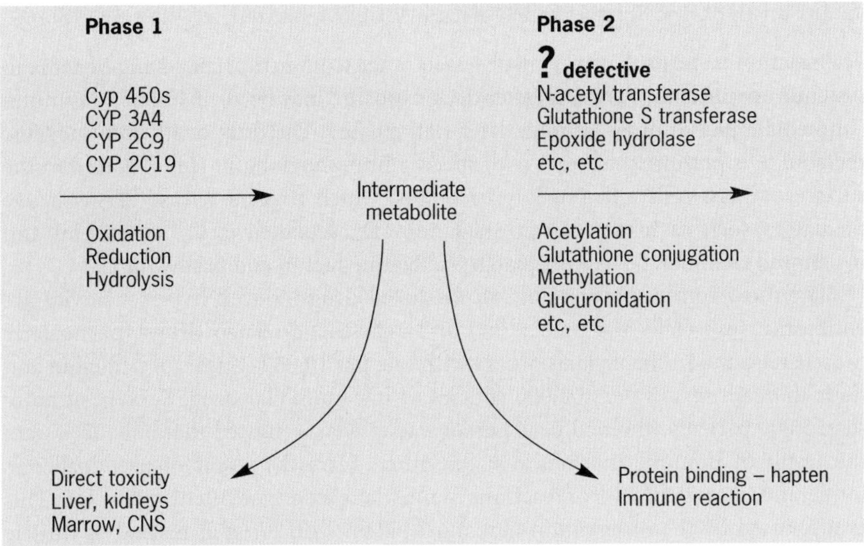

Fig 1 Metabolic drug detoxication. CNS = central nervous system.

Clinical patterns of type B reactions

Three general classes of mechanism exist: non-immunological, pseudoallergic, and true allergic. Many or any organs can be involved in these reactions.

Non-immunologic reactions are essentially chemical toxicities (type C in the formal classification). In susceptible people, chemical toxicity, such as dapsone-induced neuropathy or azathioprine-induced marrow suppression, occurs with no involvement of immune efector mechanisms.

Pseudoallergic reactions look clinically indistinguishable from type 1 (immediate) hypersensitivities (see below) with anaphylaxis, asthma, urticaria, intestinal cramps, and diarrhoea. These reactions involve chemically induced mast-cell degranulation with release of mediators. Examples are intolerances to salicylates, opiates, and muscle relaxants.

The skin is commonly involved in type B reactions and is often the earliest indicator of allergic or immune-mediated hypersensitivity reactions. The clinical pattern is an excellent indicator of the type of underlying immune effector mechanism. When the immune system reacts to an immunogen, initial activation means that helper T lymphocytes recognise the 'antigen' when it is presented in association with MHC by professional dendritic antigen-presenting cells. T cells of the CD4+ type see antigens in the context of MHC class II, while CD8+ T cells see them in association with MHC class I. The T helper cells proliferate to generate memory T cells, and they may help B lymphocytes make antibodies of different classes. This takes a minimum of seven days and often longer. To elicit the immune effector mechanisms, further exposure to the drug or immunogen is required – as a second course of the same drug or because of availability of the drug from continuous or ongoing exposure. The time when a reaction develops after exposure to a drug therefore can give important clues when it comes to identifying the culprit.

☐ TYPE I HYPERSENSITIVITY (IMMUNOGLOBULIN E-MEDIATED) REACTIONS

The reaction patterns that may involve skin range from urticaria and angioedema to systemic anaphylaxis. Reactions after drug exposure may occur in about 15 minutes (immediate phase) or 6–24 hours later (late phase). The drug or its immunogenic metabolite is presumed to react with specific immunoglobulin (Ig) E bound to the surface of mast cells and possibly basophils, which triggers release of vasoactive mediators such as histamine, prostaglandin D_2, leukotriene C_4, eosinophil and neutrophil chemotactic factors, platelet-activating factor, and bradykinin.

The most common causes of IgE-mediated drug-induced hypersensitivity are antibiotics (especially the penicillins) and anaesthetic-related drugs (particularly muscle relaxants). Anaphylaxis occurs with one per 10,000 courses of penicillin and leads to death in 1–5 per 100,000 courses of intramuscular drug. Surveys of more than 2,000 patients who had perioperative anaphylaxis showed that only 52% were the result of immune mechanisms; the others were the result of pseudoallergic intolerance. Less than 50% of reactions to muscle relaxants are mediated by IgE. This is supported by the observation that most patients (85%) who reacted to muscle relaxants had not had prior exposure to them.

☐ TYPE II HYPERSENSITIVITY REACTIONS: CYTOTOXIC/CYTOLYTIC MECHANISMS

In the skin, drug-induced type II immune hypersensitivity may manifest as pemphigus, bullous pemphigoid, or linear IgA disease. Drug-induced pemphigus can be divided into two classes. Drug-dependent pemphigus is caused by exogenous factors such as thiol group (–SH)-containing drugs (for example, D-penicillamine and captopril) and regresses once the drug is discontinued. In drug-triggered (true) pemphigus induced by non-thiol drugs (e.g. penicillins, cephalosporins, and piroxicam), the patient has the genetic predisposition for pemphigus (DRB1*0402, DRB1*1402, or DRB1*0701) and the disease does not regress after withdrawal of the drug but follows the normal natural history of the disease.

☐ TYPE III HYPERSENSITIVITY: IMMUNE COMPLEX-MEDIATED VASCULITIS

Hypersensitivity vasculitis occurs when circulating immune complexes form between IgG or IgM antibodies and antigens from exogenous sources such as bacteria (streptococci), viruses, or drugs. The immune complexes deposit within postcapillary venules, which causes vessel wall damage through activation of the complement cascade and subsequent neutrophil accumulation. Drug-induced vasculitis develops in the skin and other organs about 8–10 days after exposure to the causative drug. Vasculitis is a reaction pattern that may develop after exposure to a wide range of drugs, including antibiotics, non-steroidal anti-inflammatory drugs (NSAIDs), and cytotoxic drugs. The binding affinity of the antibody determines whether immune complexes are of the type easily cleared by the reticuloendothelial system or are soluble and persist in the circulation.

□ TYPE IV HYPERSENSITIVITY: T LYMPHOCYTE-MEDIATED REACTIONS

Type IV hypersensitivies are divided into those from topical contact and those from systemic exposure. Contact allergic drug hypersensitivity arises from topical drug preparations (such as antibiotics, antiseptics, local anaesthetics, and corticosteroids) and produces an eczematous reaction in sites of contact. Systemic T cell-mediated drug hypersensitivity underlies a variety of cutaneous drug reactions such as maculopapular eruptions ('ampicillin rash'); toxic erythemas; erythema multiforme; toxic epidermal necrolysis (TEN); and eczematous, lichenoid, and toxic pustuloderma reactions.[6]

Maculopapular eruptions/toxic erythema

This is the most common pattern of drug-induced skin eruption and can be induced by a wide range of drugs, including antibiotics, anticonvulsants, allopurinol, and NSAIDs.[7] The clinical picture can be diverse, with the rash ranging from tiny erythematous macules and papules to urticaria-like weals. This rash is differentiated from urticaria, in that individual weals last days whereas true urticarial weals last only 2–12 hours. Good evidence suggests this is a T lymphocyte-mediated process. T cells present in the skin are predominantly CD4+ cells in the dermal infiltrate but CD8+ cells in the epidermis. Antigen-specific CD8+ T cells have been cultured from lesional skin. Positive 48-hour patch tests can be elicited with the culprit drug in a proportion of cases.

Erythema multiforme and toxic epidermal necrolysis

The classic skin lesion of erythema multiforme – circular, usually slightly raised, and comprising a set of concentric rings of different colours – is the so-called target lesion. The centres are often a dusky-cyanotic hue, while the more peripheral rings are different shades of erythematous pink or white. When the process is more aggressive, the lesions blister. When 10–30% of the body surface is affected, it is called erythema multiforme major; when mucosal surfaces (buccal cavity, eyes, and genital mucosae) are involved, it is called Stevens-Johnson syndrome.[8] If the blisters become confluent and more than 30% of the skin is affected, it is referred to as TEN. In most severe cases, it may be difficult to make out the morphology of individual lesions as the involved area is a confluent mass of detaching skin. The prognosis for full-blown TEN is poor, with up to 35% mortality. A scoring system (SCORTEN) based on variables including age, extent of skin involvement, tachycardia, plasma urea, glucose, and others is helpful in predicting outcome.[9]

The immune effector mechanisms that underlie erythema multiforme involve CD4+ and CD8+ T cells. The epidermal necrolysis is caused by mass apoptosis of keratinocytes induced by increased production of the Fas-ligand, which interacts with its receptor Fas (CD95) – a member of the 'death receptor' family.[10]

Erythema multiforme responds to treatment with systemic corticosteroids, but epidermal necrolysis cannot be stopped with conventional anti-inflammatory or immunosuppressive agents. Whether or not high-dose intravenous immunoglobulin

(IVIG) can be effective is controversial, but the weight of evidence indicates that early commencement of IVIG significantly reduces mortality, with the benefit apparently related to whether the batches contain naturally occurring antibodies that neutralise Fas ligand.[10]

These reaction patterns often involve other organ systems in addition to the skin, as reflected by altered liver function tests or haematological indices. The drug hypersensitivity syndrome is characterised by rash, fever, lymphadenopathy, hepatitis, and eosinophilia. The eosinophilia reflects production of large quantities of interleukin 5 by T cells of the T helper 2 type.

Eczematous reactions

Drug-induced eczemas are often widespread, with a distribution that cannot be explained by contact with external factors. Patients often have mixed features of eczema together with urticated lesions or lichen planus-like lesions, and this can confuse the diagnostic picture. Eczematous reactions are mediated by CD4+ T cells.

Lichenoid reactions

Lichenoid reactions are so-called because they consist of small flat-topped papules that may be a dusky or mauve colour similar to that seen in spontaneously occurring lichen planus. Lichenoid reactions often come on months or even years after commencing the causal drug and can take many months to resolve after drug withdrawal. The pathogenetic mechanisms have not yet been elucidated, but it is likely to be a T cell-mediated process.

Toxic pustuloderma

These rare reactions are characterised by widespread pustules that often arise on an erythematous base. Although the inflammatory response generates polymorph neutrophil accumulation as pus, this is the result of drug-activated T lymphocytes producing large amounts of interleukin 8, which is chemotactic for neutrophils.

□ ASSESSMENT OF CAUSALITY

The key to establishing causality for a suspected ADR is a careful drug history and precise description of the clinical features. The morphology of the rash will help indicate the type of immune mechanism involved, which is relevant to possible treatment and diagnostic tests. It must be remembered that urticarial rashes, which indicate type I (IgE/mast cell) mechanisms, are characterised by individual weals of short duration (lasting only a few hours). Lesions that look like urticarial weals but last for days indicate 'toxic erythemas' or even erythema multiforme, which are mediated by T cells. Urticaria can be 'pseudoallergic', reflecting drug intolerance, in which case previous exposure may not have occurred. Normally, however, immune sensitisation requires previous exposure or at least one week of ongoing exposure.

Drawing of a figure of the times when drugs were started or withdrawn often clarifies the likely culprit (Fig 2).

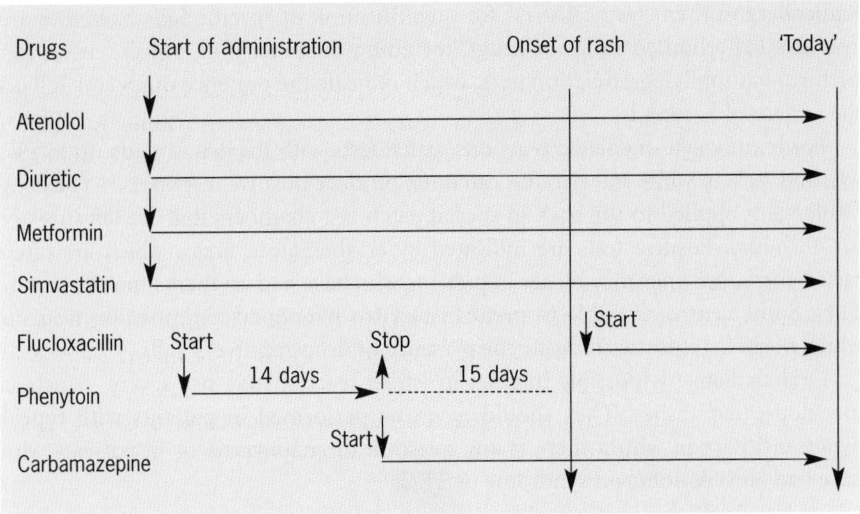

Fig 2 Drug administration time/dose relations. A patient undergoing neurosurgery for a meningioma develops fever and rash – severe erythema multiforme or toxic epidermal necrolysis (TEN) – on the date 'onset of rash'. 'Today', three days later, dermatologists are consulted. Atenolol, the diuretic, metformin, and simvastatin had been started long before. Flucloxacillin was started after the rash erupted (and so cannot be the cause). Phenytoin was started immediately after the operation for 14 days but was discontinued because of failure to control seizures. Carbamazepine was started and has continued until 'today'. Although the top four drugs must be considered, they have all been administered long term and none are notorious for this type of reaction. The most likely culprits are the anticonvulsants. Carbamazepine would be the most probable, as it was started 15 days before the onset of the erythema multiforme or TEN. Phenytoin, however, was also administered for 14 days (enough time to evoke the reaction), and it is probable that the eruption would have started sooner if it were the responsible culprit. Hypersensitivity reactions sometimes can start after withdrawal of a drug, but they usually start subsiding within a few days. If the culprit is still being administered, however, the process will be likely to be exacerbating.

Diagnostic tests

In vivo or in vitro tests may be carried out, but these are usually confined to research centres with an interest in drug allergy. The robustness and range of such tests is limited, mainly because the correct antigenic molecule, hapten, or metabolite is not known or available for most drugs. The choice of test is important and depends on the suspected immune mechanism that underlies the drug reaction. Skin testing – that is prick, intradermal, or patch testing – is usually performed six weeks to six months after resolution of the reaction.[11,12] It may, however, lead to relapse of symptoms, and, for this reason, low concentrations of the suspected agent are used initially.

Skin prick tests can be performed for immediate hypersensitivities with some drugs – particularly the penicillin family, drugs available for parenteral administration such as muscle relaxants, and anaesthetic induction agents.[12] Positive reactions develop within 15 minutes of the challenge. If there is any question of severe asthma or allergy strong enough that it may result in anaphylaxis, challenge should be performed in a setting with full cardiopulmonary resuscitation facilities. Radioallergosorbent tests (RASTs) for quantification of specific IgE antibodies are available for a limited range of drugs, including the penicillins. Some centres can perform basophil degranulation tests, which indicate the presence of specific IgE on the surface of basophils.

For lymphocyte-mediated reactions, patch tests with the drugs made up to 1%, 5%, and 10% in white soft paraffin can often produce positive responses.[11] The drug challenge is applied to the back in special patch test chambers that are left in place for 48 hours. Positive tests are indicated by erythematous areas, which are often raised and sometimes may blister in patients who have had erythema multiforme or TEN. Some centres are able to perform in vitro lymphocyte stimulation tests, in which positive responses indicate the presence of drug-reactive T cells.

Oral challenge is possible in cases in which reactions are not severe – such as maculopapular rashes. They should never be performed in patients with type I hypersensitivity in whom there is any question of anaphylaxis or in patients who have had Stevens-Johnson syndrome or TEN.

REFERENCES

1. Pirmohamed M, James S, Meakin S *et al.* Adverse drug reactions as cause of admission to hospital: prospective analysis of 18,820 patients. *BMJ* 2004;329:15–9.
2. Coombs RRA, Gell PGH. Classification of allergic reactions responsible for clinical hypersensitivity and disease. In: Gell PGH, Coombs RRA (eds), *Clinical aspects of immunology.* Oxford: Blackwell Science, 1968:576–96.
3. Park BK, Pirmohamed M, Kitteringham NR. Role of drug disposition in drug hypersensitivity: a chemical, molecular, and clinical perspective. *Chem Res Toxicol* 1998;11:969–88.
4. Friedmann PS, Lee MS, Friedmann AC, Barnetson RS. Mechanisms in cutaneous drug hypersensitivity reactions. *Clin Exp Allergy* 2003;33:861–72.
5. Cavani A, Ottaviani C, Nasorri F *et al.* Immunoregulation of hapten and drug induced immune reactions. *Curr Opin Allergy Clin Immunol* 2003;3:243–7.
6. Pichler W, Yawalkar N, Schmid S, Helbling A. Pathogenesis of drug-induced exanthems. *Allergy* 2002;57:884–93.
7. Chan HL, Stern RS, Arndt KA *et al.* The incidence of erythema multiforme, Stevens-Johnson syndrome, and toxic epidermal necrolysis. A population-based study with particular reference to reactions caused by drugs among outpatients. *Arch Dermatol* 1990;126:43–7.
8. Roujeau JC. The spectrum of Stevens-Johnson syndrome and toxic epidermal necrolysis: a clinical classification. *J Invest Dermatol* 1994;102:28S–30S.
9. Bastuji-Garin S, Fouchard N, Bertocchi M *et al.* SCORTEN: a severity-of-illness score for toxic epidermal necrolysis. *J Invest Dermatol* 2000;115:149–53.
10. Viard I, Wehrli P, Bullani R *et al.* Inhibition of toxic epidermal necrolysis by blockade of CD95 with human intravenous immunoglobulin. *Science* 1998;282:490–3.
11. Barbaud A, Goncalo M, Bruynzeel D *et al.* Guidelines for performing skin tests with drugs in the investigation of cutaneous adverse drug reactions. *Contact Dermatitis* 2001;45:321–8.
12. Laxenaire MC. Drugs and other agents involved in anaphylactic shock occurring during anaesthesia. A French multicenter epidemiological inquiry. *Ann Fr Anesth Reanim* 1993; 12:91–6.

Osteoporosis

Juliet Compston

INTRODUCTION

Osteoporosis is characterised by reduction in bone mass and disruption of bone architecture, which results in increased bone fragility and an increase in the risk of fracture. These fractures are recognised widely as a major health problem in the elderly population, leading to significant morbidity and mortality and resulting in an estimated annual cost to British health services of £1.8 billion. One in two women and one in five men older than 50 years will have a fracture because of osteoporosis during their remaining lifetime. Demographic changes over the next 50 years will result in at least a doubling in the number of these fractures.

EPIDEMIOLOGY

The incidence of osteoporotic fractures increases markedly with age; in women, the median age for Colles' fractures is 65 years and for hip fracture is 80 years. The age at which the incidence of vertebral fracture reaches a peak has been less well defined, but it is thought to be between 65 and 80 years in women. In men, no age-related increase in forearm fractures is seen, but the incidence of hip fracture rises exponentially after the age of 75 years. The prevalence of vertebral fractures increases with age in men, although less steeply than in women. The hospital-related costs of osteoporotic fractures in women exceed those attributable to stroke, myocardial infarction, and breast cancer.[1]

In recent years, a number of signalling pathways central to the regulation of bone remodelling have been characterised. These include the receptor activator of nuclear factor-kappa B (NFκB) ligand/osteoprotegerin (RANKL/OPG) pathway, which plays a major role in the regulation of osteoclast development and activity[2] and is being exploited in the development of a human monoclonal antibody to RANKL for the treatment of osteoporosis and other diseases associated with excessive bone resorption. Another is the Wnt signalling pathway, which regulates bone formation. Inactivating mutations of sclerostin, which is an inhibitor of the pathway, and activating mutations of low-density lipoprotein receptor-related protein 5 (LRP-5), a coreceptor for the pathway, are associated with high bone mass and increased bone strength.[3]

DIAGNOSIS AND RISK ASSESSMENT

Bone densitometry

Bone mass can be assessed by a number of techniques; dual energy X-ray absorptiometry (DXA) is the gold standard and provides measurements of bone mineral density in the spine and hip. According to the World Health Organization (WHO)'s classification, osteoporosis is present when the bone mineral density is 2.5 standard deviations or more below normal peak bone mass (T score ≤–2.5). Established osteoporosis is defined as a T score ≤–2.5 in association with a previous fragility fracture. The rationale of this definition is that there is an inverse relation between bone mineral density and the risk of fracture and hence measurements of bone mineral density can be used in clinical practice to predict the risk of fracture. The definition is based on data in postmenopausal women and, although probably applicable to older men, it should not be used to define osteoporosis in younger men, premenopausal women, or children.

Clinical risk factors

Although measurements of bone mineral density are useful for predicting the risk of fracture in clinical practice, it has become evident from a number of studies that the sensitivity of bone mineral density in predicting fractures is low and that, in fact, most fractures occur in women without osteoporosis as defined by the WHO. Factors that may influence the risk of fracture other than bone mineral density include falls and aspects of bone composition and structure that are not fully reflected in measurements of bone mineral density (Fig 1). In addition, some clinical risk factors are at least partially independent of bone mineral density and hence can be added to bone mineral density to improve predictions of the risk of fracture (Table 1). These include age, treatment with glucocorticoid drugs, previous history of fracture, family history of hip fracture, current smoking, alcohol abuse, and certain diseases associated with osteoporosis such as rheumatoid arthritis.[4] A WHO-supported algorithm that combines these risk factors with measurements of bone mineral density is being developed to estimate the probability of fracture and will enable intervention thresholds to be based on absolute risk rather than T scores.

Other risk factors that are associated with low bone mineral density include untreated premature menopause, other causes of hypogonadism (including treatment

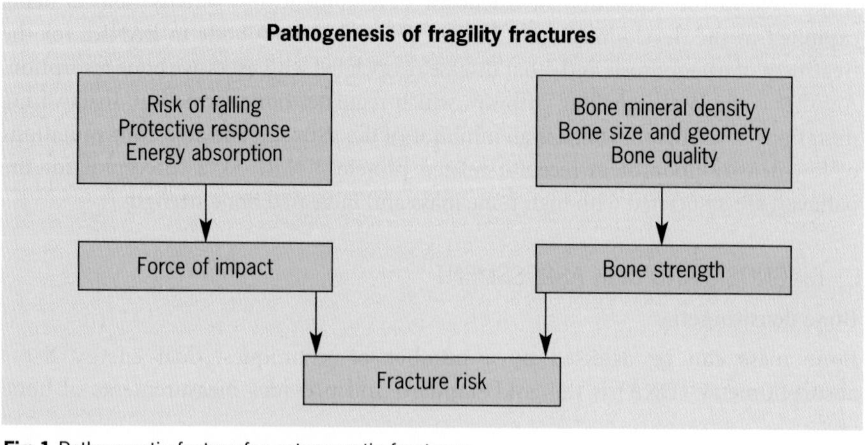

Fig 1 Pathogenetic factors for osteoporotic fractures.

Table 1 Risk factors for osteoporosis. BMD = bone mineral density. BMI = body mass index.

BMD independent	BMD dependent
• Age • Previous fragility fracture • Maternal history of hip fracture • Treatment with oral glucocorticoids • Current smoking • Alcohol intake ≥3 units/day • Rheumatoid arthritis • BMI ≤19 kg/m^2 • Falls	• Untreated hypogonadism • Malabsorption • Endocrine disease • Chronic renal disease • Chronic liver disease • Chronic obstructive pulmonary disease • Immobility • Drugs – for example, aromatase inhibitors and androgen deprivation therapy

with aromatase inhibitors or gonadotrophin-releasing hormone analogues), low body mass index, hyperthyroidism, and malabsorption (see Table 1).

Risk factors for falling are major determinants of the risk of fracture, particularly hip fracture in the elderly, and their recognition is important, as many are modifiable. They include poor visual acuity; neuromuscular weakness and incoordination; reduced mobility; cognitive impairment; and the use of sedatives, tranquillisers, and alcohol. Many environmental hazards also increase the risk of falling, such as uneven paving stones, poor lighting, and loose carpets and wires.

□ PHARMACOLOGICAL INTERVENTIONS

General considerations

Interventions approved for the prevention and treatment of osteoporosis are shown in Table 2. Most of these are approved only for the treatment of postmenopausal osteoporosis, but alendronate, etidronate, and risedronate also have licences for the prevention and treatment of glucocorticoid-induced osteoporosis, and alendronate is approved for the treatment of osteoporosis in men.

Because of their broader spectrum of antifracture efficacy, alendronate, risedronate, and strontium ranelate generally are regarded as front-line options in the prevention of fractures in postmenopausal women.[5] This distinction is important, because once a fracture occurs, the risk of a subsequent fracture at any site is increased independent of bone mineral density, and hence an intervention that covers all major fracture sites is preferable.

Strontium ranelate has a particularly strong evidence base in the very elderly (women aged ≥80 years)[6] and is the treatment of choice in frail individuals who are unable to comply with the dosing instructions for bisphosphonates. Raloxifene and ibandronate are generally considered second-line options, and the use of parathyroid hormone peptides is limited, because of their cost, to women with severe vertebral osteoporosis who are intolerant of or seem to be unresponsive to other treatments.

Table 2 Pharmacological interventions used in the prevention of osteoporotic fractures.

Intervention	Dosing regimen	Route of administration
Alendronate	• 70 mg once weekly • 5 or 10 mg once daily	• Oral
Etidronate	• 400 mg daily for two weeks every three months	• Oral
Ibandronate	• 150 mg once monthly • 3 mg once every three months	• Oral • Intravenous injection
Risedronate	• 35 mg once weekly • 5 mg once daily	• Oral
Raloxifene	• 60 mg once daily	• Oral
Strontium ranelate	• 2 g once daily	• Oral
Teriparatide	• 20 μg once daily	• Subcutaneous injection
Parathyroid hormone 1-84	• 100 μg once daily	• Subcutaneous injection

Table 3 Antifracture efficacy of pharmacological interventions for osteoporosis. HRT = hormone replacement therapy.

Intervention	Fracture		
	Vertebral	Non-vertebral	Hip
1-84 parathyroid hormone peptide	+	–	–
Alendronate	+	+	+
Etidronate	+	–	–
HRT	+	+	+
Ibandronate	+	–	–
Raloxifene	+	–	–
Risedronate	+	+	+
Strontium ranelate	+	+	+
Teriparatide	+	+	–

Reduction in the risk of fracture has been shown to occur within one year of treatment with bisphosphonates and strontium ranelate. This is particularly important in the case of vertebral fractures, as the risk of a further fracture occurring within the next 12 months after an incident vertebral fracture is 20%, emphasising the importance of prompt treatment once a fracture has occurred.[7]

Bisphosphonates

The bisphosphonates are synthetic analogues of the naturally occurring compound pyrophosphate and inhibit bone resorption.

Oral bisphosphonates generally are well tolerated. Upper gastrointestinal side-effects may occur with nitrogen-containing bisphosphonates (alendronate, risedronate, and ibandronate), particularly if the patient does not adhere to the dosing regimen. It is important therefore that patients take the drug according to the instructions, namely in the morning with a full glass of water; 30–60 minutes before food, drink, or other medications; and remaining standing or sitting upright for that time.

Ibandronate, the most recently approved bisphosphonate, is available as oral and intravenous formulations. The latter is given as an injection over 15–30 seconds every three months. An acute phase reaction may occur, particularly with the first injection, and this can result in flu-like symptoms for 24–48 hours. Antifracture efficacy has not been directly shown for this formulation or for the 150 mg once-monthly regimen, but it is assumed from a bridging study based on changes in bone mineral density.[8]

Strontium ranelate

Strontium ranelate is composed of two atoms of stable strontium, with ranelic acid as a carrier. Although its mechanism of action remains to be defined fully, some evidence suggests that it inhibits bone resorption while maintaining bone formation. Its use is associated with a substantial increase in bone mineral density in the spine and hip, although part of this increase is artefactual because of the incorporation of strontium into bone.

Strontium ranelate is taken as a single daily dose and is generally well tolerated. There are small increases in the frequency of diarrhoea, nausea, and headache and also a small increase in the risk of venous thromboembolic disease (odds ratio 1.42 (95% confidence interval 1.02 to 1.98)).

Raloxifene

Raloxifene is a selective oestrogen receptor modulator that has oestrogenic (antiresorptive) effects in the skeleton without the unwanted effects of oestrogen in the breast and endometrium. It is taken orally as a single daily dose. Adverse effects include leg oedema, leg cramps, hot flushes, and a 2–3-fold increase in the risk of venous thromboembolism. Its use is associated with a significant decrease in the risk of breast cancer.

Parathyroid hormone peptides

Recombinant human 1-34 parathyroid hormone (teriparatide) and recombinant human 1-84 parathyroid hormone peptide are administered by subcutaneous injection in daily doses of 20 μg and 100 μg, respectively. They have anabolic effects on bone, increasing bone formation and producing large increases in bone mineral density in the spine. Side-effects include nausea, headache, and dizziness; in addition, transient hypercalcaemia and hypercalciuria may occur.

Hormone replacement therapy

Because the risk–benefit balance of hormone replacement therapy (HRT) is generally unfavourable in older postmenopausal women, it is regarded as a second line-treatment option. It is, however, an appropriate option in younger postmenopausal women at high risk of fracture, particularly those with vasomotor symptoms.

Calcium and vitamin D

Available evidence does not support a role for calcium and vitamin D alone in the prevention of osteoporotic fractures except in institutionalised elderly people. Supplements of calcium and vitamin D supplements should be coprescribed with other treatments for osteoporosis, however, as the evidence base for their antifracture efficacy is derived from studies in which calcium and vitamin D were administered routinely.

Duration of therapy

The optimum duration of treatment is uncertain. There are concerns that long-term treatment with potent antiresorptives may increase bone microdamage and suppress its repair, possibly resulting in increased bone fragility. This concern has to be counterbalanced, however, by the possibility that increased bone turnover and bone loss after withdrawal of treatment may result in increased risk of fracture. The current consensus is that treatment should be continued for a minimum of five years; in those who remain at high risk (based on bone mineral density and/or incident fractures during treatment), longer treatment periods may be indicated.

Compliance and persistence

Compliance and persistence with treatment for osteoporosis are poor; about 50% of patients do not follow their prescribed treatment regimen or discontinue treatment within one year, or both.[9] Patient education is important in this respect, and nurse-led monitoring early in the course of treatment has been shown to improve compliance. Whether or not monitoring by measurement of biochemical markers of bone turnover or bone mineral density provides additional benefits has not been established.

□ FUTURE TREATMENTS

A number of new treatments are currently under development. Intravenous zoledronate given once yearly recently has been shown to reduce vertebral, non-vertebral, and hip fractures in postmenopausal women with osteoporosis and is currently being evaluated by the regulatory authorities. A human monoclonal antibody to RANKL has been developed and is now in phase III studies.[10] Other approaches being evaluated include sclerostin inhibitors, other inhibitors of the Wnt pathway, and calcium sensing receptor antagonists, which result in intermittent increases in endogenous parathyroid hormone secretion.

REFERENCES

1 Johnell O, Kanis JA. An estimate of the worldwide prevalence and disability associated with osteoporotic fractures. *Osteoporos Int* 2006;17:1726–33.

2 Lewiecki EM. RANK ligand inhibition with denosumab for the management of osteoporosis. *Expert Opin Biol Ther* 2006;6:1041–50.

3 Baron R, Rawadi G, Roman-Roman S. Wnt signaling: a key regulator of bone mass. *Curr Top Dev Biol* 2006;76:103–27.

4 Kanis JA. Diagnosis of osteoporosis and assessment of fracture risk. *Lancet* 2002;359:1929–36.

5 Poole KE, Compston JE. Osteoporosis and its management. *BMJ* 2006;333:1251–6.

6 Seeman E, Vellas B, Benhamou C *et al.* Strontium ranelate reduces the risk of vertebral and nonvertebral fractures in women eighty years of age and older. *J Bone Miner Res* 2006;21: 1113–20.

7 Lindsay R, Silverman SL, Cooper C *et al.* Risk of new vertebral fracture in the year following a fracture. *JAMA* 2001;285:320–3.

8 Delmas PD, Adami S, Strugala C *et al.* Intravenous ibandronate injections in postmenopausal women with osteoporosis: one-year results from the dosing intravenous administration study. *Arthritis Rheum* 2006;54:1838–46.

9 Compston JE, Seeman E. Compliance with osteoporosis therapy is the weakest link. *Lancet* 2006;368:973–4.

10 McClung MR, Lewiecki EM, Cohen SB *et al.* Denosumab in postmenopausal women with low bone mineral density. *N Engl J Med* 2006;354:821–31.

Inherited skin diseases: new benefits for patients

John A McGrath

Recent years have seen the molecular dissection of more than 400 monogenic disorders that have a skin phenotype. Although many of these disorders are relatively rare, the discovery of specific disease-associated genes and mutations has led to improved diagnosis, the feasibility of prenatal testing, and the development of newer forms of treatment, including pilot trials of somatic gene therapy. For common complex-trait skin diseases, genetic studies thus far have led to few direct benefits for patients, although new mutations in some proteins are beginning to emerge as major risk factors for disease susceptibility and also pave the way for the design of novel treatments for common skin diseases. This article highlights some of the recent advances relevant to the molecular discovery, diagnosis, and treatment of inherited skin diseases and how these may benefit patients.

□ DISCOVERING THE MOLECULAR BASIS OF INHERITED SKIN DISEASES

The highly visible nature of most inherited skin diseases has provided a rich resource for investigators keen to discover the genetic basis of these conditions (Fig 1). As with other inherited disorders, conventional genome-wide linkage approaches using microsatellite markers or single nucleotide polymorphisms have contributed to several key discoveries that provide insight into the pathogenesis of specific skin disorders, as well as the role of certain proteins, enzymes, and signalling molecules in health and disease.[1] Skin is a readily accessible organ, so hunting for genes through candidate gene analysis to look for insightful morphological, immunohistochemical, and biochemical clues has also made a substantial contribution towards unravelling the mysteries of many inherited skin diseases.

For rare monogenic disorders, such as skin fragility syndromes (for example, epidermolysis bullosa) and scaly skin conditions (for example, ichthyoses), the translational benefits of discovering disease-associated genes are becoming apparent: more accurate diagnoses, better genetic counselling, the feasibility of DNA-based prenatal diagnosis, and the preliminary development of newer forms of treatment, including somatic gene therapy. For more common complex traits, such as atopic dermatitis (AD) and psoriasis, the impact of molecular research on clinical management has been less dramatic, although recent characterisation of specific skin barrier defects in people with AD is beginning to influence the way we approach this very common condition. Moreover, advances in understanding of the

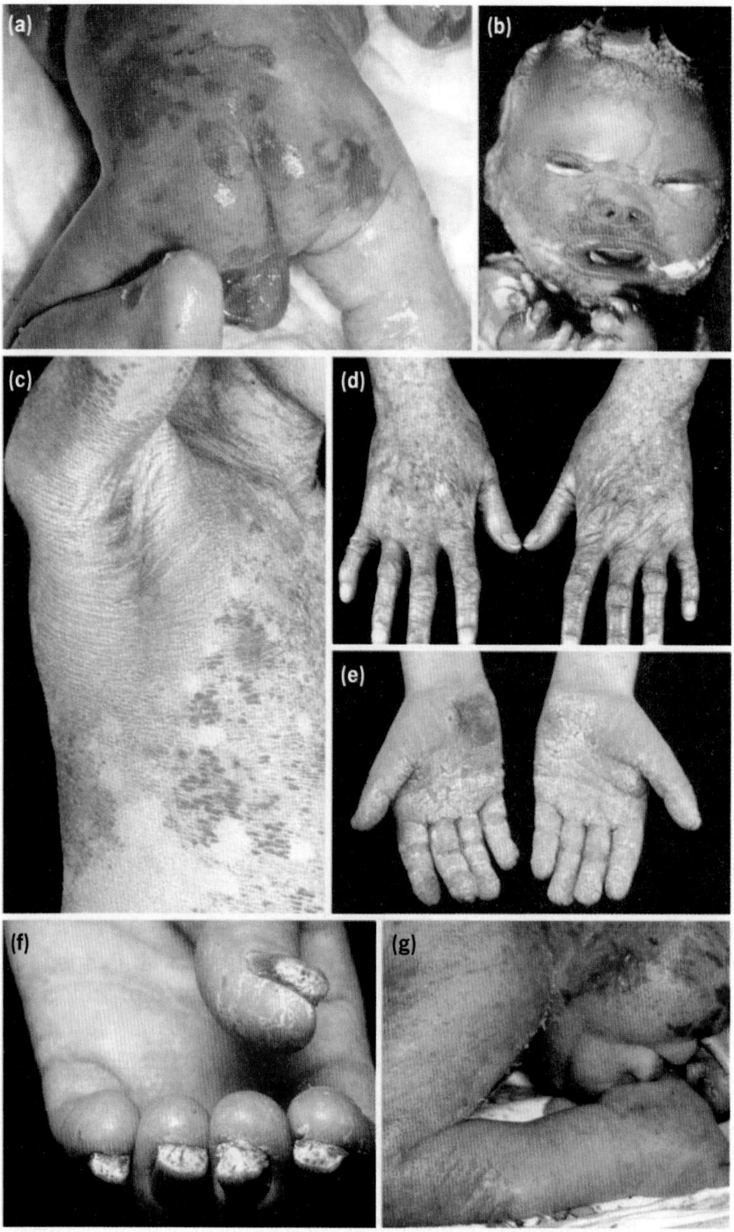

Fig 1 Recent advances in inherited skin diseases include the discovery of the molecular basis of more than 400 monogenic disorders with a skin phenotype including **(a)** Herlitz junctional epidermolysis bullosa (autosomal recessive mutations in the *LAMB3* gene, laminin-332), **(b)** harlequin ichthyosis (autosomal recessive mutations in the *ABCA12* gene, ATP-binding cassette transporter), **(c)** bullous congenital ichthyosiform erythroderma (autosomal dominant mutation in the *KRT1* gene, keratin 1), **(d)** Kindler syndrome (autosomal recessive mutations in the *KIND1* gene, kindlin-1), **(e)** Clouston's hidrotic ectodermal dysplasia (autosomal dominant mutation in the *GJB6* gene, connexin 30), **(f)** pachyonychia congenita (autosomal dominant mutation in the *KRT16* gene, keratin 16), and **(g)** ankyloblepharon-ectodermal dysplasia-clefting syndrome (autosomal dominant mutation in the *TP63* gene, transcription factor p63).

disease mechanisms in AD represent a clear example of how research on rare genetic diseases can have broader relevance to more common skin abnormalities (Fig 2).

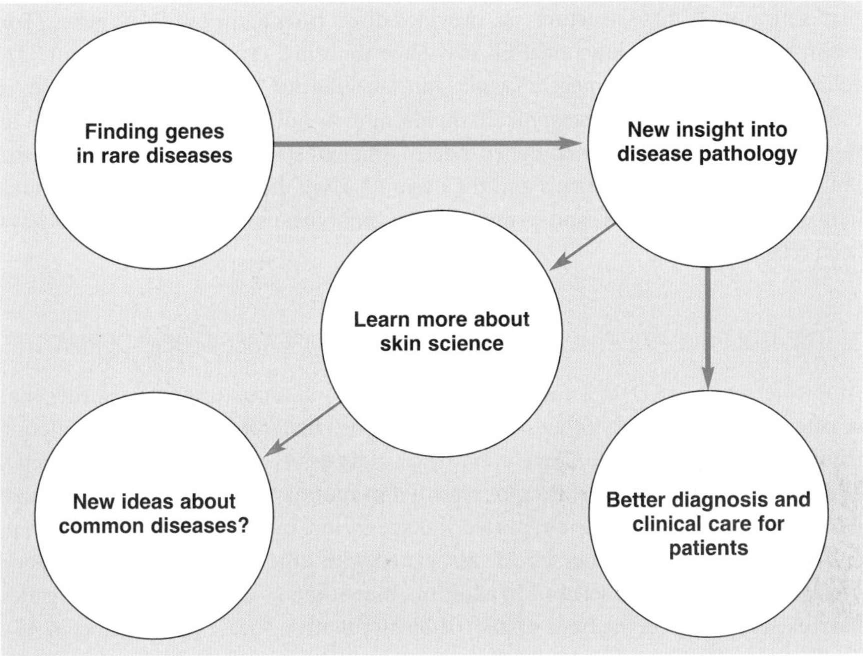

Fig 2 Many of the recent advances in understanding of inherited skin diseases have resulted from research on rare single gene disorders. Characterisation of the molecular basis of rare diseases has led to benefits for patients with these conditions, such as more accurate diagnosis, improved genetic counselling, and the feasibility of prenatal diagnosis (blue arrows). In addition, improved understanding of the pathophysiology of rare monogenic disorders has provided fresh insight into the disease's mechanisms and risk factors for more common complex traits that affect the skin (pink arrows).

□ THE MOLECULAR PATHOLOGY OF A RARE DISEASE: EPIDERMOLYSIS BULLOSA

The term epidermolysis bullosa (EB) refers to a group of inherited blistering skin diseases, some of which are among the most severe dermatological conditions. In many cases, EB presents at, or shortly after, birth. About 10,000 people in the United Kingdom (UK) have EB. The mildest and most common form is called EB simplex, and affected people typically have trauma-induced blisters on their feet during the summer months. The junctional and dystrophic forms of EB are more severe. Junctional EB can result in very extensive loss of the epidermis, and most affected people fail to survive infancy. The increased morbidity is due to overwhelming fragility of the skin and mucous membranes. Dystrophic EB varies in its severity, but most blisters are followed by scarring, and, in some cases, there is an increased risk of skin malignancy, notably squamous cell carcinoma.

The candidate gene approach has been particularly successful in establishing the molecular basis of EB. Skin biopsies taken from affected people show a spectrum of structural abnormalities in keratin intermediate filaments, the hemidesmosome-anchoring filament complexes, or the subjacent anchoring fibrils. These include aggregated keratin filaments in EB simplex, hypoplastic hemidesmosomes in junctional EB, and rudimentary anchoring fibrils in some forms of dystrophic EB. In addition, attenuated or absent immunolabelling of the skin with antibodies to proteins that contribute to these structures has provided direct clues to the candidate genes.[2] For example, patients with junctional EB may have abnormal expression of laminin-332, collagen XVII, or α6β4 integrin, while skin labelling for collagen VII frequently is reduced in patients with dystrophic EB. Epidermolysis bullosa has now been shown to result from mutations in genes that encode 10 different structural proteins close to the junction between the epidermis and the dermis.[3] More than 500 different mutations have now been described, and paradigms for genotype–phenotype correlation have been established.

□ THE MOLECULAR PATHOLOGY OF A COMMON DISEASE: ATOPIC DERMATITIS

Atopic dermatitis (AD) is a common chronic itchy inflammatory skin disorder that is often associated with other atopic conditions, including asthma and allergic rhinitis (the atopic triad). Current evidence indicates that AD is strongly genetic, with higher phenotype concordance reported in monozygotic than dizygotic twins. Genome screens for AD have reported linkage to loci on chromosomes 1q, 3q, 3p, and 17q, as well as other loci for AD associated with other atopic manifestations or increased levels of IgE in serum.[4] In addition, more than 20 different candidate genes have been assessed on the basis of knowledge of putative disease mechanisms in AD.

The locus on 1q is of particular interest to dermatologists because it encompasses the epidermal differentiation complex set of genes, including the profilaggrin gene (*FLG*) that encodes for filaggrin – a natural moisturising substance that contributes to the integrity of the skin barrier. A genetic abnormality in the profilaggrin gene has long been suspected as the basis of the semi-dominant condition ichthyosis vulgaris – a dry scaly skin disorder that affects about one in 200 people and frequently co-occurs clinically with AD. Sequencing of the *FLG* gene, however, has been difficult technically because of the almost identical nucleotide sequences of the filaggrin repeat units. In 2006, however, these longstanding laboratory obstacles were overcome and loss of function mutations in *FLG* finally were identified in patients with ichthyosis vulgaris (Fig 3).[5] Mutations in *FLG* have also been shown to be a major risk factor for AD, AD that persists into adulthood, and asthma associated with AD but not for asthma alone.[6] These findings do not indicate that AD is entirely a structural disorder of the skin barrier: other abnormalities, perhaps that involve innate and adaptive immune responses, are certainly likely to be of pathogenic relevance in some individuals. The association of *FLG* mutations with other allergic diseases, however, emphasises the clinical significance of exposure to cutaneous antigens in the development of systemic allergy.

□ DIAGNOSING INHERITED SKIN DISEASES

Common diseases such as AD or psoriasis are usually relatively straightforward to diagnose clinically, but similar clinical features of extensive skin erosions and blisters

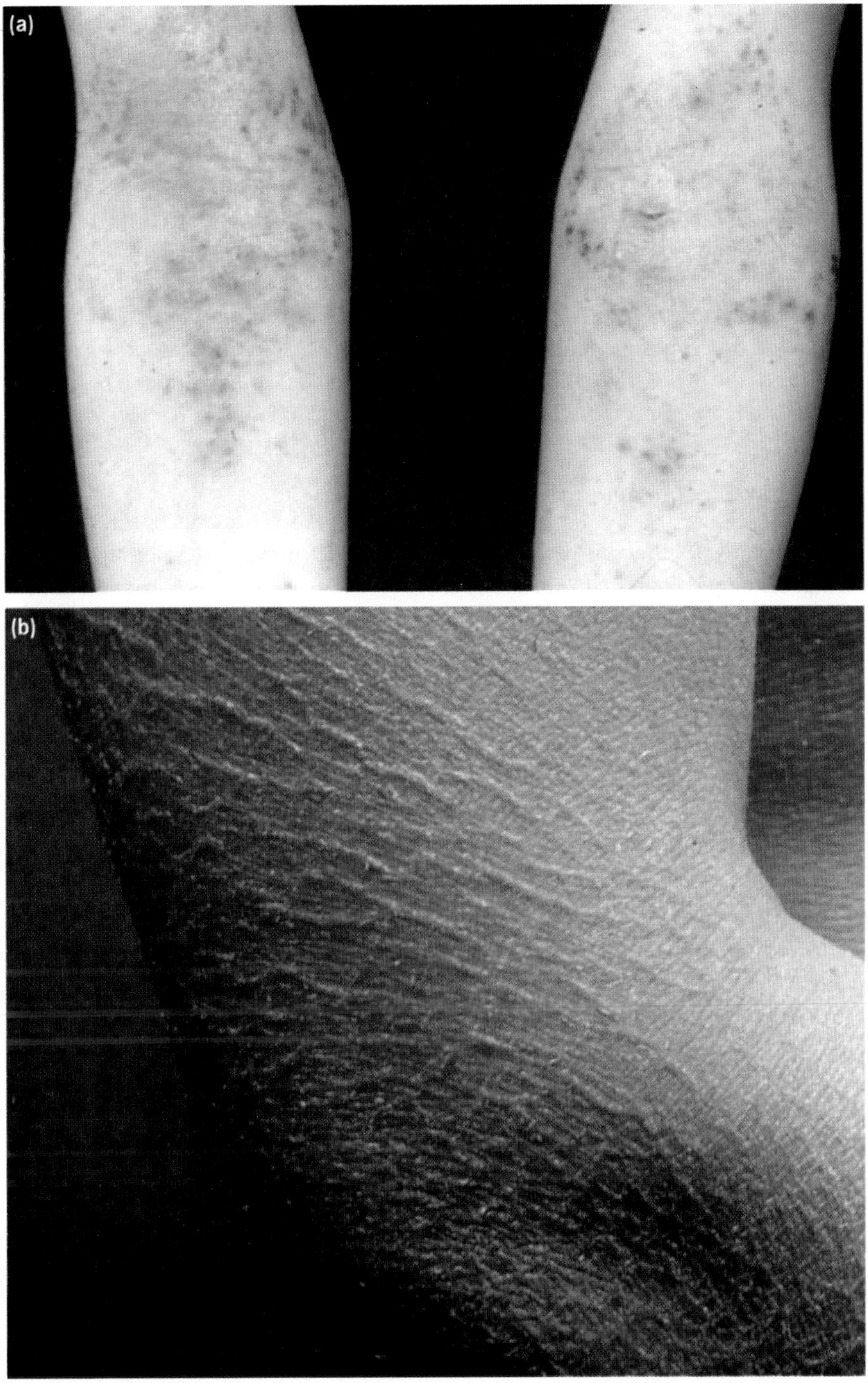

Fig 3 Clinical relevance of the recent discovery of mutations in the filaggrin gene *FLG*: **(a)** mutations in *FLG* are a major risk factors for susceptibility to atopic dermatitis as well as asthma associated with atopic dermatitis and **(b)** mutations in *FLG* are the cause of the semi-dominant disorder ichthyosis vulgaris.

in rare diseases such as EB can reflect diverse underlying pathologies with different prognoses ranging from spontaneous improvement to neonatal death. The autosomal recessive forms of EB are usually associated with loss of function mutations on both alleles of the relevant gene. This leads to low or absent levels of the corresponding messenger RNA (mRNA) and protein. Immunolabelling with antibodies to the mutated protein in patients' skin, therefore, typically, shows a marked reduction or complete ablation of staining at the dermal–epidermal junction. A panel of antibodies against the various target proteins in EB is readily available, and immunostaining of skin sections takes less than one day to perform. As such, it is possible to make rapid diagnosis of EB. Immunohistochemical skin tests are also becoming established for other inherited skin diseases – for example, labelling of the epidermis in neonates with congenital red scaly skin can be useful for diagnosis of Netherton's syndrome and some variants of lamellar ichthyosis.

□ PRENATAL DIAGNOSIS OF INHERITED SKIN DISEASES

Since the early 1980s, considerable progress has been made in developing prenatal testing for severe inherited skin disorders (Fig 4).[7] Ultrastructural examination of fetal skin biopsies was initially established in a limited number of conditions, such as bullous congenital ichthyosiform erythroderma and the junctional and dystrophic forms of EB. The first skin biopsies were performed with the aid of a fetoscope to visualise the fetus; however, improvements in sonographic imaging mean that biopsies of fetal skin are now taken under ultrasound guidance. Samples initially could be examined only by light microscopy and transmission electron microscopy, but the development of a number of monoclonal and polyclonal antibodies to various components of the basement membrane during the mid-1980s led to the development of immunohistochemical tests to help complement ultrastructural analysis in establishing an accurate diagnosis, especially in cases of EB.

Nevertheless, as the molecular basis of an increasing number of inherited skin diseases has been elucidated, analysis of fetal skin gradually has been superseded by DNA-based diagnostic screening with fetal DNA from amniotic fluid cells or chorionic villus sampling (CVS). Fetal skin samples are usually taken at 16–20 weeks' gestation, whereas CVS is performed at 10–12 weeks. Analysis of fetal DNA is also more feasible than tests involving fetal skin sampling in many more disorders. Current research is trying to develop less invasive methods of prenatal testing, such as analysis of free fetal DNA in the maternal circulation, although this has yet to be applied clinically for inherited skin diseases. Advances in three-dimensional ultrasonography have also led to earlier diagnosis of some severe forms of congenital ichthyosis in which the gene defect is not known and structural changes on fetal skin biopsy develop only during a late stage of pregnancy.

□ PREIMPLANTATION GENETIC DIAGNOSIS/HAPLOTYPING

Preimplantation genetic diagnosis (PGD) is an alternative method of prenatal testing that obviates the need for termination of pregnancy. The technique is based

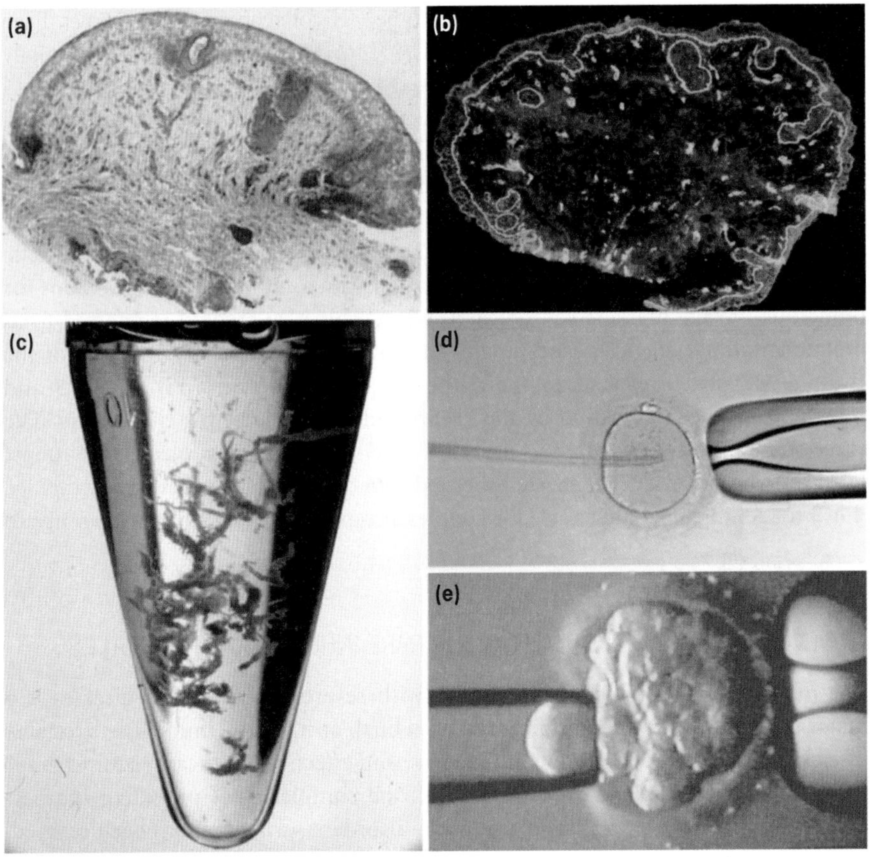

Fig 4 Advances in reproductive technology have led to more options for the prenatal diagnosis of inherited skin diseases: **(a)** fetal skin biopsy (here shown with normal appearance at 18 weeks' gestation) has been feasible for more than 25 years, **(b)** immunolabelling of fetal skin biopsies (here shown with normal appearances for type IV collagen staining at 18 weeks' gestation) has been useful in the diagnosis of inherited blistering skin diseases, **(c)** chorionic villi (illustrated here after removal of maternal decidua) can be sampled at the end of the first trimester and used for direct analysis of fetal DNA, **(d)** earlier diagnosis through preimplantation genetic diagnosis is now becoming a more widely available option (this figure shows the introduction of a single sperm cell via a cannula into an egg (intracytoplasmic sperm injection)), and **(e)** preimplantation genetic diagnosis (this figure illustrates sampling of a single blastomere from a 72 hour old embryo).

on DNA analysis of single blastomeres extracted from embryos after in vitro fertilisation. First successfully performed for cystic fibrosis in 1990, PGD subsequently has been applied in many other diseases, with pregnancy rates of about 25% per cycle leading to the birth of several hundred unaffected healthy children. Preimplantation genetic diagnosis for a family at risk of one particular inherited skin disorder – skin fragility ectodermal dysplasia syndrome – also has been established. The laboratory approach involves nested polymerase chain reaction (PCR) amplification to amplify DNA from a single embryonic cell with direct mutation analysis of the plakophilin 1 gene (*PKP1*). Other assays, including a sensitive single cell semi-duplex PCR assay that involves two highly polymorphic dinucleotide repeat microsatellite markers close to the type VII collagen gene (*COL7A1*), have also been designed and are licensed by the UK Human Fertilisation and Embryology Authority (HFEA) for diagnosis of recessive dystrophic EB.

Nevertheless, it has taken considerable time to optimise the established tests, which has severely limited their clinical application. Recent advances in single cell PCR technology, however, have led to the introduction of a new approach based on whole genome amplification of DNA from single blastomeres by multiple displacement amplification (MDA). This increases the amount of DNA template from a single cell from about 6 pg to 6 μg, after which multiplex PCR reactions for numerous linkage markers can be carried out. This new method is referred to as preimplantation genetic haplotyping (PGH).[8] Specific PGH assays for two of the laminin-332 genes relevant to the pathogenesis of junctional EB (*LAMA3* and *LAMB3*) have been approved by the HFEA and are available for clinical use. The successful application of MDA as part of the PGD protocol now means that robust PGH tests for several other severe inherited skin diseases can be developed rapidly, thus broadening personal choice for couples at reproductive risk of a wide range of genetic diseases.

☐ DEVELOPING NEW TREATMENTS FOR RARE INHERITED SKIN DISEASES

The optimal management of individuals with severe inherited skin diseases is a major challenge. Many conditions present at birth and require immediate specialist assessment and intervention. Comprehensive and effective healthcare requires input from a multidisciplinary team. In the UK, the complexity of providing the best possible care for people with inherited skin disorders such as EB has been realised, and a framework for national centres for EB was established in 2003. Supported centrally by the National Health Service, specialist units in the north and south of England now provide expert local care as well as appropriate diagnostic tests.

At present, however, there is no effective treatment for EB or other forms of inherited skin disease. Gene, protein, and cell therapy approaches are all being assessed in animal models or in vitro skin cultures (Fig 5). Thus far, however, only one successful trial of a test area of somatic gene therapy in one patient (who had autosomal recessive junctional EB because of mutations in the *LAMB3* gene) has been reported.[9] The affected person had had repeated skin blistering that made skin stem cells (holoclones) hard to identify. Suitable stem cells eventually were isolated from the skin on the palm, cultured, and then transduced with a retroviral vector that expressed the *LAMB3* complementary DNA (cDNA). Follow up over one year showed sustained normal levels of functional laminin-332, with no evidence of blisters, infections, inflammation, or immune response. Retroviral integration site analysis showed that the regenerated epidermis (which maintained its palmar characteristics despite being grafted onto the thigh) was sustained by transduced stem cells. In general, gene replacement strategies are appropriate for recessive disorders, but mutations result in dominant-negative interference in a large number of dominant skin diseases, so gene therapy is predominantly directed at silencing the mutant allele. Although not yet clinically relevant, recent advances in small interfering RNA (siRNA) technology are providing a basis for introducing this technology for disorders that result from heterozygous mutations in keratins 6a, 6b, 16, and 17, such as pachyonychia congenita.[10]

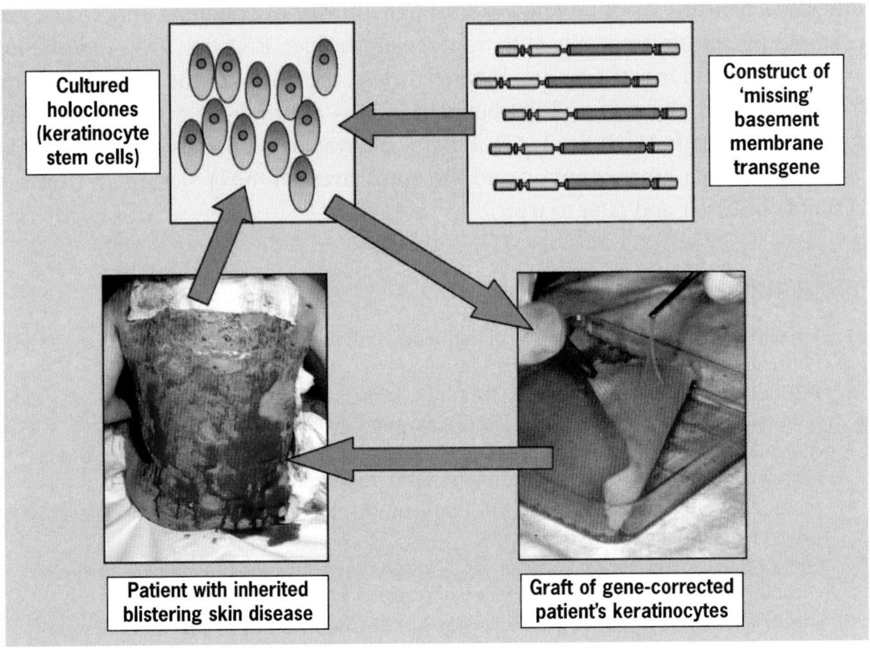

Fig 5 Principles of somatic gene therapy for an autosomal recessive inherited blistering skin disease in which blisters result from loss of expression of a basement membrane protein. A skin biopsy from the patient is cultured and stem cells (holoclones) are transduced with the appropriate transgene. Skin grafts are then prepared so that gene-corrected autologous keratinocytes can be grafted back onto the patient's skin.

☐ DEVELOPING NEW TREATMENTS FOR COMMON SKIN DISEASES

The current management of AD involves topical and systemic treatments that aim to restore transepidermal water loss (emollient creams or ointments) or reduce inflammation (corticosteroids, azathioprine, ciclosporin, etc). Although helpful for many patients, the existing treatment options may have side-effects, such as skin atrophy or systemic immunosuppression. The recent finding that the defective skin barrier in many people with AD is due to a very common premature termination codon (PTC) mutation in the *FLG* gene, however, raises the possibility of a new approach based on avoidance of degradation of *FLG* mRNA transcripts containing PTCs. The specific mutation in *FLG* – p.R501X – represents an attractive target for small molecule approaches that modify post-transcriptional mechanisms that lead to 'readthrough' of nonsense mutations and therefore stabilise expression of mRNA. This type of pharmacological manipulation is already in phase II clinical trials for genetic disorders such as cystic fibrosis and Duchenne muscular dystrophy using a compound called PTC-124 (a 1,2,4-oxadiazole compound developed by PTC

Therapeutics, New Jersey, USA). The functional properties of PTC-124 are similar to the aminoglycoside antibiotic gentamicin (which was first shown to enhance PTC readthrough in mdx mice),[11] but the two compounds are chemically distinct, and PTC-124 does not exhibit any antibiotic characteristics. Aside from this approach, other mechanisms of obtaining readthrough of PTCs containing mRNAs – for example by transfecting cells with suppressor transfer RNA (tRNA) – are being assessed, albeit in in vitro models.[12] Nevertheless, the results of the clinical trials of PTC-124 in cystic fibrosis and Duchenne muscular dystrophy may be very relevant to individuals with AD. Indeed, AD could be an even better disease to target in this way as it is much more common and the outer layers of the epidermis will almost certainly be easier and safer to treat.

REFERENCES

1 Irvine AD, McLean WH. The molecular genetics of the genodermatoses: progress to date and future directions. *Br J Dermatol* 2003;148:1–13.

2 Fassihi H, Wong T, Wessagowit V, McGrath JA, Mellerio JE. Target proteins in inherited and acquired blistering skin disorders. *Clin Exp Dermatol* 2006;31:252–9.

3 Aumailley M, Has C, Tunggal L, Bruckner-Tuderman L. Molecular basis of inherited skin-blistering disorders, and therapeutic implications. *Expert Rev Mol Med* 2006;8:1–21.

4 Morar N, Willis-Owen SA, Moffatt MF, Cookson WO. The genetics of atopic dermatitis. *J Allergy Clin Immunol* 2006;118:24–34.

5 Smith FJ, Irvine AD, Terron-Kwiatkowski A *et al.* Loss-of-function mutations in the gene encoding filaggrin cause ichthyosis vulgaris. *Nat Genet* 2006;38:337–42.

6 Palmer CN, Irvine AD, Terron-Kwiatkowski A *et al.* Common loss-of-function variants of the epidermal barrier protein filaggrin are a major predisposing factor for atopic dermatitis. *Nat Genet* 2006;38:441–6.

7 Fassihi H, Eady RA, Mellerio JE *et al.* Prenatal diagnosis for severe inherited skin disorders: 25 years' experience. *Br J Dermatol* 2006;154:106–13.

8 Renwick PJ, Trussler J, Ostad-Saffari E *et al.* Proof of principle and first cases using preimplantation genetic haplotyping – a paradigm shift for embryo diagnosis. *Reprod Biomed Online* 2006;13:110–9.

9 Mavilio F, Pelligrini G, Ferrari S *et al.* Correction of junctional epidermolysis bullosa by transplantation of genetically modified epidermal stem cells. *Nat Med* 2006;12;1397–402.

10 Hickerson RP, Smith FJ, McLean WH *et al.* SiRNA-mediated selective inhibition of mutant keratin mRNAs responsible for the skin disorder pachyonychia congenita. *Ann N Y Acad Sci* 2006;1082:56–61.

11 Barton-Davis ER, Cordier L, Shoturma DI, Leland SE, Sweeney HL. Aminoglycoside antibiotics restore dystrophin function to skeletal muscles of mdx mice. *J Clin Invest* 1999; 104:375–81.

12 Sako Y, Usuki F, Suga H. A novel therapeutic approach for genetic diseases by introduction of suppressor tRNA. *Nucleic Acids Symp Ser (Oxf)* 2006;50:239–40.

☐ SKIN AND BONES SELF-ASSESSMENT QUESTIONS

Drug allergies

1 Adverse drug reactions involving the skin:
 (a) Are type B idiosyncratic reactions
 (b) Are mediated by immunological hypersensitivity mechanisms
 (c) Never occur with first exposure to a provoking drug
 (d) Are due to increased metabolic detoxication of the drug
 (e) Are predictable by HLA typing

2 Adverse drug reactions:
 (a) Account for up to 7% of all hospital admissions
 (b) Are always due to the expected pharmacological effect of the drug
 (c) Are classified into types 1–4
 (d) Are thought to be due to impaired detoxication of the drug
 (e) Are most commonly induced by NSAIDs

3 With respect to adverse drug reactions comprising urticaria, asthma, or anaphylaxis:
 (a) They are due to drug 'intolerance' in 80% of cases
 (b) They are mediated by type 1 hypersensitivity mechanisms
 (c) They require treatment with systemic steroids
 (d) Causality is confirmed by prick test challenge with the drug
 (e) They are diagnosed by lymphocyte proliferation tests

4 Adverse drug reactions of the Stevens–Johnson or toxic epidermal necrolysis pattern:
 (a) Are associated with 35% mortality
 (b) Are predisposed to by infection with HIV
 (c) Are usually not associated with multi-system involvement
 (d) Are best treated with high-dose systemic steroids
 (e) Are mediated by drug-specific IgG antibodies

Osteoporosis

1 The following agents are approved for the treatment of osteoporosis in postmenopausal women:
 (a) Alendronate
 (b) Pamidronate
 (c) Strontium ranelate
 (d) Teriparatide

2 The following risk factors for fracture are independent of bone mineral density:
 (a) Premature menopause
 (b) Glucocorticoid treatment
 (c) Previous fracture

3 The following agents have been shown to reduce vertebral and non-vertebral fractures, including hip fractures:
(a) Alendronate
(b) Risedronate
(c) Ibandronate
(d) Raloxifene
(e) Strontium ranelate

Inherited skin diseases: new benefits for patients

1 With respect to the skin protein filaggrin:
(a) Filaggrin is a natural moisturiser that contributes to the formation of an intact skin barrier
(b) Mutations in the gene for filaggrin are the cause of the semi-dominant disorder ichthyosis vulgaris
(c) Mutations in the gene for filaggrin are a major risk factor for atopic dermatitis
(d) Mutations in the gene for filaggrin are a major risk factor for asthma associated with atopic dermatitis
(e) Mutations in the gene for filaggrin are a major risk factor for asthma that is not associated with atopic dermatitis

2 Prenatal diagnosis for inherited skin diseases:
(a) Usually involves assessment of fetal skin biopsies
(b) Has been performed to exclude eczema or psoriasis
(c) Most commonly involves analysis of fetal DNA at the end of the first trimester
(d) Is most frequently performed to test for rare forms of severe inherited skin blistering (epidermolysis bullosa)
(e) Includes reports of successful genetic diagnosis before implantation

3 In considering gene therapy for inherited skin diseases:
(a) Clinical trials have not yet been attempted in patients
(b) Strategies for recessive diseases most commonly involve gene replacement
(c) Strategies for dominant diseases may involve silencing of mutant alleles
(d) Skin stem cells are mainly located in the interfollicular epidermis
(e) Gene therapy is clearly superior to protein or cell therapies

Renal disease

Treatment of antineutrophil cytoplasm antibody-associated systemic vasculitis

Wai Y Tse and Dwomoa Adu

□ INTRODUCTION

Wegener's granulomatosis, microscopic polyangiitis, renal-limited vasculitis, and Churg-Strauss syndrome are small-vessel vasculitides that are associated with antibodies to the neutrophil cytoplasmic antigens proteinase 3 and myeloperoxidase. The systemic vasculitides were once fatal diseases with 80% mortality at one year, but the introduction of prednisolone and cyclophosphamide improved outcomes, and patient survival at five years is now greater than 80%.[1] The challenges clinicians now face include finding better and safer ways to induce and maintain remission and reduce relapses. Other challenges include optimising the treatment of refractory cases and avoiding treatment-related morbidity and toxicity.

□ CLASSIFICATION AND CLINICAL FEATURES

In an attempt to overcome the problems of classification, the Chapel Hill consensus definitions were drawn up; these base the classification of vasculitis on the size of vessels involved (Table 1).[2]

Table 1 Classification of vasculitis according to predominant size of involved vessel.

Predominant size of involved vessel	Positive for ANCA	Negative for ANCA
Small	• Wegener's granulomatosis • Microscopic polyangiitis • Renal-limited vasculitis • Churg-Strauss syndrome	• Henoch–Schönlein purpura • Cryoglobulinaemia • Cutaneous leucocytoclastic vasculitis
Medium		• Polyarteritis nodosa • Kawasaki disease
Large		• Giant-cell arteritis • Takayasu's arteritis

ANCA = antineutrophil cytoplasmic antibodies.

Many patients develop their disease on a background of non-specific constitutional symptoms such as malaise, weight loss, fever, myalgia, arthralgia, and night sweats. Most clinical features are a consequence of necrotising vasculitis.

Patients with Wegener's granulomatosis and Churg-Strauss syndrome also develop granulomatous inflammation. Patients with microscopic polyangiitis almost always have glomerulonephritis, and, rarely, the disease may be limited to the kidneys. Wegener's granulomatosis typically affects the upper and lower respiratory tracts. Many organs can be affected in patients with systemic vasculitis, including the upper respiratory tract, lungs, kidneys, skin, and peripheral nerves. The clinical features are detailed by Jennette and Falk.[3]

☐ DIAGNOSIS

Diagnosis is based on typical clinical features, biopsy, and the presence of antineutrophil cytoplasmic antibodies (ANCAs). These antibodies have specificity for myeloperoxidase or proteinase 3 and can be detected by enzyme-linked immunosorbent assay (ELISA). In indirect immunofluorescence tests, anti-proteinase 3 antibodies lead to a cytoplasmic staining pattern (cANCA) and antimyeloperoxidase antibodies to a perinuclear staining pattern (pANCA). A combination of testing with ELISA and indirect immunofluorescence is recommended, as this increases specificity, although at the cost of a 10% reduction in sensitivity.

☐ MONITORING OF DISEASE ACTIVITY

It is important to differentiate the manifestations of active disease, which requires immunosuppression, from manifestations that are the consequence of damage from scarring or treatment. The Birmingham vasculitis activity score (BVAS)[4] and vasculitis damage index (VDI)[5] were developed to aid treatment decisions, as well as to facilitate clinical trials. The BVAS is designed to include 64 clinical and radiological items in 10 organ systems, whereas damage is measured by the VDI, which scores 64 damage items grouped into 11 organ systems. A number of prospective studies have shown that relapses are preceded by a rise in the titre of ANCAs, and some investigators have suggested that clinical relapses can be pre-empted by increasing treatment after a rise in ANCAs. In some patients, titres of ANCAs correlate with disease severity, while in others they do not. Although an increase in the titre of ANCAs is not specific for a relapse, this should prompt careful re-evaluation of the patient for clinical evidence of active disease. Patients in whom ANCAs persist seem to be at greater risk of relapse, unlike those who are persistently negative for ANCAs. Patients with Wegener's granulomatosis and those who have antibodies to proteinase 3 are at increased risk of relapse. We do not advocate initiating or escalating treatment solely on the basis of titres of ANCA because of the risk of overtreatment with immunosuppressive drugs.

☐ TREATMENT

The management of ANCA-associated systemic vasculitis (AASV) is complex. Several studies have been conducted to determine the optimal route of administration of cyclophosphamide, duration of induction therapy, adjunctive therapy, maintenance therapy, and treatment of relapses. Many of these studies are conducted by the European Vasculitis Study Group (EUVAS; www.vasculitis.org).

Early non-systemic disease

Methotrexate has been used as an alternative to cyclophosphamide in the induction of remission in patients with Wegener's granulomatosis who do not have severe organ damage. The non-renal Wegener's granulomatosis treated alternatively with methotrexate (NORAM) trial was undertaken by EUVAS to determine whether methotrexate could replace cyclophosphamide in the early treatment of AASV.[6] Patients with newly diagnosed AASV with serum creatinine levels <150 μmol/l and without critical organ manifestations were randomised to receive standard oral cyclophosphamide (2 g/kg/day) or oral methotrexate (20–25 mg/week) together with prednisolone. The rate of remission in patients treated with methotrexate was about 90% and was not inferior to that in patients treated with cyclophosphamide, who had a remission rate of 94%. Remission, however, was delayed by about two months in the methotrexate group and the relapse rate was also higher, although the difference did not reach statistical significance. Methotrexate in combination with prednisolone thus can induce remission in patients with limited disease. Its use is contraindicated in patients with renal impairment.

Generalised renal disease

In the cyclophosphamide versus azathioprine during remission in ANCA-associated vasculitis (CYCAZAREM) trial by EUVAS, 155 patients with newly diagnosed generalised vasculitis and serum creatinine levels <500 μmol/l were treated with oral cyclophosphamide for 3–6 months until remission was induced.[7] They were then randomised to receive azathioprine or a lower dose of cyclophosphamide for up to 12 months followed by a switch to azathioprine. No significant difference was seen in relapse rates, which were 15.5% in the azathioprine group and 13.7% in the cyclophosphamide group. There were also no differences in renal function, BVAS, or score on the VDI. The duration of exposure to cyclophosphamide when inducing remission may be reduced safely to 3–6 months, and azathioprine is an effective drug for the maintenance of remission.

Intravenous pulse cyclophosphamide offers the potential advantage of lower cumulative dosage and hence adverse effects. A meta-analysis of randomised controlled trials that compared intravenous pulse cyclophosphamide with oral cyclophosphamide showed that intravenous pulse cyclophosphamide was as effective as oral cyclophosphamide in inducing remission and less toxic but possibly at the expense of more relapses.[8] No differences in end-stage renal failure or deaths were seen between the two regimens.

In the cyclophosphamide daily oral versus pulsed (CYCLOPS) study by EUVAS, 160 patients with newly diagnosed, untreated, generalised AASV with an entry creatinine of 150–500 μmol/l were randomised to treatment with daily oral or pulse cyclophosphamide.[9] After remission, patients in both arms of the study were switched to azathioprine (2 mg/kg) in conjunction with a tapering steroid regimen. An interim analysis showed equal efficacy with the two regimens but at a lower cumulative dose of cyclophosphamide in those who received pulse cyclophosphamide.

Severe renal disease

Preliminary studies suggested that plasma exchange improved the outcome of dialysis-dependent patients with AASV compared with standard drug therapy alone. The methylprednisolone versus plasma exchange as additional therapy for severe ANCA-associated glomerulonephritis (MEPEX) study by EUVAS randomised patients with AASV and levels of serum creatinine >500 μmol/l to treatment with adjunctive plasma exchange (seven sessions in the first two weeks) or three pulses of intravenous methylprednisolone in addition to standard therapy with prednisolone and cyclophosphamide. Preliminary analysis suggested that plasma exchange was more effective in recovering renal function than methylprednisolone.[10]

□ EMERGING TREATMENTS

Mycophenolate mofetil

Mycophenolate mofetil has been used in small, non-randomised trials as a remission-inducing and remission-maintaining agent in patients with AASV with variable results.[11] It holds promise as a potential alternative to azathioprine as a remission maintenance agent, and this is currently being tested in the mycophenolate mofetil versus azathioprine for maintenance therapy in ANCA-associated systemic vasculitis (IMPROVE) study by EUVAS.

Tumour necrosis factor alpha (TNF-α) antagonists

Etanercept is a protein that comprises two p75 TNF-α receptors fused to the F_c portion of a human monoclonal antibody. It binds to soluble TNF. The Wegener's granulomatosis etanercept trial (WGET) was a randomised, placebo-controlled trial in which 180 patients with Wegener's granulomatosis treated with glucocorticoids plus cyclophosphamide or methotrexate were randomised to etanercept or placebo.[12] The mean follow up was 27 months. No significant differences in the rates of sustained remission were seen between the etanercept and control groups (69.7% and 75.3%, respectively). Disease flares were common in both groups, with 118 flares in the etanercept group and 134 in the control group. During the study, 56.2% of patients in the etanercept group and 57.1% of those in the control group had at least one severe or life-threatening adverse event or died. Of concern, solid cancers developed in six patients in the etanercept group and none in the control group (p=0.01). All patients who developed cancer had also received cyclophosphamide, which may have increased their risk of malignancy. The findings of this study do not support the use of etanercept in the treatment of patients with Wegener's granulomatosis.

Infliximab is a chimeric monoclonal antibody that binds to TNF-α. Pilot studies suggest it may be of benefit in patients with AASV, but randomised controlled studies are required to establish its role in the treatment of these disorders.

Rituximab

The safe and effective use of the anti-B-cell treatment rituximab (anti-CD20) in resistant AASV has been reported in small series.[13] The Immune Tolerance Network is recruiting 200 patients with Wegener's granulomatosis or microscopic polyangiitis into a prospective, randomised, controlled, double-blind trial of rituximab in patients with AASV (www.immunetolerance.org/RAVE/). This study will investigate whether B-cell depletion with rituximab can induce remission and, in addition, can tolerise patients to the ANCA antigens myeloperoxidase and proteinase 3.

Leflunomide

Leflunomide is an inhibitor of de novo pyrimidine synthesis and has anti-inflammatory effects through inhibition of TNF-α and interleukin 1β. In an open-label study of 20 patients with Wegener's granulomatosis, leflunomide was substituted for cyclophosphamide after successful induction.[14] During a median follow up of 21 months, one major relapse required treatment with cyclophosphamide and eight minor relapses were treated successfully by increasing the dose of leflunomide. A multicentre, randomised, controlled trial is comparing leflunomide with methotrexate after induction with cyclophosphamide.

Deoxyspergualin

Deoxyspergualin blocks the transcriptional activation of κ light chain expression during the development of B lymphocytes and the development of cytotoxic T cells. Deoxyspergualin was effective for the induction of remission in 20 patients with active refractory AASV (19 with Wegener's granulomatosis) in one multicentre pilot trial.[15] A clinical response was seen in 70% of patients, and six of 20 patients achieved complete remission. A prospective, multicentre, controlled trial is underway for those with chronic persistent disease despite conventional immunosuppression.

Antithymocyte globulin

Antithymocyte globulin is a T cell-depleting polyclonal antibody directed against surface antigens of activated T cells. The treatment of refractory systemic vasculitis with antithymocyte globulin (SOLUTION) study by EUVAS found antithymocyte globulin to be effective in inducing remission in 13/15 patients with active, refractory Wegener's granulomatosis unresponsive or intolerant to cyclophosphamide.[16] Two patients died: one because of pulmonary haemorrhage and the other because of sepsis.

☐ TREATMENT-RELATED TOXICITY

A major problem in the management of patients with vasculitis is treatment-related toxicity. Although cyclophosphamide is effective at inducing and maintaining remission, its use is associated with adverse effects such as bone marrow suppression, infection, infertility, haemorrhagic cystitis, and malignancy. In the CYCAZAREM trial, 55% of patients had neutropenia and severe adverse events occurred in 26% of patients. Infections remain a major cause of death and morbidity in patients with vasculitis.

□ PROGNOSIS

Adverse prognostic factors include increasing age and poor renal function. Patients with Wegener's granulomatosis are more likely to relapse than those with microscopic polyangiitis. Similarly, patients with antiproteinase 3 antibodies are more likely to relapse than those with antimyeloperoxidase antibodies.

□ CONCLUSION

The recent randomised controlled trials provide evidence-based guidance for the treatment of AASV. The treatment protocols are summarised on www.vasculitis.org. It is important to avoid the long-term use of cyclophosphamide, as toxicity is dependent on cumulative dosage. The BVAS and VDI permit separation of disease activity, which requires treatment, and damage, which does not, and are useful in management. In patients with Wegener's granulomatosis, evidence shows that cotrimoxazole can reduce the recurrence of upper airways disease, possibly by reducing nasal carriage of staphylococci. This has the advantage of providing prophylaxis for infections caused by *Pneumocystis* and *Nocardia* species. Despite real advances in management, the outcome in patients with systemic vasculitis is still not good. New treatment strategies are needed to improve the outcome from these disorders.

REFERENCES

1 Fauci AS, Haynes BF, Katz P *et al.* Wegener's granulomatosis: prospective clinical and therapeutic experience with 85 patients for 21 years. *Ann Intern Med* 1983;98:76–85.

2 Jennette JC, Falk RJ, Andrassy K *et al.* Nomenclature of systemic vasculitides. Proposal of an international consensus conference. *Arthritis Rheum* 1994;37:187–92.

3 Jennette JC, Falk RJ. Small-vessel vasculitis. *N Engl J Med* 1997;337:1512–23.

4 Luqmani RA, Bacon PA, Moots RJ *et al.* Birmingham vasculitis activity score (BVAS) in systemic necrotizing vasculitis. *QJM* 1994;87:671–8.

5 Exley AR, Bacon PA, Luqmani RA *et al.* Development and initial validation of the vasculitis damage index for the standardized clinical assessment of damage in the systemic vasculitides. *Arthritis Rheum* 1997;40:371–80.

6 De Groot K, Rasmussen N, Bacon PA *et al.* Randomized trial of cyclophosphamide versus methotrexate for induction of remission in early systemic antineutrophil cytoplasmic antibody-associated vasculitis. *Arthritis Rheum* 2005;52:2461–9.

7 Jayne D, Rasmussen N, Andrassy K *et al.* A randomized trial of maintenance therapy for vasculitis associated with antineutrophil cytoplasmic autoantibodies. *N Engl J Med* 2003; 349:36–44.

8 de Groot K, Adu D, Savage CO. The value of pulse cyclophosphamide in ANCA-associated vasculitis: meta-analysis and critical review. *Nephrol Dial Transplant* 2001;16:2018–27.

9 de Groot K, Jayne D, Tesar V *et al.* Randomised controlled trial of daily oral versus pulse cyclophosphamide for induction of remission in ANCA-associated systemic vasculitis. *Kidney Blood Press Res* 2005;28:195 (Abstract 103).

10 Gaskin G, Jayne D. Adjunctive plasma exchange is superior to methylprednisolone in acute renal failure due to ANCA-associated glomerulonephritis. *Am Soc Nephrol* 2002;13:2A–3A.

11 Nowack R, Gobel U, Klooker P *et al.* Mycophenolate mofetil for maintenance therapy of Wegener's granulomatosis and microscopic polyangiitis: a pilot study in 11 patients with renal involvement. *J Am Soc Nephrol* 1999;10:1965–71.

12 Wegener's Granulomatosis Etanercept Trial (WGET) Research Group. Etanercept plus standard therapy for Wegener's granulomatosis. *N Engl J Med* 2005;352:351–61.

13 Keogh KA, Wylam ME, Stone JH, Specks U. Induction of remission by B lymphocyte depletion in eleven patients with refractory antineutrophil cytoplasmic antibody-associated vasculitis. *Arthritis Rheum* 2005;52:262–8.

14 Metzler C, Fink C, Lamprecht P, Gross WL, Reinhold-Keller E. Maintenance of remission with leflunomide in Wegener's granulomatosis. *Rheumatology (Oxford)* 2004;43:315–20.

15 Birck R, Warnatz K, Lorenz HM *et al.* 15-deoxyspergualin in patients with refractory ANCA-associated systemic vasculitis: a six-month open-label trial to evaluate safety and efficacy. *J Am Soc Nephrol* 2003;14:440–7.

16 Schmitt WH, Hagen EC, Neumann I *et al.* Treatment of refractory Wegener's granulomatosis with antithymocyte globulin (ATG): an open study in 15 patients. *Kidney Int* 2004;65:1440–8.

Polycystic kidney disease – then and now

Albert CM Ong

☐ A HISTORICAL PERSPECTIVE

Polycystic kidney disease (PKD) was first recognised in 1757 by the Italian anatomist, Domenico Galeazzi, and later by the French pathologists Jean Cruveilhier (1829) and Pierre Rayer (1841), who described it as 'cystic transformation' and 'cystic degeneration,' respectively. The term 'polycystic kidney disease' was actually coined by another French physician, Felix Lejars (1888), who defined it as a clinical entity for the first time. An important observation was that the disease could be transmitted within families by dominant or recessive transmission. Daalgard's landmark study in 1957 indicated that PKD was common, with an estimated incidence of one in 1000. In 1984, it was recognised that the dominant variety (autosomal dominant polycystic kidney disease (ADPKD)) could be caused by mutations in more than one gene – these were named *PKD1* and *PKD2*. Both genes were finally identified in 1994 and 1996, respectively. The very rare recessive form of PKD (autosomal recessive PKD (ARPKD)) usually presents in infants and is the result of mutations in a single gene, *PKHD1*, which was identified in 2002. We thus now know all three genes that cause significant PKD in man. In this paper, I will focus primarily on ADPKD and review how the identification of *PKD1* and *PKD2* has advanced clinical diagnosis, prognosis, and treatment of this condition.

☐ AUTOSOMAL DOMINANT POLYCYSTIC KIDNEY DISEASE

Important cause of kidney failure

Autosomal dominant polycystic kidney disease (OMIM 173910) is one of the most common human monogenic diseases, with an incidence of one in 400 to one in 1,000 live births. It accounts for about 10% of treated end-stage renal disease (ESRD) in the UK and is the fourth most common cause of ESRD (Fig 1[1]). Worldwide, ADPKD may affect 5–10 million people, which makes it the single most common monogenic cause of ESRD. The defining feature of ADPKD is the presence of focal cysts in both kidneys, which progressively develop and enlarge over many years, typically resulting in ESRD by the fifth decade (Fig 2).

More than a kidney disease

Although cystic renal disease is the major cause of morbidity, the occurrence of non-renal cysts, most notably in the liver (occasionally resulting in clinically

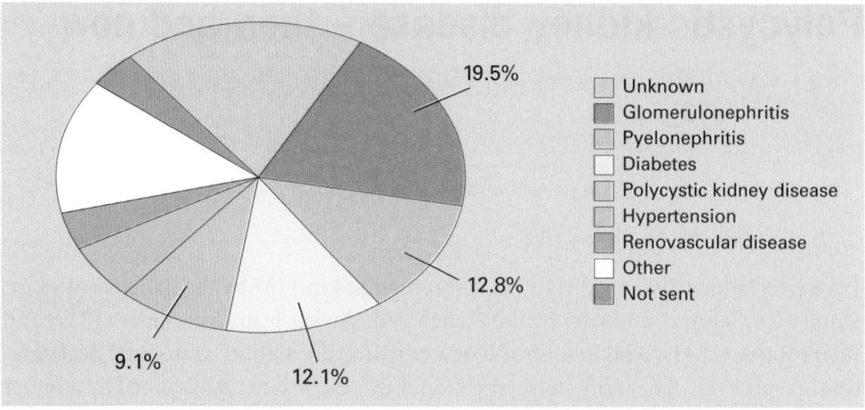

Fig 1 Primary renal diagnosis in prevalent patients on renal replacement therapy in England and Wales in 2004.[1]

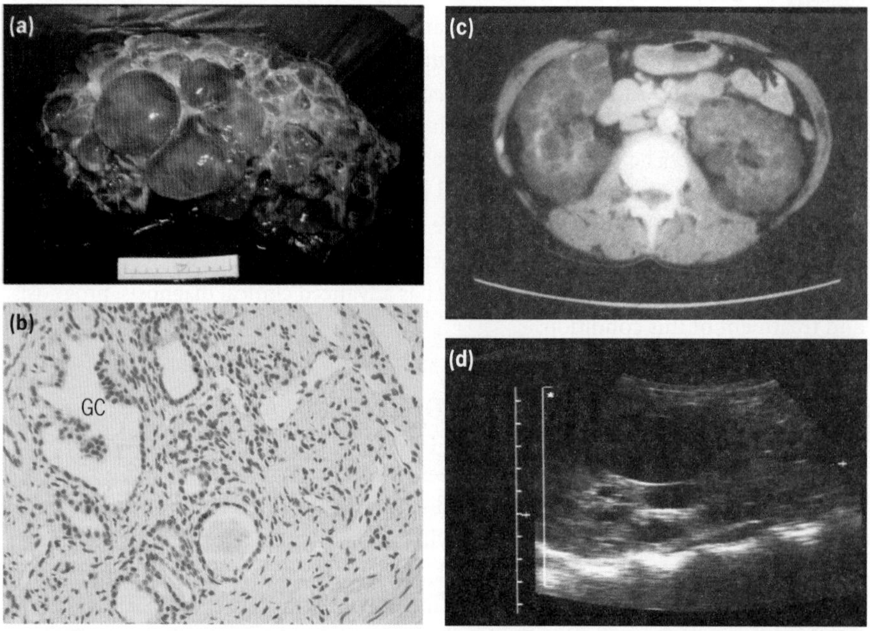

Fig 2 Kidneys from patients with polycystic kidney disease (PKD) at different stages of disease: **(a)** end-stage polycystic kidney disease, showing gross enlargement of the kidney and numerous fluid-filled cysts, **(b)** tissue section stained with a marker of proliferating cells (proliferating cell nuclear antigen (PCNA)) – a marked increase in proliferating cells (brown nuclei) can be seen in some normal and mildly dilated tubular segments, and a single glomerular cyst (GC) can also be visualised, **(c)** computed tomogram showing the presence of multiple cysts in both kidneys, and **(d)** ultrasound scan of a patient aged five years with very early onset (VEO) PKD, showing the multiple cysts of different sizes.

significant polycystic liver disease) and pancreas, is well documented. The prevalence of non-cystic abnormalities, including intracranial aneurysms (ICAs), mitral valve prolapse, and diverticular disease, is also increased in patients with ADPKD.

Two-gene cause

Mutations in *PKD1* (chromosome region 16p13.3) is the most common cause of ADPKD (about 86% of cases), with most of the remainder due to changes in *PKD2* (4q22). Patients with mutations in *PKD1* and *PKD2* have indistinguishable renal and extrarenal phenotypes: they were only recognised as distinct diseases by genetic linkage analysis in the late 1980s.[2] *PKD1* is a complex gene with 46 exons, which generates a large transcript (about 14 kb) that contains a long, open-reading frame predicted to encode a protein of 4302 amino acids named polycystin-1 (Fig 3). Characterisation of the structure of the gene and identification of mutations has been complicated by genomic duplication of the 5' region of *PKD1* (to exon 33), such that about six copies of *PKD1*-like pseudogenes are located in 16p13.1. The *PKD2* gene has 15 exons, generates a transcript of about 5 kb, and encodes polycystin-2 – a protein of 968 amino acids that has strong homology to the transient receptor potential (TRP) family of non-selective calcium channels (see Fig 3). Both polycystin proteins are expressed ubiquitously, which is consistent with ADPKD being a systemic disease. Good evidence suggests that they form a functional protein complex in the kidney and other tissues.

Gene locus effect

Mutations in *PKD2* produce a significantly milder disease in terms of older age at diagnosis, lower prevalence of hypertension, and later age at onset of ESRD (54.3 years

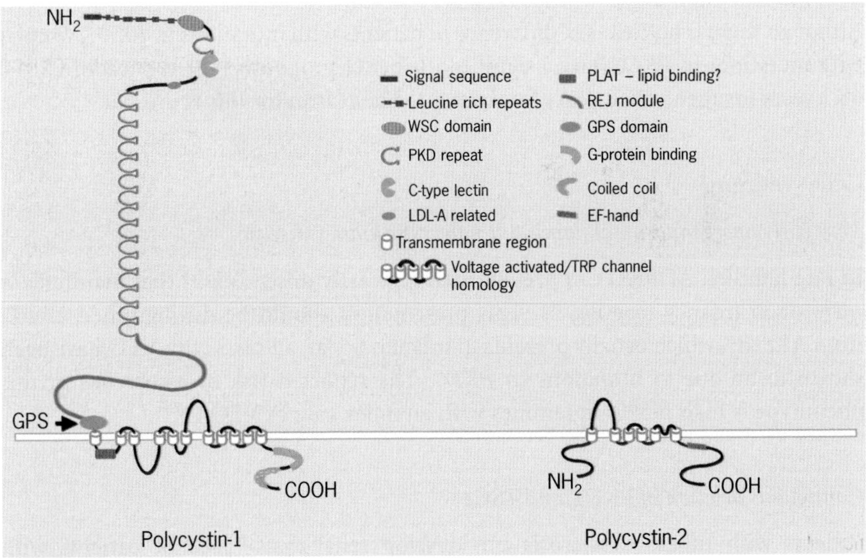

Fig 3 Predicted structure and topology of polycystin-1 and polycystin-2 – the proteins involved in autosomal dominant polycystic kidney disease (PKD). A number of protein-, carbohydrate-, and lipid-binding functional domains of both proteins are depicted. Polycystin-1 has a predicted large extracellular N-terminal domain. A G-protein coupled receptor proteolytic site (GPS) may allow polycystin-1 to be cleaved into two halves that remain tethered by non-covalent bonds. Polycystin-2 is highly homologous to transient receptor potential (TRP) channel proteins. Both proteins interact via a coiled coil domain in their C-termini to form a functional complex. LDL = low-density lipoprotein; PLAT = polycystin/lipoxygenase/α-toxin; REJ = receptor for egg jelly; WSC = cell-wall integrity and stress-response component 1.

for mutations in *PKD1* *v* 74.0 years for mutations in *PKD2*). Consistent with this milder phenotype, there seems to be an enrichment of patients with mutations in *PKD2* among patients with ADPKD who present late with ESRD (after the age of 63 years).

Allelic heterogeneity

Both *PKD1* and *PKD2* exhibit marked allelic heterogeneity, with about 200 different mutations in *PKD1* and more than 50 different mutations in *PKD2* described. Unlike *PKD2*, *PKD1* is also highly polymorphic, with at least 71 changes described so far. Most mutations are private (that is, unique to a single family), which indicates that a significant level of new mutation is occurring. For *PKD1*, mutations 5' to the median are associated with more severe disease (average age at onset of ESRD: 53 years for 5' mutations *v* 56 years for 3' mutations) and a significantly greater risk of developing ICAs. This association is not related to the type of mutation and may be due to the proposed cleavage of polycystin-1 into two different proteins via a G-protein coupled receptor proteolytic site (GPS) (see Fig 3), with mutations to each half having potentially different phenotypic consequences. As yet, no clear phenotype–genotype correlations have been reported for *PKD2*.

The effect of sex

Although there is no clear sex difference in patients with mutations in *PKD1*, women with mutations in *PKD2* have a significantly better prognosis (age at onset of ESRD: 68.1 years for men *v* 76.0 years for women). The reason for this is unclear.

Gene syndromes

Very early onset autosomal dominant polycystic kidney disease

In rare families, ADPKD can present with very early onset (VEO) that manifests *in utero* or in infancy (see Fig 2). This presentation should be distinguished clearly from ARPKD, which usually presents in infancy. So far, all cases with VEO have been shown to be due to mutations in *PKD1*. The reported risk of recurrence of this phenotype is high (45%) in families with an index case of VEO PKD.[3]

Contiguous deletion of PKD1 *and* TSC2

Patients with tuberous sclerosis can develop renal cysts (50% of patients with mutations in *TSC2* and 12.5% of those with mutations in *TSC1*); however, in 5% of patients with mutations in *TSC2*, early-onset PKD can be the dominant presentation. In the vast majority of these cases, contiguous gene deletions of both *PKD1* and *TSC2* have been found.[4] This most probably indicates a synergistic role between polycystin-1 and tuberin (the protein encoded for by *TSC2*) in the development of cysts: tuberin may play a role in trafficking polycystin-1 to the lateral cell membrane in renal epithelial cells.

Bilineal inheritance of mutations in PKD1 *and* PKD2

A family with bilineal inheritance of germline mutations in *PKD1* and *PKD2* has been described.[5] Although the patients had more severe disease than those with either mutation alone, the difference is not dramatic – that is, not every renal tubular cell gives rise to a cyst. The effect of a transheterozygous mutation in either gene seems to act as a modifying factor for the other in terms of the risk of cyst development or the hastening of its progression rather than an effect on cyst initiation itself.

Familial intracranial aneurysms

The prevalence of ICAs in patients with ADPKD is 8% compared with 2% in the general population. In a proportion of families affected by ADPKD (caused by mutations in *PKD1* or *PKD2*), there is cosegregation of ICA rupture and PKD that affects at least two other first-degree relatives (an example is shown in Fig 4). The youngest patient with PKD reported to have rupture of ICA is 15 years. As described above, patients with more 5' mutations in *PKD1* are at significantly greater risk of developing ICAs (see Fig 4).[6]

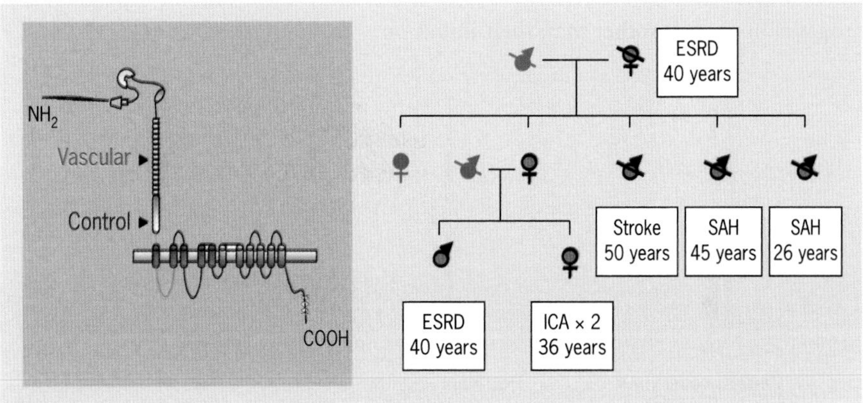

Fig 4 Pedigree affected by PKD, with an aggregation of ruptured and unruptured intracranial aneurysms (ICAs). This is an example of a three-generational family affected by mutations in *PKD1*, with at least four family members with PKD and associated rupture of or surgery for ICAs. The median mutation position in this family and other similar pedigrees maps more to the 5' end of the *PKD1* gene (*vascular*) compared with pedigrees with no vascular history (*control*) and would truncate the polycystin-1 protein earlier.

Polycystic liver disease

Polycystic liver disease (PCLD) can be a marked feature in some patients with otherwise typical ADPKD. This phenotype is not related to genotype and has a marked preponderance in women. Isolated PCLD without renal cysts can be due to autosomal dominant polycystic liver disease (ADPLD, OMIM 174050). This disease is due to mutations in two other genes –*SEC63* and *PKRCSH.*

Overlap connective tissue disorder

Several families affected by mutations in *PKD1* with a cosegregating overlap connective tissue disorder (OCTD) – that is, Marfanoid habitus (and other cardiovascular abnormalities) – have been described. In some, linkage to the genes for Marfan's syndrome, *FBN1* (fibrillin) and *FBN2*, has been excluded.

Mutational mechanisms – one hit or two?

Fewer than 1% of tubular cells that carry a germline mutation in *PKD1* or *PKD2* have been estimated to give rise to cysts. The focal nature of cyst formation and its heterogeneity has given rise to the proposal of a 'two-hit' mechanism for ADPKD (consisting of a germline mutation to one allele and a somatic mutation to the other) (Fig 5). Consistent with this notion, cells isolated from individual cysts in the kidney and liver show evidence for clonality and a high rate of somatic mutations. Experimentally, a unique *Pkd2* knockout mouse (*Pkd2*^{WS25} mutant) that has an unstable allele (prone to inactivation by recombination) develops progressive cystic disease in a manner consistent with a two-hit model. Questions remain, however, as to whether a two-hit mechanism is the only means to generate a cyst and, indeed, whether these somatic events may be later events more important for expansion and progression of cysts rather than their initiation.

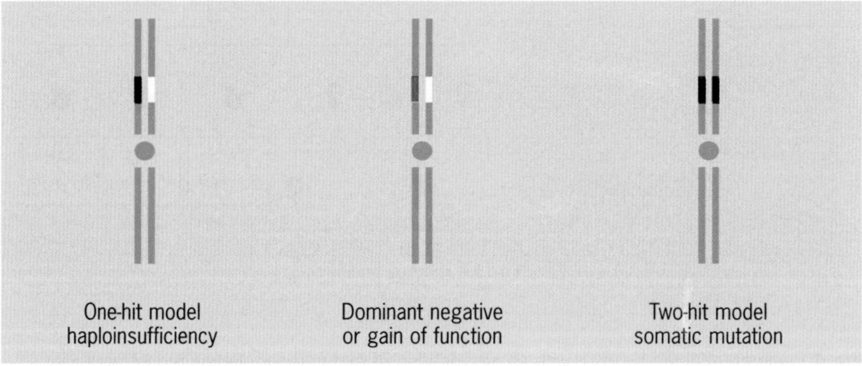

Fig 5 Mutational mechanisms that underlie initiation of cysts in patients with autosomal dominant polycystic kidney disease. The presence of a germline null mutation (black) in *PKD1* or *PKD2* is necessary but not sufficient for cysts to arise from every cell. A one-hit model is consistent with the presence of a normal allele (white), whereas a two-hit model requires a somatic null mutation (black) to disrupt the normal allele. Alternatively, a germline mutant allele (red) could exert a phenotypic change in the presence of a normal allele (white) via a dominant negative or gain-of-function mechanism.

A decrease in (loss of a single allele or haploinsufficiency) or increase in (transgenic expression) dosage of polycystin-1 may itself result in cyst formation. In addition, haploinsufficient *Pkd2* mice have reduced survival (not due to renal failure), which indicates that a dosage reduction of polycystin-2 itself can exert a phenotypic load. Recent studies have shown that *Pkd1*$^{+/-}$ and *Pkd2*$^{+/-}$ kidney tubular cells are hyperproliferative (see Fig 2).[7]

In summary, there seem to be multiple mechanisms that could underlie formation of cysts. Development of cysts requires a germline mutation, but beyond this, the likelihood of cyst formation is influenced by a number of different factors that could include somatic genetic events at the other (normal) allele, mutations at the other gene associated with ADPKD, and possibly a wide array of other genetic loci (for example, *TSC2*). In effect, these loci act as modifiers of disease presentation in patients with ADPKD. Environmental or genetic factors that modulate the rate of somatic mutation or DNA repair could modify the disease phenotype. Beyond the genetic events, stochastic factors probably also influence whether a cell that is haploinsufficient for a mutation associated with ADPKD is diverted into a cystogenic pathway. Another factor that could modify the cystic phenotype is the presence of partially functional (mutant) polycystin-1 protein, or a non-functional mutant protein could act in a dominant-negative manner. Finally, non-cystic manifestations of PKD, such as ICAs, are likely to be related to haploinsufficiency rather than a 'two-hit' model.

Polygenic disorder

Intrafamilial variability

A wide range of intrafamilial phenotypic variability has been described in large families affected by ADPKD and more recently for those with mutations in *PKD1* and *PKD2*. The phenomenon of genetic anticipation in families affected by ADPKD was first postulated in 1925, with the description of babies with VEO often born to relatively asymptomatic parents. No evidence for dynamic unstable mutations in *PKD1* or *PKD2*, however, has been found.[8]

The causes of this variability are largely non-allelic and could include modifying genes, environmental factors, or stochastic events (Fig 6). For cases with VEO, it is difficult to envisage (although impossible to exclude) that somatic mutations to *PKD1* could be the underlying reason for increased disease severity *in utero*.

A number of studies have attempted to define the possible role of modifying genes (heritability) in determining renal outcome. An informative study in 1995 by Geberth *et al* of 74 parent–offspring pairs in which the age of renal death of both was known showed a wide Gaussian distribution of values around zero. Furthermore, no difference was seen in the median age of renal death between two decades (1950–1971 and 1975–1985), which thus excluded the effect of secular trend as a major confounding factor. Another study by Persu *et al* (2004) that included sibling pairs compared the age of ESRD between 56 pairs of siblings and nine pairs of monozygotic twins and calculated the intraclass correlation coefficient (ICC) within both groups. The ICC, which compares the similarity within pairs of sibling to that between pairs of siblings, was significantly higher for twins (0.92) than siblings (0.49). Discordance in the renal phenotype between a pair of dizygotic twins who carried the same mutation in *PKD1* has been reported in one family.[8] This could imply that foetal environment does not play a major role in determining the cystic phenotype compared with genetic factors.

The possible influence of modifying genes (heritability) in families affected by mutations in *PKD1* also has been addressed recently in two large studies. Heritability

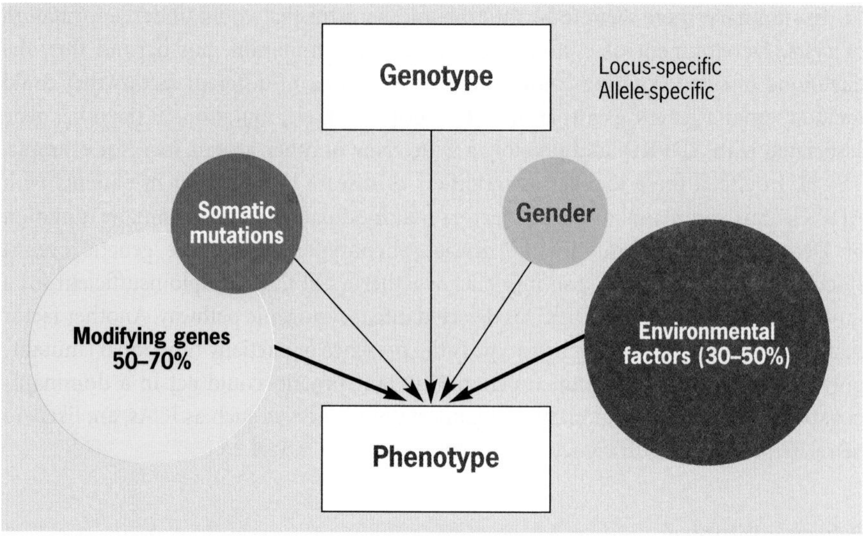

Fig 6 Factors that could determine the severity of the cystic phenotype in an individual who inherits a germline mutation in *PKD1* or *PKD2*. Although autosomal dominant polycystic kidney disease (ADPKD) is a monogenic disease, multiple factors such as sex, modifying genes, and environmental factors ultimately influence the consequences of inheriting a particular mutation. Genetic background may interact with environmental triggers to determine the rate of somatic mutations or its downstream consequences. In this regard, ADPKD could be regarded as a polygenic disease.

for the age of ESRD was estimated at 43–78%; however, the number of potential modifiers, their allele frequency, and their relative effect with respect to determining loss of renal function is not clear. Paterson *et al* calculated that a genome-wide scan to look for a single modifier locus will require very large cohorts to be powered adequately and thus will necessitate international collaboration.[9] These studies also point to the likely significance of (unknown) environmental contributory factors to the phenotype associated with ESRD. These factors could include urinary tract infections in men and the number of pregnancies in women but require verification in larger scale populations.

A different experimental approach that seeks to address this issue has been to utilise whole genome quantitative trait loci (QTL) mapping in inbred rodent models of PKD to map major modifier gene loci.[10] In theory, this approach allows environmental factors to be controlled for, which thus allows the contribution of genetic factors to be paramount. The evolutionary significance of any rodent modifier genes for PKD could then be tested in human pedigrees.

A number of studies have examined the association between candidate gene polymorphisms (for example, the genes for angiotensin-converting enzyme (*ACE)* and endothelial nitric oxide synthase (*eNOS*)) and kidney function. Overall, these findings have proved to be inconclusive and contradictory. As discussed above, similar studies in the future will need to be powered adequately to reach any meaningful conclusions.

Development of orthologous models

The identification of *PKD1* and *PKD2* has facilitated the generation of animal models of disease (higher to lower vertebrates) to investigate how the disease starts and progresses, especially from the earliest stages. To date, at least 12 mouse mutants have been reported;[2] unfortunately, almost all are lethal to embryos in the recessive state. Nevertheless, hypomorphic, unstable, or conditional null alleles also have been described and have led to more useful models for studying progression of disease.

This promising approach will also enable new candidate drugs to undergo preclinical testing with more relevant orthologous models. So far, it has facilitated the rapid clinical translation of vasopressin type 2 receptor (V2R) antagonists for human ADPKD after they showed dramatic efficacy in a mouse model of *PKD2*.[11] The pathological role of vasopressin on cyst expansion was unexpected but may relate to its role in mobilising cyclic adenosine monophosphate (cAMP) in the epithelial cells of cysts.

Polycystins, calcium, and cilia

Studies in even more simple organisms such as biflagellar green algae (*Chlamydomonas*), fruitflies (*Drosophila*), and nematodes (*Caenorhabditis elegans*) have led to a greater appreciation of the potential roles of polycystin-1 and polycystin-2 in basic or essential cellular functions.[12] One key function that seems to be common from flies up to man is the regulation of intracellular calcium ions (Ca^{2+}) – a major messenger molecule. Much effort is currently going into developing understanding of how this occurs. An unexpected insight into the pathogenesis of PKD came from studies of mating behaviour in *C. elegans* and flagellar motility in *Chlamydomonas*. These studies showed the functional importance of a previously neglected organelle – the non-motile or primary cilium – in the pathogenesis of PKD (Fig 7). Both polycystin proteins have been localised to this organelle (albeit not exclusively), and some evidence suggests that they may transduce mechanosensory Ca^{2+} signals that originate from ciliary bending.

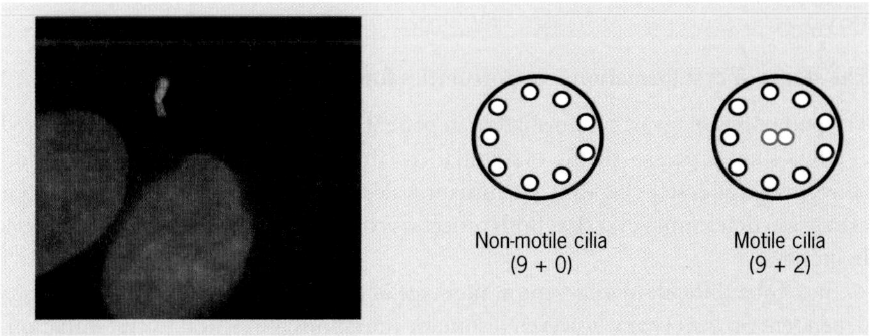

Fig 7 Abnormalities in the structure or function of primary cilia may be the underlying cause of different forms of cystic disease, including autosomal dominant polycystic kidney disease (ADPKD). The left panel shows a solitary primary cilium (red) arising from the apical surface of one of two (blue nuclear stain) cultured human renal cells. Almost all cell types in the body express primary cilia. They are also known as non-motile or '9+0' cilia, because they lack the central doublet pair of microtubules normally found in motile or '9+2' cilia (right panel).

Is genetic testing feasible?

The identification of *PKD1* and *PKD2* has allowed techniques to be developed for mutation screening within individuals and families, especially where the diagnosis is in doubt. Although technically challenging, the rate of detection of mutations in these genes approaches 90% in the most experienced centres. It seems unlikely, however, that large-scale routine detection of mutations will be performed in pedigrees affected by ADPKD, as there is a high rate of new mutations, most mutations are 'private', mutation 'hot spots' are lacking, and the allele-specific effects on ESRD are weak. At present, prenatal genetic diagnosis is also not performed routinely due to the late-onset nature of the disease and the tremendous phenotypic variability within families. The indications for mutation screening could change if effective new treatments become available, however, as it then would be advantageous to make the diagnosis early.

Can we predict which patients will progress to end-stage renal disease?

The Consortium of Radiologic Imaging Studies of Polycystic Kidney Disease (CRISP) recently reported the results of a three-year follow up of 232 patients with creatinine clearance ≥70 ml/min by magnetic resonance imaging (MRI).[13] The study showed that it was possible with MRI to derive a distinct growth signature curve for each individual at an early stage of renal dysfunction. Secondly, the baseline total kidney volume usefully predicted the annual rate of increase in volume independent of age – kidneys >1500 ml were associated with more rapid deterioration of GFR than smaller kidneys. In a follow-up study, kidneys in patients with mutations in *PKD1* were found to be significantly larger and contained more cysts than those from patients with mutations in *PKD2*; however, the rate of cyst growth did not differ significantly between the two genotypes. These results arguably support the idea that genotype determines the number of cysts but not the process of cyst growth. The latter may be influenced by sex – that is, kidneys from men were larger and grew faster than kidneys from women.

The stages of cyst formation – opportunities for intervention

The pathophysiology of cyst formation in patients with ADPKD could be considered as a two-stage process – that is, cyst initiation (the birth of cysts) and cyst expansion (the growth of cysts) (Fig 8). Cyst initiation determines cyst number, whereas cyst expansion determines cyst size. Both processes contribute to the total burden of cysts in kidneys.

It may be difficult to intervene at the stage of cyst initiation (a process that seems dependent on genotype); however, if somatic mutations are critical to cyst initiation, approaches that prevent damage to the DNA or promote repair of DNA may be useful. Alternatively, if haploinsufficiency (gene dosage) is critical to the function of a polycystin complex, strategies to influence protein–protein interactions or membrane targeting may work. Regardless of the molecular mechanism, an antiproliferative strategy could be effective, as an increase in tubular proliferation seems to

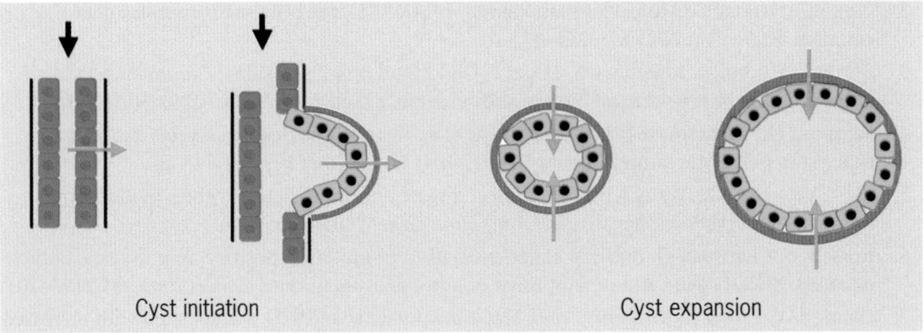

Fig 8 The different stages of cyst formation. The process of cyst formation can be divided into two stages: cyst initiation and cyst expansion. The black arrows indicate the direction of tubular fluid flow, and the orange arrows indicate the direction of reabsorption of tubular fluid. Cysts arise focally from any part of the nephron. At this stage, an increase in cell number (yellow) and basement membrane thickening (red) is detectable. Eventually, these small outpouchings separate from the tubular lumen and become enclosed hollow spheres lined by a monolayer of cells. Cyst enlargement occurs mainly by cell division and fluid secretion.

precede cyst formation in the kidneys of patients with ADPKD (see Fig 2). The processes that underlie cyst expansion are also likely to involve cell proliferation, although changes in fluid secretion may play a more important role at this stage (see Fig 8). Other features of diseased kidneys in patients with ADPKD include interstitial inflammation and fibrosis, although it is unclear whether these occur early or late in the disease process.

Currently, three compounds are being tested in national or international clinical trials for ADPKD. Most interest has centred around tolvaptan, a small molecule antagonist of the V2R that was developed initially for the treatment of hyponatraemia and syndrome of inappropriate antidiuretic hormone (SIADH). Two other compounds, sirolimus (rapamycin) and somatostatin, are also being tested in smaller studies. Tolvaptan and somatostatin are likely to target proliferation and fluid secretion, whereas sirolimus is likely to affect cell proliferation. Nevertheless, it seems likely that a combination of drugs rather than a single agent will be needed to treat patients with ADPKD effectively. The timing of intervention, its duration and intensity, and potential differences in efficacy between genotypes are important issues that will need to be resolved. In addition, different agents will be needed to treat hepatic cysts and the vascular complications of ADPKD.

☐ ACKNOWLEDGEMENTS

Work in the author's laboratory was supported by the Wellcome Trust, Polycystic Kidney Disease Foundation (USA), Research Councils UK, and Medical Research Council.

REFERENCES

1 Ansell D, Feest T, Rao R *et al.* Chapter 4: All patients receiving renal replacement therapy in the United Kingdom in 2004. In: *The Renal Association UK Renal Registry: the Eighth Annual Report, December 2005.*

2 Ong AC, Harris PC. Molecular pathogenesis of ADPKD: the polycystin complex gets complex. *Kidney Int* 2005;67:1234–47.

3 Zerres K, Rudnik-Schöneborn S, Deget F. Childhood onset autosomal dominant polycystic kidney disease in sibs: clinical picture and recurrence risk. *J Med Genet* 1993;30:583–8.

4 Sampson JR, Maheshwar MM, Aspinwall R *et al.* Renal cystic disease in tuberous sclerosis: role of the polycystic kidney disease 1 gene. *Am J Hum Genet* 1997;61:843–51.

5 Pei Y, Paterson AD, Wang KR *et al.* Bilineal disease and trans-heterozygotes in autosomal dominant polycystic kidney disease. *Am J Hum Genet* 2001;68:355–63.

6 Rossetti S, Chauveau D, Kubly V *et al.* Association of mutation position in polycystic kidney disease 1 (PKD1) gene and development of a vascular phenotype. *Lancet* 2003;361:2196–201.

7 Chang MY, Parker E, Ibrahim S *et al.* Haploinsufficiency of Pkd2 is associated with increased tubular cell proliferation and interstitial fibrosis in two murine Pkd2 models. *Nephrol Dial Transplant* 2006;21:2078–84.

8 Peral B, Ong AC, San Millán JL *et al.* A stable, nonsense mutation associated with a case of infantile onset polycystic kidney disease 1 (PKD1). *Hum Mol Genet* 1996;5:539–42.

9 Paterson AD, Magistroni R, He N *et al.* Progressive loss of renal function is an age-dependent heritable trait in type 1 autosomal dominant polycystic kidney disease. *J Am Soc Nephrol* 2005;16:755–62.

10 Guay-Woodford LM. Murine models of polycystic kidney disease: molecular and therapeutic insights. *Am J Physiol Renal Physiol* 2003;285:F1034–49.

11 Torres VE, Wang X, Qian Q *et al.* Effective treatment of an orthologous model of autosomal dominant polycystic kidney disease. *Nat Med* 2004;10:363–4.

12 Ong AC, Wheatley DN. Polycystic kidney disease – the ciliary connection. *Lancet* 2003;361:774–6.

13 Grantham JJ, Torres VE, Chapman AB *et al.* Volume progression in polycystic kidney disease. *N Engl J Med* 2006;354:2122–30.

Acute tubular necrosis – is there any hope of a treatment?

John Firth

□ INTRODUCTION

Acute renal failure, now referred to in enlightened circles as acute kidney injury, is a common clinical problem. Depending on the definition used, it affects about 5% of acute hospital admissions, with the vast majority of cases being due to renal dysfunction caused by something in the spectrum between 'prerenal' renal failure at the milder end and 'acute tubular necrosis' at the other end. Morbidity and mortality are high, particularly if acute tubular necrosis severe enough to require renal replacement treatment to sustain life is associated with other organ failure, yet we have no specific treatment for the condition. What are the best hopes for useful specific treatments in the future?

□ PATHOPHYSIOLOGY OF ACUTE TUBULAR NECROSIS

The development of rational and effective strategies for the treatment of any condition clearly depends on an understanding of pathogenesis, which in the case of acute tubular necrosis undoubtedly is complex (Fig 1).[1,2]

Vascular and endothelial abnormalities

An enormous amount of experimental and clinical evidence indicates that disturbance of renal perfusion is important in the initiation and perpetuation of acute tubular necrosis, as are abnormalities of endothelial function:

- □ Intrarenal vasoconstriction typically is observed, and the renal vessels show enhanced sensitivity to vasoconstrictors such as norepinephrine and endothelin, with blocking of the latter shown to lessen abnormalities in some model systems.
- □ Autoregulation of renal perfusion is impaired, which can be ameliorated by the use of intrarenal calcium channel blockers in some models.
- □ Congestion in the outer medullary region of the kidney is associated with upregulation of adhesion molecules in the area, and blocking of their action can protect against acute ischaemic injury in some models.

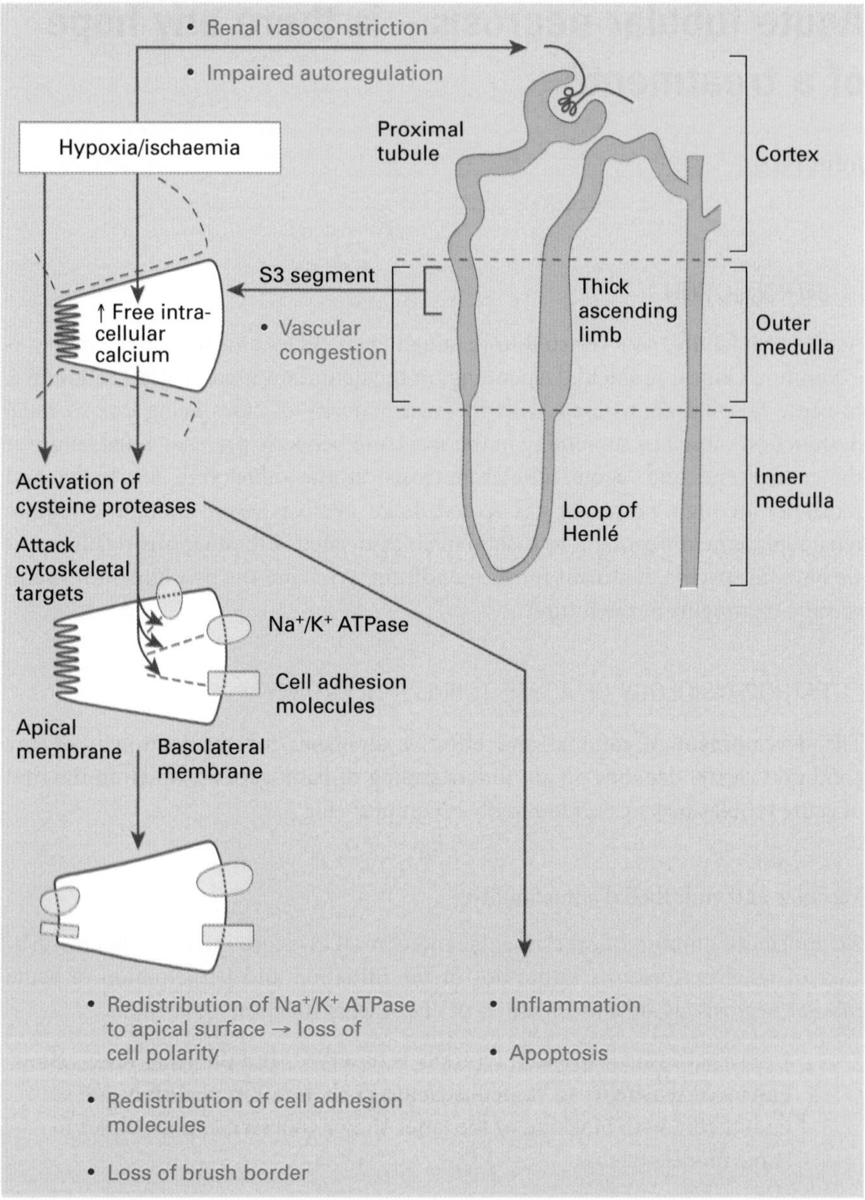

Fig 1 Pathophysiological processes involved in acute tubular necrosis. Note that the relative importance of each of these processes will undoubtedly differ in different patients or different experimental models and will vary within a single patient or experimental model at different times.

- A variety of endothelial functions are impaired, perhaps because of oxidant injury, which results in a tilt of the delicate balance between production of vasodilators and production of vasoconstrictors towards the latter.

Mechanisms of tubular damage

As the term implies, acute tubular necrosis is characterised by necrosis of tubular cells, with those in the S_3 segment of the proximal tubule, which lies in the congested outer medullary region, most typically affected, but the use of the word 'necrosis' is misleading if it is taken to imply that this is the specific mechanism of cell death in all circumstances. It is also worth emphasising that cell necrosis, when it does occur, is the obvious end stage of a process, not the beginning, and therapeutic benefit is most likely to arise from an understanding of early events. Renal biopsies taken from patients with acute tubular necrosis often reveal foci of inflammation, but not much attention has been given to these in the past – 'just one of those things that we see sometimes' being a typical comment at a meeting on biopsy. However, a significant inflammatory element to acute ischaemic renal injury has been recognised recently. Careful analysis is beginning to tease apart a range of changes that occur in response to renal ischaemia and/or reperfusion:

- Increases in intracellular concentrations of calcium, probably in response to hypoxia, have a variety of consequences, including activation of calpain and other cysteine proteases.
- Cysteine proteases attack a number of targets within the cell, which leads to loss of normal polarity, with Na^+/K^+ ATPase and integrins that are usually located only at the basolateral membrane being translocated to the cytoplasm and the apical surface. Among other things, this loss of polarity causes the tubule to be unable to transport sodium in its normal manner.
- Activation of various different cysteine proteases leads to the triggering of pathways that lead to inflammatory processes and cell death by apoptosis.
- Viable cells and those that have died from apoptosis or necrosis are shed into the tubular lumen.

These processes are all subject to complex modulatory influences – for example, in various experimental systems, inhibition of inducible nitric oxide synthase (iNOS) is protective, as can be induction of vascular endothelial nitric oxide synthase (eNOS).

The consequences for tubular function

The various sorts of tubular damage can have several effects on function. At different times and in different models, the following have been observed (Fig 2):

- failure of sodium reabsorption in the proximal tubule, which leads to increased distal delivery and activation of the tubuloglomerular feedback mechanism to cut down glomerular blood flow and filtration rate; this was famously termed 'acute renal success' because failure to repress glomerular filtration if the tubules are unable to reabsorb sodium would lead to loss of all the body's sodium within a matter of hours

- back-leak of filtrate from the tubular lumen into the peritubular interstitium, from where it is reabsorbed into the blood
- tubular blockage by casts, which are more than simply dead leaves stuck in the rainwater pipes, as inhibition of the active process of integrin-mediated adhesion can attenuate their effects in some experiments.

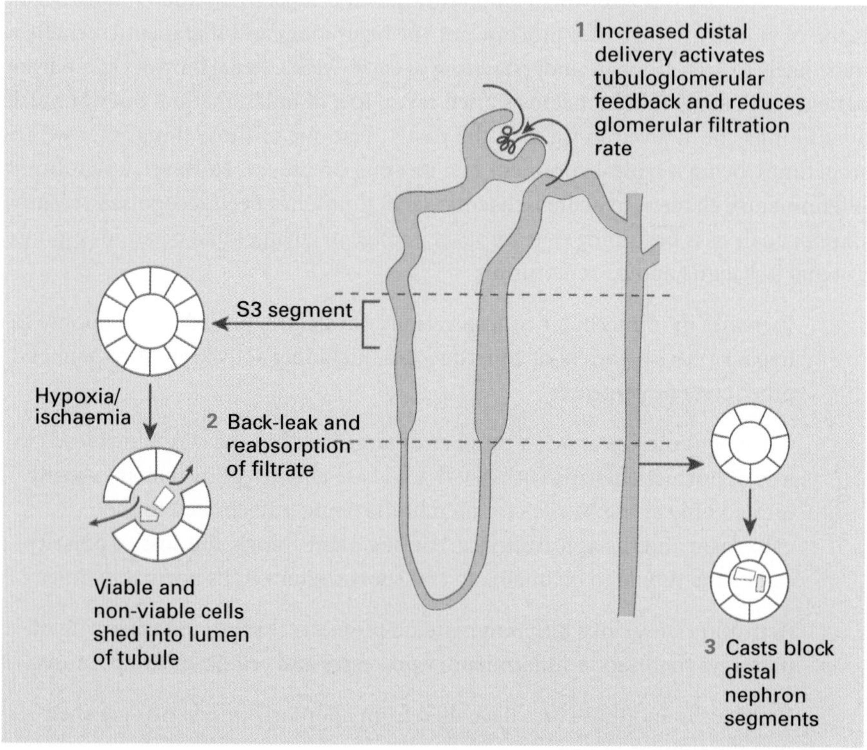

Fig 2 Possible mechanisms of filtration failure in acute tubular necrosis. Note that the relative importance of each of these processes will undoubtedly differ in different patients or different experimental models and will vary within a single patient or experimental model at different times.

□ 'TREATMENTS' THAT DO NOT WORK OR DO SO VERY RARELY

No major recent advances have been made in the clinical approach to patients with acute renal failure. The priorities remain the treatment of life-threatening complications, optimisation of intravascular volume, removal and avoidance of nephrotoxins, exclusion of urinary obstruction and renal inflammatory disease, and – for the very many patients with acute tubular necrosis – vigorous treatment of the precipitating condition followed by timely introduction of renal replacement therapy if required. Beyond this, nothing else is proved to work, with evidence over the past decade swinging firmly against benefit from two drugs previously commonly advocated – diuretics and dopamine.

The use of diuretics, most typically the loop diuretic furosemide, was based mainly on the logic that inhibiting sodium transport would cut tubular oxygen demand – surely a good thing if the tubules were ischaemic – and that encouraging diuresis would 'flush out' casts that were causing tubular obstruction. These effects may be real, but they have limited clinical consequence. A recent meta-analysis of the use of furosemide to prevent or treat acute renal failure considered nine randomised controlled trials that incorporated a total of 849 patients and found that doses of up to about 2 g/day did not have any clinically useful outcome: in particular, renal recovery or patient survival were not altered.[3]

Dopamine in a low or 'renal' dose was advocated on the basis that by acting locally in the kidney it would specifically and beneficially improve renal blood flow at a time when this was reduced. Even if we allow ourselves to forget compelling arguments that this is not a full and proper explanation of the basis of any action that dopamine has on renal function in the context of acute renal failure, the fact remains that good quality studies have now shown that it is not effective in the prevention or treatment of acute renal failure in the clinical contexts in which it used to be recommended.[4]

□ WHAT ARE THE PROSPECTS FOR THE FUTURE?

One treatment will not fit all

The term acute tubular necrosis is used clinically to mean – in a context of circulatory shock, sepsis, or nephrotoxins, or their combination – that the kidney stops working properly in a manner that is not immediately remedied by restoration of a stable and relatively normal circulation, treatment of sepsis, and removal of toxins. The complexity of the renal response to injury that has been described above means it would be naive in the extreme to think that a single pathophysiological mechanism will be crucial in all cases. One might as well describe a condition of 'breathlessness' and look for a single useful treatment. If we accept that acute tubular necrosis may be caused by different mechanisms of injury in different parts of the kidney in different patients, or even within a single patient at different times, it follows that our best hope of developing useful treatments must depend on our ability to find ways of finding out what is going on, or likely to be going on, in the particular kidneys of a particular patient at a particular time.

What is going on in the particular kidneys of a particular patient at a particular time?

It remains a sad fact that we have no better method of determining what is happening to a patient's kidneys in routine clinical practice than bladder catheterisation for hourly monitoring of urinary output. An increasing level of serum creatinine tells us that the kidneys stopped working normally some time ago. We badly need the renal equivalent of the electrocardiogram to give warning of and localise ischaemic damage, but the kidney is less generous with its secrets than the heart and we do not have such a technique. What might help us? Perhaps one or more of knowledge of a patient's genetic predisposition, biomarkers specific to particular pathways of injury, and improved imaging techniques could be helpful.

Genetic predisposition

Sepsis is one of the most common causes of acute tubular necrosis. It is becoming increasingly clear that an individual's response to sepsis depends to some extent on their genetic predisposition.[5] It might be possible in the future, therefore, to say that patient 1 but not patient 2 is particularly vulnerable to process X, Y, or Z but not process A, B, or C in their kidneys, which would be a step along the road to rational treatment.

Biomarkers specific to particular pathways of injury

Literature is vast on a wide variety of urinary and/or serum markers of renal injury, increases of each being reported as an early warning sign that all is not well with the kidney. The current new kid on the block is called, reasonably enough, kidney injury molecule 1 (KIM-1). This is a type 1 membrane protein with extracellular immunoglobulin and mucin domains, which may function as a regulatory molecule for flow-induced calcium signalling and whose expression on proximal tubular cells and shedding into the urine increases rapidly and substantially in response to tubular injury.[6] This and all its predecessors are of limited clinical utility, however, as evidenced by the fact that none have found their way into routine practice. Their presence indicates that damage to the kidney is occurring, but not why, and without knowing why it is not possible to devise potentially useful interventions. How might we do better than this?

Increased knowledge of the various necrotic, apoptotic, and inflammatory processes involved in renal injury undoubtedly will provide useful information as to which genes are likely to be upregulated or downregulated if particular processes are active, and a transcriptomic approach might tell us which genes actually are upregulated or downregulated in a particular patient at a particular time.[7] In simple terms, these techniques allow the levels of all types of messenger RNA within a cell or tissue sample to be measured. They are proving to be enormously powerful in oncological practice, with particular characteristic signatures of gene expression allowing clinically useful subdivision of disease entities previously considered homogeneous for treatment purposes.

Improved imaging techniques

The nephron is a complicated three-dimensional structure, and failure of any part of it for any reason could destroy the function of the whole. In the context of acute renal failure, imaging now is used primarily to exclude urinary obstruction and sometimes to assess perfusion and arterial or venous patency. No routinely available imaging techniques will allow dissection of processes going on in particular areas within the substance of the kidney, yet this is almost certainly what we will need to dissect out the variety of conditions now clustered under the heading of 'acute tubular necrosis'. Is there any prospect of this in the future?

Fig 3 shows a montage of pictures generated by magnetic resonance imaging (MRI) and angiographic techniques: the degree of detail is stunning and would have been impossible to achieve only a few years ago. Notwithstanding recent concerns about the administration of gadolinium to patients with renal impairment, new MRI techniques that use probes specific for ischaemia, inflammation, or other cellular processes may allow analysis of what is happening within regions of the kidney, even to the point where we might be able to say 'in this patient now…X is going on…in region Y' and use this as a basis for a rational attempt at treatment.

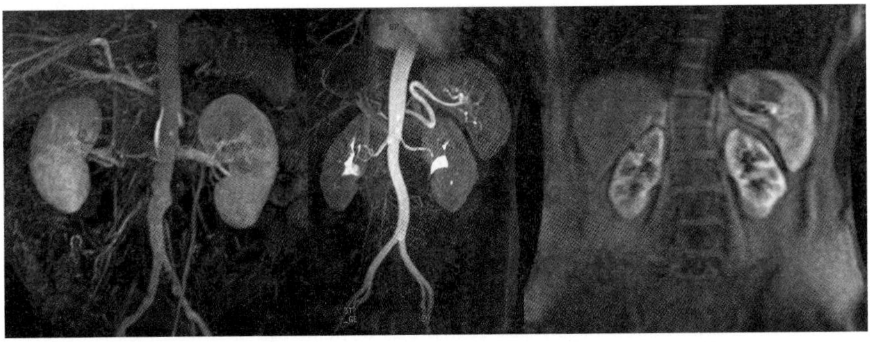

Fig 3 Series of magnetic resonance and angiographic images of the kidneys showing the quality of spatial resolution now obtainable.

Treatments that might work

It is possible to predict anything except the future, but given that, and what we know of pathogenesis, what might work?

Vasoactive substances

There is little doubt that ischaemia drives some aspects of acute tubular necrosis in some instances – in which case, attempts to improve renal perfusion may be helpful. As stated above, dopamine – a drug with a variety of effects – has been tried and tested and found wanting (at least when applied indiscriminately to all patients with the diagnosis of acute tubular necrosis), but this does not mean that all vasoactive substances must be doomed to failure. Fenoldopam – a potent dopamine A-1 receptor agonist – seems worthy of further study; a recent meta-analysis of randomised controlled trials that incorporated 1,290 patients with or at risk of acute kidney injury showed that those who received the drug had reduced risk for acute kidney injury (odds ratio (OR) 0.43 (95% confidence interval 0.32 to 0.59)), reduced need for renal replacement therapy (0.54 (0.34 to 0.84)), and reduced risk of death in hospital (0.64 (0.45 to 0.91)).[8]

Growth factors and stem cells

Recovery from acute tubular necrosis depends on regeneration of cells, and a wealth of evidence from animal experiments shows that a variety of growth factors can speed up this process and lead to more rapid recovery of renal function. One regimen of recombinant human insulin-like growth factor-I was found to be ineffective in the circumstances of one multicentre clinical trial, and use of some other growth factors in patients has been restrained by safety concerns. These do not mean that the principle is flawed, however, and the impressive results obtained in animal studies mean that further attempts to treat acute tubular necrosis with growth factors will be made. A surprise to many in the renal world will be the possibility that a drug that nephrologists know well – erythropoietin – may be useful in preventing apoptosis within and supporting regeneration of the kidney, as well as of red blood cells: given six hours after insult in an ischaemic injury model, it can significantly reduce tissue injury and subsequent renal dysfunction.[9]

Growth factors have already delivered enormous clinical benefits, few more dramatic than that produced by erythropoietin for the treatment of renal anaemia. From my time as a trainee nephrologist just more than 20 years ago, I can remember several patients, each younger than I was at the time, who died of an intractable combination of anaemia and iron overload from multiple transfusions. We now debate whether the target haemoglobin should be 11 g/dl or 12.5 g/dl.

The possibility of introducing a cell that would have the capacity to reconstitute damage into a damaged organ has enormous appeal, but a note of caution with regard to stem cells seems appropriate. They have not yet really delivered in any major sphere of medicine, and the view that simply injecting them into an acutely damaged kidney will be useful is not realistic.[10]

REFERENCES

1. Schrier RW, Wang W, Poole B, Mitra A. Acute renal failure: definitions, diagnosis, pathogenesis, and therapy. *J Clin Invest* 2004;114:5–14.
2. Goligorsky MS. Whispers and shouts in the pathogenesis of acute renal ischaemia. *Nephrol Dial Transplant* 2005;20:261–6.
3. Ho KM, Sheridan DJ. Meta-analysis of frusemide to prevent or treat acute renal failure. *BMJ* 2006;333:420–5.
4. Kellum JA, Decker JM. Use of dopamine in acute renal failure: a meta-analysis. *Crit Care Med* 2001;29:1526–31.
5. Jaber BL, Pereira BJ, Bonventre JV, Balakrishnan VS. Polymorphism of host response genes: implications in the pathogenesis and treatment of acute renal failure. *Kidney Int* 2005;67:14–33.
6. Han WK, Bailly V, Abichandani R, Thadhani R, Bonventre JV. Kidney injury molecule-1 (KIM-1): a novel biomarker for human renal proximal tubule injury. *Kidney Int* 2002;62: 237–44.
7. Yuen PS, Jo SK, Holly MK, Hu X, Star RA. Ischemic and nephrotoxic acute renal failure are distinguished by their broad transcriptomic responses. *Physiol Genomics* 2006:25;375–86.
8. Landoni G, Biondi-Zoccai GG, Tumlin JA *et al.* Beneficial effect of fenoldopam in critically ill patients with or at risk of acute renal failure: a meta-analysis of randomized clinical trials. *Am J Kidney Dis* 2007;49:56–68.
9. Johnson DW, Pat B, Vesey DA *et al.* Delayed administration of darbepoetin or erythropoietin protects against ischemic acute renal injury and failure. *Kidney Int* 2006;69:1806–13.
10. Duffield JS, Park KM, Hsiao LL *et al.* Restoration of tubular epithelial cells during repair of the postischemic kidney occurs independently of bone marrow-derived stem cells. *J Clin Invest* 2005;115:1743–55.

☐ RENAL DISEASE SELF-ASSESSMENT QUESTIONS

Treatment of antineutrophil cytoplasm antibody-associated systemic vasculitis

1 Systemic vasculitis:
- (a) Can accompany infection
- (b) Can be associated with malignancy
- (c) Can be associated with the use of non-steroidal anti-inflammatory drugs (NSAIDs) such as ibuprofen
- (d) Is always associated with the presence of circulating anti-neutrophil cytoplasmic antibodies (cANCAs)
- (e) Only affects arteries and not veins

2 Microscopic polyangiitis:
- (a) Is characterised by the presence of a pauci-immune vasculitis in the kidneys
- (b) Is often associated with constitutional symptoms
- (c) Can be associated with pulmonary haemorrhage
- (d) Can present as mononeuritis multiplex
- (e) Is often associated with the presence of perinuclear anti-neutrophil cytoplasmic antibodies (pANCAs)

3 Systemic Wegener's granulomatosis:
- (a) Is characterised by the presence of granuloma and small-vessel vasculitis
- (b) Is often associated with constitutional symptoms
- (c) Can be associated with pulmonary haemorrhage
- (d) Can present as mononeuritis multiplex
- (e) Is often associated with the presence of cANCAs

4 Churg–Strauss syndrome:
- (a) Is characterised by the presence of granuloma and small-vessel vasculitis
- (b) Is associated with eosinophilia
- (c) Is associated with constitutional symptoms
- (d) Can present with gastrointestinal symptoms
- (e) Is often associated with the presence of pANCAs

5 Classic polyarteritis nodosa:
- (a) Is a small-vessel vasculitis
- (b) Is associated with the presence of glomerulonephritis
- (c) Is rarely associated with hypertension
- (d) Is associated with the presence of microaneurysms
- (e) Is often associated with the presence of ANCAs

Polycystic kidney disease – then and now

1 Autosomal dominant polycystic kidney disease (ADPKD):
  (a) Is the second most common cause of end-stage renal disease (ESRD) in the United Kingdom (UK)
  (b) Has an incidence of one in 1,000 births
  (c) Typically leads to ESRD by the fifth decade
  (d) Is more severe in women with mutations in *PKD2* than men with mutations in *PKD2*
  (e) Due to mutations in *PKD1* is associated with larger kidney volumes than that due to mutations in *PKD2*

2 Regarding the genetics of ADPKD:
  (a) Mutations in three genes have been implicated
  (b) There is a clear mutation hot spot in *PKD1* but not in *PKD2*
  (c) The age of onset of ESRD is closer in monozygotic twins than in dizygotic twins
  (d) 25% of patients with ADPKD have a family history of subarachnoid haemorrhage
  (e) Mutations are detected in >80% of unselected patients with ADPKD

3 Extrarenal manifestations of ADPKD include the following:
  (a) Polycystic ovaries
  (b) Inguinal hernia
  (c) Uterine prolapse
  (d) Mitral valve prolapse
  (e) Diverticular disease

Acute tubular necrosis – is there any hope of a treatment?

1 The following part of the tubule is the main site of damage in patients with acute tubular necrosis:
  (a) Bowman's capsule
  (b) S3 part of proximal convoluted tubule
  (c) Loop of Henle
  (d) Medullary thick ascending limb
  (e) Distal convoluted tubule

2 The following statements are true:
  (a) In a normal kidney, Na/K ATPase is localised at the apical tubular membrane
  (b) In a normal kidney, integrins are located at the apical tubular membrane
  (c) Renal ischaemia provokes necrosis but not apoptosis of tubular cells
  (d) Increased intracellular levels of calcium are an early step in the processes that lead to acute tubular necrosis
  (e) Activation of calpain is an early step in the processes that lead to acute tubular necrosis

3 The following are thought to play a significant role in the reduction of glomerular filtration rate caused by acute tubular necrosis:
(a) Increase in glomerular ultrafiltration coefficient
(b) Back-leak of filtrate through damaged tubules into the renal interstitium
(c) Activation of tubuloglomerular feedback by increased distal delivery of solute
(d) Tubular blockage by casts
(e) Oedema of the renal papilla

Rheumatology

New biologics for rheumatoid arthritis

Kimme L Hyrich

□ INTRODUCTION

Rheumatoid arthritis (RA) is a disease characterised by chronic inflammation and destruction of the synovial joints that leads to marked disability. With an estimated prevalence of 1% in adults, the potential social and economic impact of this disease is tremendous. The condition is also associated with a reduction in life expectancy, with standardised mortality ratios approximately twice those of the general population. Leading causes of death include cardiovascular disease, malignancy, and infection.

□ TRADITIONAL TREATMENT

The goals of treatment for RA are to control pain and other symptoms, slow down or arrest the destruction of cartilage and bone, minimise physical disability, and maximise quality of life. The focus of modern treatment has been disease-modifying antirheumatic drugs (DMARDs), which are used to control disease activity and slow the progression of joint destruction. The gold standard is methotrexate. Others include sulphasalazine, gold, and leflunomide. The success of each has been variable, and, to date, no single drug has had the ability to consistently and completely stop the underlying inflammatory process. These drugs have also been associated with an array of associated toxicities. Some side-effects, such as rash or nausea, are benign and disappear after the drug has been discontinued. The potential for life-threatening infections, or even malignancies, however, exists for many of these drugs. This has prompted the continued search for safer and more effective treatments for RA.

□ NEW BIOLOGIC THERAPIES

The treatment of RA has recently undergone a transformation. The paradigm of new treatments has shifted from general immunosuppressive agents towards treatments targeted at key components of the immune response. The underlying cause of RA remains unknown, although the disease is accepted to result from an inappropriate activation of immune cells, an accumulation of CD4+ T cells in the rheumatoid synovium, and the secretion of proinflammatory cytokines, including tumour necrosis factor (TNF), interleukin (IL)-1, and IL-6. The net result is activation of osteoclasts, fibroblasts, and chondroctyes and the secretion of matrix metalloproteinases and other effector molecules, which results in the destruction of cartilage and bone.[1]

Anti-TNF agents

Tumour necrosis factor is a soluble, 17 kD protein composed of three identical subunits. Its functions are mediated through cell surface receptors (designated type I (p55) and type II (p75)) that are expressed on numerous cell types. Some of these receptors are cleaved from the cell surface and are known as soluble TNF receptors. High levels of TNF have been demonstrated in the synovial fluid of patients with RA and are present in early and established disease. In addition, blockade of TNF results in downregulation of other proinflammatory cytokines, including IL-1 and IL-6, which makes it an attractive target for directed therapies.[2]

Three anti-TNF agents are currently available and licensed for use in patients with RA. Etanercept is a soluble p75 TNF receptor fusion protein that contains a genetic fusion of a recombinant soluble p75 TNF receptor and the F_c portion of human immunoglobulin G (IgG). It is self-administered by weekly or twice-weekly injections. Infliximab is a monoclonal chimeric (75% human–25% murine (mouse)) antibody. The antibody consists of a human IgG1 F_c region combined with a murine variable (antigen-binding) region, which is specific for TNF. After an initial loading phase, it is administered every eight weeks by intravenous infusion. Concern about the development of human antichimeric antibodies (HACA) means that the drug should be coprescribed with methotrexate. Adalimumab is a humanised monoclonal anti-TNF antibody that is administered subcutaneously on a fortnightly basis.

The efficacy of these agents has been studied in more than 6000 patients in randomised controlled trials (RCTs) that have included patients with established, usually methotrexate-resistant, RA, as well as in those with early disease (defined as disease duration shorter than three years).[3] Although head-to-head trials have not been undertaken with these drugs, their efficacy seems to be roughly equivalent, with about 60% of patients showing at least a 20% improvement in disease activity as defined by the American College of Rheumatology response score – a composite measure of seven core outcomes in RA. Fewer than 40% of patients, however, achieved the more substantial response of a 70% improvement. All drugs slow radiological progression of the disease, and they may prevent new erosions in early disease in a greater proportion of patients than methotrexate in methotrexate-naive patients. In the UK, the drugs are currently approved for patients with established RA who have persistent disease activity despite treatment with at least two DMARDs, one of which should be methotrexate.[4]

Reassuringly, no increase in serious adverse events compared with placebo was observed during early RCTs. Small increases were reported in the risk of infusion reactions with infliximab and the risk of injection site reactions with etanercept and adalimumab, although neither was a common reason to discontinue treatment. With more widespread use of these drugs, however, spontaneous pharmacovigilance has highlighted certain potential safety concerns, including serious infections, tuberculosis, malignancy, and heart failure.

Despite the detrimental effects of TNF in patients with RA, it plays a key role in the body's defence against infective pathogens. Although infections were not increased during RCTs, postmarketing reports of several serious infections have continued research in this area. Recent data from the British Society for Rheumatology's large biologics register, however, have shown that the drugs do not seem to increase the overall risk of infection compared with traditional DMARD therapy,[5] which, in part, may be related to the already increased risk of infection in patients with RA. There may be, however, an increase in susceptibility to certain types of infection, including skin and soft tissue infections and those due to intracellular pathogens, including *Salmonella* and *Listeria* species. Current guidelines state that the drug should be stopped temporarily in the presence of infection and avoided in those at high risk of infection. Patients are also advised to avoid high-risk foods, such as raw eggs, unpasteurised dairy products, and paté.

Postmarketing surveillance has also heightened the awareness of an association between the use of anti-TNF drugs and the development of tuberculosis.[6] Tumour necrosis factor is known to play a key role in the formation and maintenance of granulomas after mycobacterial infection, and blockade of this cytokine may result in reactivation of the infection. The British Thoracic Society has published screening guidelines for patients about to start anti-TNF drugs. These guidelines stress that tuberculin testing may be unreliable in patients already receiving immunosuppressant treatment and highlight the importance of pretreatment chest X-rays and adequate history of exposure.[7]

The relation between anti-TNF drugs and the development of certain malignancies, particularly lymphoma, remains controversial. A recent meta-analysis of RCTs of infliximab and adalimumab (not etanercept) suggested a threefold increase in the rate of all malignancies in patients who received active treatments compared with placebo-treated patients.[8] This risk seemed to be concentrated in patients who received high doses of anti-TNF drugs (equivalent to ≥6 mg/kg every eight weeks), which is higher than the recommended dose of 3 mg/kg for the management of RA. The rate of malignancy was also lower than expected in the placebo arm, which may have falsely elevated the risk in the treated arms. In addition, all patients with severe RA are well recognised to already have an increased risk of non-Hodgkin's lymphoma, which correlates with cumulative disease activity. The patients most likely to receive anti-TNF treatment therefore may already be at increased risk. Further follow up of treated patients is needed to address this issue further.

Clinical trials of etanercept and infliximab in patients with severe (New York Heart Association Class 3 or 4) heart failure did not show any benefit in the case of etanercept and, in fact, showed an increased risk of death or hospitalisation in the patients who received the highest doses of infliximab.[9] The drugs therefore are contraindicated in patients with a history of severe congestive heart failure and should be used with caution in patients with mild CHF. The effects of these agents on other cardiac conditions, primarily ischaemic heart disease, are unknown but of intense interest given the high frequency of atherosclerotic heart disease in patients with RA.

Other potential reported toxicities include reports of demyelinating disease, aplastic anaemia, interstitial lung disease, and the induction of a lupus-like syndrome. Small numbers of reports, however, prevent more robust estimates of risk. In the United Kingdom (UK) and other European countries, national registers of patients receiving anti-TNF drugs have been established in order to study these potential longer term risks.

B-cell depleting treatments

There remains keen interest in the importance of the B cell in the pathogenesis of RA. In addition to stimulating production of autoantibodies, including rheumatoid factor and anti-cyclic citrullinated peptide (CCP) antibodies, this cell also may be involved in antigen presentation, T-cell activation, and the secretion of proinflammatory cytokines. The most striking evidence for its role in the pathogenesis of RA has been the success of B-cell-depleting treatments in controlling the symptoms of RA.[10]

Rituximab is a chimeric anti-CD20 monoclonal antibody that has been used most widely in patients with non-Hodgkin's lymphoma. CD20 is expressed on B cells from the pre-B-cell stage to the pre-plasma-cell stage. Treatment with rituximab results in depletion of circulating B cells, primarily through antibody-dependent cell-mediated cytotoxicity. Clinical trials of this drug have been undertaken in patients with methotrexate-resistant RA, as well as anti-TNF-resistant RA. The drug shows similar efficacy to the anti-TNF drugs, with a 20% improvement in signs and symptoms of RA according to the American College of Rheumatology criteria (ACR20) in 55–70% of patients who had failed methotrexate and 50% of anti-TNF treatment failures. The drug is currently licensed in the UK, in combination with methotrexate, for anti-TNF-resistant RA.

The recommended dose is two 1,000 mg infusions administered two weeks apart. The drug is administered with 100 mg intravenous methylprednisolone. Patients should also receive weekly methotrexate cotherapy to increase efficacy. After an initial course of therapy, B cells are depleted for a variable length of time, typically 5–14 months. The return of synovitis does not always correlate with the return of B cells, with many patients remaining symptom free for a much longer period. The timing of retreatment is not yet clear. Other than infusion reactions, particularly with the first dose, there have been no reports of an increase in serious adverse events during clinical trials in patients with RA. Serum levels of immunoglobulin and levels of antitetanus toxoid and antipneumococcal polysaccharide antibodies are not affected significantly. Interestingly, significant decreases in serum levels of rheumatoid factor, which subsequently increase again with the return of more severe clinical disease, are reported in patients who respond to the drug.

On the horizon

Newer agents awaiting licences or final-phase clinical trials include a fully humanised anti-CD20 monoclonal antibody (ocrelizumab), the cytotoxic T lymphocyte-associated antigen abatacept, and an inhibitor of IL-6 (tocilizumab). Abatacept modulates the CD80/86 and CD28 costimulatory signal required for full T-cell activation. It is administered by monthly intravenous infusion and, as for rituximab, has been studied in patients who have failed methotrexate and in those who have failed anti-TNF. Efficacy is again similar to the anti-TNF drugs. Clinical trials have not shown any increased risk of serious adverse events when the drug is used alone or in combination with methotrexate. When the drug was combined with etanercept, however, an increase in serious adverse events was observed,[11] and, as such, these biologic agents, at least at this point in time, should not be combined. Early studies suggest that tocilizumab, a humanised anti–interleukin-6 (IL-6) receptor antibody, has promise as a new agent for the management of methotrexate-resistant RA. Again, 61–74% of patients achieve ACR20. However, suggestions of moderate but reversible increases in transaminases and bilirubin, as well as increases in total cholesterol, high-density lipoprotein cholesterol, and triglycerides, among patients who receive active treatment warrant further investigation.[12] As for the anti-TNF agents, intense post-marketing surveillance will be needed for all of these agents once licences are granted.

□ CONCLUSIONS

The introduction of directed biologic treatments has offered hope for patients with chronic DMARD-resistant RA. Studies in patients with early disease suggest they are at least as effective as standard treatments and may confer an additional benefit in terms of radiological progression. The agents have not proved to be an immunologic panacea, however, with only a minority of patients achieving complete remission and about 30% of patients not showing any significant response at all, thus driving the continued search for more effective treatments. New agents are arriving at a fast pace and continue to teach us more about the underlying pathophysiology of this condition. The long-term safety of all of these new treatments remains unclear, however, and further research clearly is warranted.

REFERENCES

1 Choy EH, Panayi GS. Cytokine pathways and joint inflammation in rheumatoid arthritis. *N Engl J Med* 2001;344:907–16.
2 Feldmann M, Maini RN. Discovery of TNF-alpha as a therapeutic target in rheumatoid arthritis: preclinical and clinical studies. *Joint Bone Spine* 2002;69:12–8.
3 Scott DL, Kingsley GH. Tumor necrosis factor inhibitors for rheumatoid arthritis. *N Engl J Med* 2006;355:704–12.
4 Ledingham J, Deighton C. Update on the British Society for Rheumatology guidelines for prescribing TNF-alpha blockers in adults with rheumatoid arthritis (update of previous guidelines of April 2001). *Rheumatology (Oxford)* 2005;44:157–63.
5 Dixon WG, Watson K, Lunt M *et al.* Rates of serious infection, including site-specific and bacterial intracellular infection, in rheumatoid arthritis patients receiving anti-tumor necrosis factor therapy: results from the British Society for Rheumatology Biologics Register. *Arthritis Rheum* 2006;54:2368–76.
6 Askling J, Fored CM, Brandt L *et al.* Risk and case characteristics of tuberculosis in rheumatoid arthritis associated with tumor necrosis factor antagonists in Sweden. *Arthritis Rheum* 2005;52:1986–92.
7 British Thoracic Society Standards of Care Committee. BTS recommendations for assessing risk and for managing *Mycobacterium tuberculosis* infection and disease in patients due to start anti-TNF-alpha treatment. *Thorax* 2005;60:800–5.
8 Bongartz T, Sutton AJ, Sweeting MJ *et al.* Anti-TNF antibody therapy in rheumatoid arthritis and the risk of serious infections and malignancies: systematic review and meta-analysis of rare harmful effects in randomized controlled trials. *JAMA* 2006;295:2275–85.
9 Sarzi-Puttini P, Atzeni F, Shoenfeld Y, Ferraccioli G. TNF-alpha, rheumatoid arthritis, and heart failure: a rheumatological dilemma. *Autoimmun Rev* 2005;4:153–61.
10 Dass S, Vital EM, Emery P. Rituximab: novel B-cell depletion therapy for the treatment of rheumatoid arthritis. *Expert Opin Pharmacother* 2006;7:2559–70.

11 Nogid A, Pham DQ. Role of abatacept in the management of rheumatoid arthritis. *Clin Ther* 2006;28:1764–78.

12 Maini RN, Taylor PC, Szechinski J *et al.* Double-blind randomized controlled clinical trial of the interleukin-6 receptor antagonist, tocilizumab, in European patients with rheumatoid arthritis who had an incomplete response to methotrexate. *Arthritis Rheum* 2006;54:2817–29.

Systemic lupus erythematosus: a problem with B cells

Jonathan CW Edwards and Maria J Leandro

☐ SUMMARY

For several decades, there has been a consensus that systemic lupus erythematosus ('lupus') results from of a failure of B-cell regulation, with tissue damage mediated by a variety of autoantibodies through both type III and type II hypersensitivity pathways. A disturbance of signals involved in clearance of nuclear material, particularly in complement pathways, was long suspected. In the past few years, specific hypotheses that go a considerable way towards explaining how B-cell regulation may become disturbed have emerged. The recent introduction of B-cell depletion therapy for patients with autoimmune disease has provided a way of probing such hypotheses, and this approach promises to be of major benefit to patients.

☐ HISTORICAL PERSPECTIVE

Since at least the 1960s, the clinicopathological manifestations of systemic lupus have been attributed to the effects of multiple populations of autoantibodies. Many features – such as arthritis, rash, proteinuria and neutropenia – mimic the syndrome of 'serum sickness', which is known to be mediated by circulating antigen-antibody complexes and thus falls within the definition of type III hypersensitivity. Other features – such as haemolytic anaemia, neonatal heart block in children of women positive for anti-Ro antibodies (Sjögren's syndrome antigen (SSA)) and anti-phospholipid syndrome – are consistent with direct effects of antibodies on cells or biochemical pathways and thus fall, at least partly, within the definition of type II hypersensitivity.

Histopathological studies of lupus emphasised, from the earliest times, the presence of necrosis, with the concept of fibrinoid necrosis of collagen underlying the old term 'collagen vascular disease'. An important distinction between the necrosis found in lesions in patients with lupus and those in other situations is that 'fibrinoid' necrosis, although typically eosinophilic (like fibrin), is often basophilic in patients with lupus, indicating release of DNA into the tissue matrix. Nuclear material is also seen as haematoxyphil bodies and the lupus erythematosus (LE) cell phenomenon. Recent discussion has latched on to apoptosis, but it is probably best simply to note that nuclear material from dead cells gets into places it normally does not. This, with the presence of antinuclear antibodies, led early on to the idea that dysregulation of nuclear clearance might be important in lupus.

The association of lupus with both primary genetic and secondary consumptive defects in complement raised the possibility that abnormal nuclear clearance might involve complement dysfunction. Complement is also of interest because it is crucial to the selection process that normally allows expansion of antimicrobial B cells and removal of autoreactive B cells.[1] Complement dysfunction might be expected to weaken immune responses to pathogens and facilitate the formation of autoantibodies on a broad front. Complement also protects against infection, so there have been, since the 1970s, several reasons for seeing lupus as a disease of complement malfunction.

The historical picture of lupus was probably not far off the mark, but two uncertainties stood out. Firstly, the precise mechanisms by which immune complexes caused tissue injury were unclear. Secondly, the way, or ways, in which complement deficiencies or other factors might dysregulate antibody production so as to allow the production of many autoantibodies, often against nuclear material, needed to be understood.

☐ BETTER UNDERSTANDING OF EFFECTOR MECHANISMS

The detailed mechanisms of immune complex-mediated injury are still incompletely understood, but one major clarification has occurred, based partly on basic studies in mice and partly on clinical studies in man.[2] It is now appreciated that complexes can cause disease through two quite different processes. Until recently, most people have had a picture of immune complexes causing disease by deposition, usually in relation to an endothelial or epithelial (or interposed) basement membrane. This occurs in the glomerulus and at the dermoepidermal junction in patients with lupus (the 'lupus band'). Choroidal deposition may explain raised intracranial pressure in patients with acute cerebral lupus. It is less clear, however, how it would explain arthritis or serositis.

As far back as 1983,[3] immune complexes were known to be able to stimulate cytokine production by macrophages through immunoglobulin Fc receptors. These receptors were subsequently shown to be central to immune complex-mediated disease in mice, and in the mid 1990s, with renewed interest in immune complexes in rheumatoid disease, it became clear that activation of macrophages by immune complexes through Fc receptors might be an important stimulus for the production of tumour necrosis factor (TNF) in patients with autoimmune rheumatic disease. The Fc receptor FcγRIIIa was specifically implicated, as it is selectively expressed in the limited group of tissues affected by macrophage activation in rheumatoid arthritis and, in most cases also in lupus: synovium, serosae, bone marrow, alveoli, lymph node and spleen, salivary glands, hepatic sinusoids (Kuppfer cells), ocular sclera and restricted sites in the dermis that correspond to the sites of rheumatoid nodules.[2]

These findings suggest that the serum sickness syndrome involves two mechanisms. The dominant mechanism is activation of macrophages (and perhaps mast cells) by small complexes that can access tissue partly because of their molecular radius and partly because they are too small to be cleared by complement. The second mechanism, which may come into play only if complement is overloaded or malfunctioning, is deposition of large complexes that accumulate in filtering structures if they are not cleared by complement. The first mechanism, which is the only one expected in rheumatoid disease, involves cytokine release, which explains the increases in C-reactive protein. The second, which is more specifically associated with lupus, may or may not engage the production of cytokines, and thus primarily causes problems through abnormal vascular permeability.

□ AUTOANTIBODY PRODUCTION AS A CHAIN REACTION

A further development in understanding of the role of autoantibodies, which triggered the use of B-cell depletion therapy in patients with rheumatoid arthritis and those with lupus, was the suggestion that autoantibody production might be self-driving.[4] In a normal immune response, the presence of antibody fuels the production of more antibody, and the process subsides when antigen is consumed. Although this has advantages, it has the weakness that, in autoimmunity, autoantibody production may become unstoppable once allowed to start.

Antibody facilitates further antibody production through two mechanisms. Firstly, antibody on the surface of antigen-presenting cells facilitates endocytosis of antigen and its presentation to T cells capable of providing help to B cells recognising the same antigen. In the case of the B cell, surface antibody mediates presentation and acquisition of help via a single cooperative relationship. This mechanism should fail for autoantigens because no relevant T cells should be available. Secondly, if antibody attaches to antigen to form a complex that can acquire complement C3d, the complexed antigen can give a survival signal back to the B cell. Uncomplexed antigen, in contrast, may give a negative signal, and this may be a major mechanism for ensuring that autoreactive B cells do not normally survive long enough to make antibody.

In the late 1990s, it was proposed that both of these feedback mechanisms, which should not be available for B cells making autoantibodies, might be engaged inappropriately by autoantibodies to certain specific antigens, including anti-IgG F_c (rheumatoid factors) and the lupus autoantibodies anticomplement C1q and anti-DNA.[4] There are possible explanations for the production of antiacetylcholine receptor antibodies and the antilectin antibodies of Crohn's disease and sarcoidosis.[4] It was suggested that for these particular autoantigens autoreactive B cells could potentially become self-perpetuating by subverting normal control mechanisms. This gave rise to the idea that depletion of B cells might remove these clones and thus allow the immune system to return to normality.

The mechanism by which anti-C1q antibodies might drive their own production is based on the well-established observation that anti-C1q antibodies can activate complement (generating C3d) under conditions that do not apply to other antigens. Possible mechanisms by which anti-DNA antibodies might subvert regulation became apparent through a variety of new findings. It had been appreciated that anti-DNA B cells might endocytose a combination of DNA and nucleic acid binding proteins such as ribonucleoproteins, histones, etc – the extractable nuclear antigens. Nucleoprotein peptides might then be presented to T cells, which at least might be expected to recognise microbial nucleoproteins. More recent data suggest that T-cell responses to self-nucleoproteins might occur, perhaps because of cross reactivity with conserved sequences. A further potential mechanism then became available when it was recognised that DNA binds directly to toll-like receptor (TLR)-9, which is present on B cells.[5] This allows immune complexes containing DNA to give an extra survival signal to anti-DNA B cells. DNA can also bind C1q directly, making the situation apparently even more precarious. Most recently, it was found that nucleoproteins can also engage TLR-7.[6]

Much more needs to be understood about the ways in which autoreactive B cells recognising these disease-associated autoantigens may subvert the normal regulatory rules. However, the central concept, in providing the incentive for B-cell depletion therapy, has already provided a powerful new tool for studying exactly these mechanisms in human disease.

☐ OTHER ROLES FOR B CELLS?

Despite the wealth of evidence for antibody-mediated effector mechanisms in lupus, there has been an odd tendency since the mid 1990s to suggest that the idea that B cells might be involved in diseases such as lupus is somehow novel. Moreover, the suggestion is made that B cells are important not because they produce antibody but because they present antigen to T cells and secrete cytokines. Antigen presentation by B cells, or even the secretion of soluble factors, is hardly novel. MHC class II was first identified as a 'B-cell marker' before being discovered on other cells. Antigen presentation and cytokine production by B cells is integral to, rather than distinct from, antibody production. The situation is further confused by the fact that evidence for B cells having a pathogenic effect independent of antibody comes largely from mice with a Fas defect that overrides the normal antibody-dependent selection process described above.

In simple terms, it seems illogical to suggest that removing B cells has an effect by preventing presentation of antigen to T cells and thereby preventing the provision of help to B cells that by definition are no longer there! Moreover, as indicated below, the experimental evidence indicates that the benefits of B-cell depletion relate to absence of autoantibody rather than absence of B cells.

☐ B-CELL DEPLETION THERAPY

B-cell depletion therapy was made possible by the development of the anti-CD20 monoclonal antibody rituximab for the treatment of B-cell lymphoma. Rituximab is used successfully as monotherapy in several autoimmune diseases, but B-cell depletion is unreliable with rituximab monotherapy in patients with lupus, so it is chiefly used together with cyclophosphamide. Even so, depletion in lupus is relatively brief: typically 4–6 months.

Although benefits from B-cell depletion have been described in more than 20 autoantibody-associated conditions, proof of concept rests on controlled trials in rheumatoid arthritis.[7] Open studies in lupus were started in Germany by Tony and extended by Leandro, Looney, Eisenberg and van Vollenhoven.[8–10] The consensus is that it is difficult to attribute to chance the degree of improvement achieved in most patients with doses that achieve greater than 95% depletion of circulating B cells. Resolution of haematological and renal manifestations for periods of four or more years after a cycle of treatment has been seen. Van Vollenoven's group has shown histological resolution of renal disease. The pharmacodynamics seem broadly similar to those in rheumatoid arthritis.

The original rationale for B-cell depletion did not require selectivity for disease-associated cells. The justification, as in lymphoma, was that as long as disease-associated cells were cleared, and did not reappear, removal of all normal cells for a period, with recovery from stem cells, was acceptable. Use of rituximab in lymphoma confirmed that this approach was clinically viable, with little decrease in levels of circulating immunoglobulin. It is now clear, however, that current protocols rarely, if ever, clear disease-associated B cells permanently in patients with autoimmune disease. The strategy remains useful because of the serendipitous finding that autoantibody levels tend to decrease more significantly after rituximab than protective antibody levels. In patients with lupus, this selective decrease is consistently found for anti-DNA and antinucleosome antibodies but not for antibodies to extractable nuclear antigens such as Ro and ribonucleoprotein. This may have some clinical implications, but these are not yet well defined.

Pharmacodynamic studies of B-cell depletion are most easily interpreted in rheumatoid arthritis because disease can be monitored by C-reactive protein. Inflammation subsides not immediately with B-cell depletion but with the decrease in autoantibody and returns when autoantibody returns. (No major or consistent benefit has been seen from B-cell depletion in autoantibody-negative conditions.) The situation in lupus is more difficult to analyse because even a quasilinear index of disease is not available. Nevertheless, improvement broadly follows the decline in autoantibodies and relapse is correlated with return of autoantibodies rather than just B cells;[11] this really is to be expected, as there is little or no evidence of effector mechanisms in the tissue pathology of (human) lupus other than through antibody.

□ CONCLUSION

In summary, the historical view of lupus as a complex disease mediated by autoantibody remains valid. The nature of the inflammatory effector mechanisms has been clarified and the way in which aberrant signalling involving systems such as complement and toll-like receptors may drive the immunopathology is beginning to become clear. The results of B-cell depletion therapy are consistent with the established model, and further use of this treatment may shed light on details of pathogenesis, which may in turn lead to further refinement of treatment strategies.

REFERENCES

1 Fearon DT, Carter RH. The CD19/CR2/TAPA-1 complex of B lymphocytes: linking natural to acquired immunity. *Annu Rev Immunol* 1995;13:127–49.

2 Edwards JC, Cambridge G. B-cell targeting in rheumatoid arthritis and other autoimmune diseases. *Nat Rev Immunol* 2006;6:394–403.

3 Nardella FA, Dayer JM, Roelke M, Krane SM, Mannik M. Self-associating IgG rheumatoid factors stimulate monocytes to release prostaglandins and mononuclear cell factor that stimulates collagenase and prostaglandin production by synovial cells. *Rheumatol Int* 1983;3:183–6.

4 Edwards JC, Cambridge G, Abrahams VM. Do self-perpetuating B lymphocytes drive human autoimmune disease? *Immunology* 1999;97:1868–76.

5 Boule MW, Broughton C, Mackay F *et al.* Toll-like receptor 9-dependent and -independent dendritic cell activation by chromatin-immunoglobulin G complexes. *J Exp Med* 2004;199:1631–40.

6 Lau CM, Broughton C, Tabor AS *et al.* RNA-associated autoantigens activate B cells by combined B cell antigen receptor/toll-like receptor 7 engagement. *J Exp Med* 2005;202:1171–7.

7 Edwards JC, Szczepanski L, Szechinski J *et al.* Efficacy of B-cell-targeted therapy with rituximab in patients with rheumatoid arthritis. *N Engl J Med* 2004;350:2572–81.

8 Leandro MJ, Edwards JC, Cambridge G, Ehrenstein MR, Isenberg DA. An open study of B lymphocyte depletion in systemic lupus erythematosus. *Arthritis Rheum* 2002;46:2673–7.

9 Anolik JH, Campbell D, Felgar RE *et al.* The relationship of FcgammaRIIIa genotype to degree of B cell depletion by rituximab in the treatment of systemic lupus erythematosus. *Arthritis Rheum* 2003;48:455–9.

10 van Vollenhoven RF, Gunnarsson I, Welin-Henriksson E *et al.* Biopsy-verified response of severe lupus nephritis to treatment with rituximab (anti-CD20 monoclonal antibody) plus cyclophosphamide after biopsy-documented failure to respond to cyclophosphamide alone. *Scand J Rheumatol* 2004;33:423–7.

11 Cambridge G, Leandro MJ, Teodorescu M *et al.* B cell depletion therapy in systemic lupus erythematosus: effect on autoantibody and antimicrobial antibody profiles. *Arthritis Rheum* 2006;54:3612–22.

New developments in spondyloarthritis

Antoni Chan, Simon Kollnberger and Paul Bowness

□ INTRODUCTION

The spondyloarthritides are the second most common group of inflammatory arthitides and comprise ankylosing spondylitis (AS), reactive arthritis, the axial arthritis associated with inflammatory bowel disease and psoriasis, enthesitis-associated juvenile idiopathic arthritis, and undifferentiated spondyloarthropathy. The combined prevalence of the spondyloarthritides approaches 1% of the population.

The spondyloarthritides share an HLA-B27 association (Table 1) and a predilection for specific tissue sites, including the axial skeleton (Fig 1), large peripheral joints, entheses (attachments of ligament or joint capsule to bone), and anterior uveal tract. Although the aetiology of the spondyloarthritides is unknown, recent studies have confirmed and started to elucidate the predominant genetic effect in AS and have shown a key role for tumour necrosis factor alpha (TNF-α) in the inflammatory process. This review will summarise this knowledge, describe the dramatic recent advances in treatment, and argue the need for earlier diagnosis of these conditions.

Table 1 HLA-B27 associations of the spondyloarthritides.

Disease	Approximate frequency of HLA-B27 (%)
Ankylosing spondylitis	96
Undifferentiated spondyloarthropathy	70
Reactive arthritis	30–70
Colitis-associated spondyloarthritis	33–75
Psoriatic spondyloarthritis	40–50
Juvenile enthesitis-related arthritis	70
Acute anterior uveitis	50–70
Cardiac conduction defects with aortic incompetence	Up to 88

□ PATHOGENESIS OF SPONDYLOARTHRITIDES

Genetics

Although 95% of patients with AS have long been known to carry HLA-B27, it has recently become increasingly clear that other genes, not yet all identified, make major contributions. The predisposition to AS is largely genetic, as demonstrated by

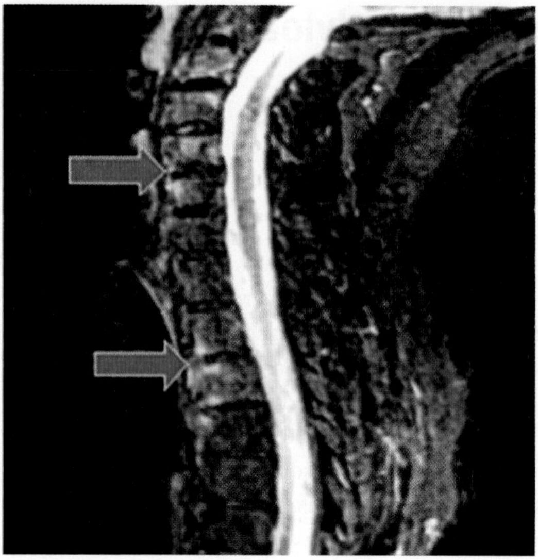

Fig 1 Magnetic resonance imaging scan (sagittal fat-suppressed STIR) of cervical and thoracic spine showing Romanus lesions (arrowed) indicative of enthesal inflammation in ankylosing spondylitis.

the high risk of recurrence among close relatives of patients. Heritability studies in twins show a concordance rate in HLA-B27-positive monozygotic twin pairs of 63% and in dizygotic twin pairs of 23%.[1] Data from risk of recurrence studies in twins suggest that the heritability of AS is greater than 92% and that HLA-B27 accounts for less than half of the polygenic genetic contribution. As only 2–8% of people positive for HLA-B27 develop AS, other major histocompatibility complex (MHC) and non-MHC genes are likely to influence susceptibility to spondyloarthritis – modelling suggests perhaps five other genes. In addition, the allelic variation in HLA-B27 itself also contributes to the variation in susceptibility to AS.

Additional HLA associations have been reported with HLA-B*60, HLA-DR1, and HLA-DR2. At least one further gene on chromosome 6 is likely to predispose to AS. Candidates that have been investigated include the tumour necrosis factor (*TNF*) locus; MHC class I chain-related gene A (*MICA*); and the genes for transporters with antigen processing (*TAP*), low molecular weight polypeptide (*LMP*), and heat shock protein (*HSP*).

Evidence for the involvement of non-MHC genes in the predisposition to AS comes from whole-genome scans of families with affected sibling pairs. These confirmed the linkage with HLA on chromosome 6 and identified six other regions with moderate linkage to disease outside the MHC on chromosomes 1, 2, 9, 10, 16, and 19. The strongest linkage was to chromosome 16q, and the magnitude of the genetic effect of this region (measured by the statistic λ) is estimated to be equivalent in magnitude to the genetic effect of HLA-DRB1 in patients with rheumatoid arthritis. Further gene mapping will be needed to determine the genes involved in this region of chromosome 16.

A linkage to the cytochrome P450 *CYP 2D6* gene (debrisoquine hydroxylase) on chromosome 22 has also been shown; however, the relative risk is only 2.1 and as 6% of the population in the UK have a poor-metaboliser phenotype, the role of this gene in susceptibility to AS is probably small. On chromosome 2q13, the *IL-1* gene cluster – which encodes IL-1a, IL-1b, and the natural antagonist IL-1RA – has been shown to be linked with AS in genome-wide studies. This has been further confirmed by studies showing over-representation of the IL-1 receptor antagonist (IL-1RA) variable number of tandem repeat polymorphism (VNTR) allele 2 in patients with AS. More recently, a strong association with haplotypes of the *IL-1B* gene and another member lying close to *IL-1RN* (termed *IL-1F10*) has been shown. Although the *IL-1* gene complex is the most significant non-MHC susceptibility locus identified, the significance of this remains uncertain, as allele 2 is reported to be associated with increased production of IL-1RA, which could inhibit the proinflammatory response of IL-1.

Genetic associations have also been found in other forms of spondyloarthritides. In enteropathic arthritis, there are associations between type 1 arthropathy (which is self-limiting, pauciarticular, and associated with flares of disease) and HLA-B*27, HLA-B*35, and HLA-DRB1*0103. Type 2 arthropathy (which is polyarticular, symmetric, persistent, and not related to activity) is associated with HLA-B44. In psoriatic arthritis, associations with TNF promoter polymorphisms, variants of the *TAP* gene, and *CARD15* have been reported.

HLA-B27, homodimers and disease pathogenesis

Confirmation of the critical role of HLA-B27 in disease pathogenesis has come from studies of HLA-B27 transgenic rats, which develop a multisystem disease with large joint and spinal arthritis, orchitis, colitis, and psoriaform lesions. One immunological function of HLA-B27 is to bind antigenic peptides together with beta 2-microglobulin (β2m) for presentation to the T-cell receptor (TCR) of CD8+ cytotoxic T cells. Cell transfer experiments in the rat model, however, have not shown a key role for CD8 T cells.

We have shown that HLA-B27 heavy chains form disulphide-bonded β2m-free homodimers called $B27_2$. We have proposed that they play a pathogenic role in AS through interactions with immune receptors other than TCR (the 'homodimer hypotheis'). $B27_2$ are expressed on the cell surface of leucocytes from patients and B27 transgenic rodents and bind several immunomodulatory molecules, including members of the killer cell immunoglobulin-like receptor (KIR) family (Fig 2). The KIR are expressed on certain natural killer (NK), T and NK T cells. The only cognate KIR for HLA-B27 is the three domain KIR3DL1; however, $B27_2$ also binds KIR3DL2, which has been previously shown to bind only to HLA-A3 and A11. We have recently shown that patients with AS have expanded populations of KIR3DL2-positive NK and CD4 T cells in their peripheral blood and joints (Fig 3).[2] This intriguing finding is of potential pathogenic significance and has led us to propose a new model of pathogenesis, which is illustrated in Fig 4. A triggering stimulus – for example, infection with intracellular bacteria – thus results in increased expression of cell-surface $B27_2$ homodimers on antigen-presenting cells. $B27_2$ is engaged by NK (or leucocyte immunoglobulin-like receptors (LILR)) receptors on other immune cells that consequently initiate or perpetuate inflammation.

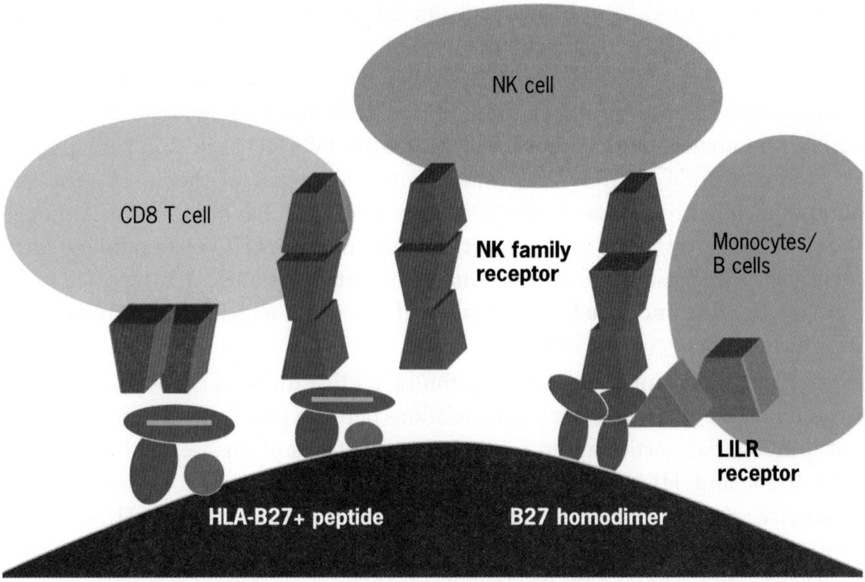

Fig 2 Recognition of different forms of HLA-B27 by natural killer (NK) receptors and leucocyte immunoglobulin like receptors. $B27_2$ = HLA-B27 heavy chain homodimer; LILR = leucocyte immunoglobulin-like receptors.

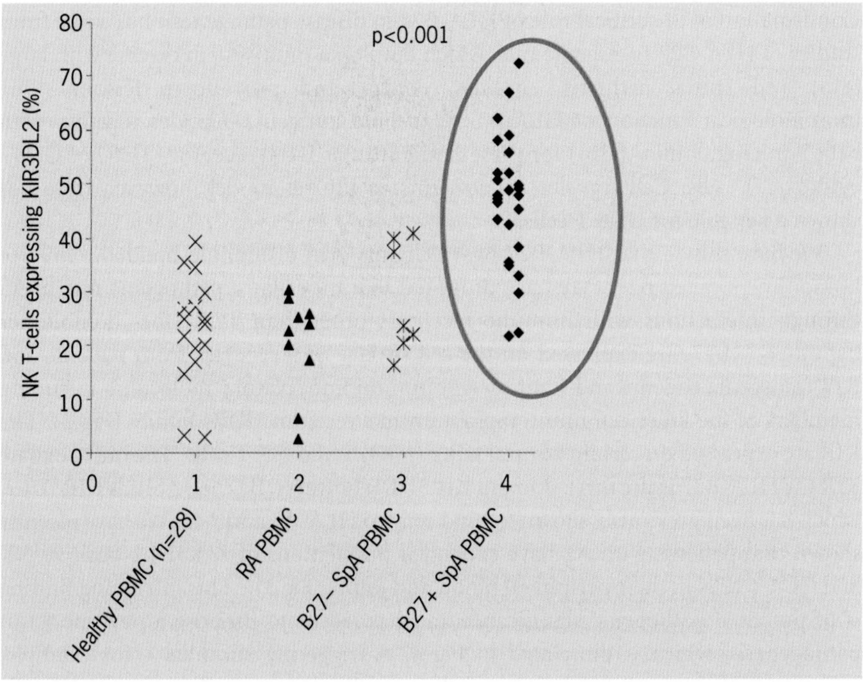

Fig 3 Expansion of KIR3DL2-positive natural killer (NK) cells in the peripheral blood of patients with ankylosing spondylitis. Fluorescent activated cell sorting analysis using a monoclonal antibody to KIR3DL2 is shown. PBMC = peripheral blood mononuclear cell; RA = rheumatoid arthritis; SpA = spondyloarthropathy. Adapted from Chan *et al*[2] with permission.

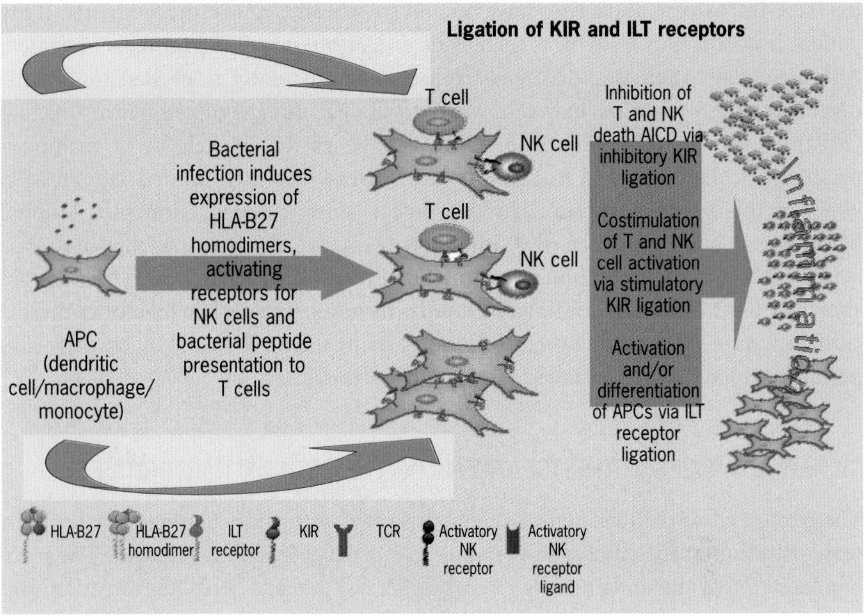

Fig 4 Model suggesting pathogenic role of HLA-B27 heavy chain homodimer in spondyloarthritis. AICD = activation-induced cell death. APC = antigen-presenting cell. DC = dendritic cell. ILT = immunoglobulin-like transcripts. KIR = killer cell immunoglobulin-like receptor. NK = natural killer. TCR = T-cell receptor.

□ THE NEED FOR EARLY DIAGNOSIS OF THE SPONDYLOARTHRITIDES

With the advent of effective treatments that are potentially disease modifying (see below), earlier diagnosis of AS becomes ever more important. The average time from onset of symptoms to diagnosis is currently longer than five years,[3,4] and a therapeutic window of opportunity may be missed. Recent advances in this area have concentrated on optimising the diagnostic utility of clinical features and investigations. As back pain is ubiquitous, the criteria for the inflammatory back pain found in patients with spondyloarthritides have been refined by Rudwaleit (Box 1).[5] People with two or more of the criteria have a positive likelihood ratio of 3.7; for those with four criteria, the likelihood ratio rises to 12.4.

In patients with inflammatory back pain, it is useful to obtain the HLA-B27 status. If psoriasis or inflammatory bowel disease is not present, a patient negative

Box 1 New criteria for diagnosis of inflammatory back pain.

Two or more of the following criteria should be present in an adult younger than 50 years:

- Morning stiffness >30 minutes
- Improvement with exercise but not with rest
- Awakening during the second half of the night (with back pain)
- Alternating buttock pain

for HLA-B27 is very unlikely to have AS and we would not investigate further. If the patient is positive for HLA-B27, further investigation, usually imaging, is indicated. Although plain radiology of the sacroiliac joints currently is needed for formal diagnosis of AS, changes may take years to appear. Magnetic resonance imaging (MRI) of the sacroiliac joints therefore can be extremely helpful in making a presumptive diagnosis and in assessment of disease activity. Limited sagittal MRI views of the whole spine similarly can detect 'shiny corners' (Romanus lesions) before overt changes are seen on X-ray – and again give objective evidence of disease activity that is likely to respond to treatment with anti-TNF agents. Such findings are shown in Fig 1. A number of imaging studies have suggested a key role for enthesitis (inflammation of the attachment of tendon or ligament to bone) as an early and perhaps primary site of pathology in spondyloarthritides.

□ NEW ADVANCES IN THE TREATMENT OF THE SPONDYLOARTHRITIDES

The greatest advance in the management of spondyloarthritides undoubtedly has been demonstration of the efficacy of the anti-TNF-α drugs in their treatment. The place of non-steroidal anti-inflammatory drugs (NSAIDs) perhaps needs re-evaluation, and bisphosphonates and new agents such as imitinib may also have a role.

Anti-TNF-α agents

Anti-TNF-α agents have been shown to be effective in the treatment of AS in numerous randomised controlled trials.[6–10] Infliximab (a chimeric anti-TNF immunoglobulin (Ig) G1 monoclonal antibody), adalumimab (a fully humanised anti-TNF monoclonal antibody), and etanercept (a recombinant soluble TNF receptor IgG1 fusion protein) are all markedly superior to placebo in the treatment of active AS. More than 50% of patients who received infliximab had a 50% improvement in scores on the Bath ankylosing spondylitis disease activity index (BASDAI) compared with 9% of controls at 12 weeks.[7] Remission was achieved in 20% of patients who received infliximab compared with none in controls. Infliximab has also been effective in the treatment of other types of spondyloarthropathies, including undifferentiated spondyloarthropathy. In the European, multicentre, ankylosing spondylitis study for the evaluation of recombinant infliximab therapy (ASSERT), 61% of patients in the infliximab group had a 20% decrease in the original ankylosing spondylitis assessment score (ASAS) compared with 19% of patients in the placebo group ($p<0.001$). Patients who received infliximab also showed significant improvements in scores on the BASDAI and functional and metrology indices and in the physical component summary score of the short form (SF)-36. Adverse events were reported with equal frequency in the two groups.

Similarly, in patients with AS, decreases of 20% in the original ASAS were seen in 59% of patients who received etanercept compared with 9% in the placebo control group at week 12 and in 57% and 22% of patients, respectively, at week 24 ($p<0.0001$ for both).[8] Gorman *et al* showed that 80% of patients who received etanercept achieved 20% improvement in ASAS at four months compared with 30%

of those who received placebo (p=0.004).[9] Adalimumab (a humanised anti-TNF monoclonal antibody) was recently shown to have comparable clinical efficacy in treating AS, with benefit also shown on MRI.[10]

Re-evaluation of the role of NSAIDs

The traditional mainstay of treatment for AS has been physical therapy and the use of NSAIDs. Although the use of NSAIDs has been shown to be effective in the control of pain and stiffness in patients with active AS, there previously was little evidence that usage altered the rate of paraspinal ossification. A recent study, however, compared the continuous use of NSAIDs with 'on-demand' use over a period of 24 months and showed more pronounced disease progression in the latter group.[11] Twice as many patients in the on-demand group scored moderate to high levels of spinal joint damage at two years compared with patients in the continuous treatment group. No significant difference was seen in adverse events between the two groups. This evidence of benefit needs to be weighed against evidence of the increased gastrointestinal, cardiovascular, and cerebrovascular morbidity and mortality now clearly associated with the use of NSAIDs. It is likely that risk–benefit analysis will need to be performed on an individual basis, and it is possible that the anti-TNF agents may prove to be safer in patients with AS than long-term use of NSAIDs.

A role for bisphosphonates?

One small randomised controlled trial has shown pamidronate to be efficacious in the treatment of AS; other studies of bisphosphonates are ongoing. Although our clinical experience is that bisphosphonates benefit only a minority of patients with AS, they may be worth trialling on an individual basis, given that patients with AS are known to have reduced bone density and are at increased risk of fractures.

New drugs, including imatinib

An uncontrolled pilot study of six patients has recently been reported to show benefit with imatinib.[12] This tyrosine kinase inhibitor is effective in patients with chronic myeloid leukaemia, but it is also known to have activity against other kinases, including macrophage colony-stimulating factor.

□ CONCLUSIONS AND FUTURE WORK

The efficacy of anti-TNF-α treatment in patients with spondyloarthritides is one of the most remarkable medical success stories of the last decade, especially given the lack of effective pre-existing disease-modifying treatments. Future work will include prospective studies to assess the disease-modifying affects of anti-TNF treatment, most likely including both MRI and sequential X-ray imaging, as well as functional and disease activity scoring. New study methods, including a non-inferiority design, may well be introduced more widely, because the high efficacy of current best treatments will make it increasingly difficult to demonstrate further improvements. We predict that the future may see the use of biomarkers as well as more detailed genetic analysis to make earlier and more accurate diagnoses. A deeper understanding of pathogenesis will be obtained by further work on the biology of HLA-B27 –in the transgenic rat model and in patients – and this hopefully will ultimately yield more precise treatments.

REFERENCES

1 Brown MA, Kennedy LG, MacGregor AJ *et al.* Susceptibility to ankylosing spondylitis in twins: the role of genes, HLA, and the environment. *Arthritis Rheum* 1997;40:1823–8.

2 Chan AT, Kollnberger SD, Wedderburn LR, Bowness P. Expansion and enhanced survival of natural killer cells expressing the killer immunoglobulin-like receptor KIR3DL2 in spondylarthritis. *Arthritis Rheum* 2005;52:3586–95.

3 Bollow M, Hermann KG, Biedermann T *et al.* Very early spondyloarthritis: where the inflammation in the sacroiliac joints starts. *Ann Rheum Dis* 2005;64:1644–6.

4 Braun J, Sieper J. Early diagnosis of spondyloarthritis. *Nat Clin Pract Rheumatol* 2006:2:536–45.

5 Rudwaleit M, Metter A, Listing J, Sieper J, Braun J. Inflammatory back pain in ankylosing spondylitis: a reassessment of the clinical history for application as classification and diagnostic criteria. *Arthritis Rheum* 2006;54:569–78.

6 Braun J, Sieper J. Biological therapies in the spondyloarthritides – the current state. *Rheumatology (Oxford)* 2004;43:1072–84.

7 Braun J, Brandt J, Listing J *et al.* Treatment of active ankylosing spondylitis with infliximab: a randomised controlled multicentre trial. *Lancet* 2002;359:1187–93.

8 Davis JC Jr, Van Der Heijde D, Braun J *et al.* Recombinant human tumor necrosis factor receptor (etanercept) for treating ankylosing spondylitis: a randomized, controlled trial. *Arthritis Rheum* 2003;48:3230–6.

9 Gorman JD, Sack KE, Davis JC Jr. Treatment of ankylosing spondylitis by inhibition of tumor necrosis factor alpha. *N Engl J Med* 2002;346:1349–56.

10 van der Heijde D, Kivitz A, Schiff MH *et al.* Efficacy and safety of adalimumab in patients with ankylosing spondylitis: results of a multicenter, randomized, double-blind, placebo-controlled trial. *Arthritis Rheum* 2006;54:2136–46.

11 Wanders A, Heijde D, Landewe R *et al.* Nonsteroidal antiinflammatory drugs reduce radiographic progression in patients with ankylosing spondylitis: a randomized clinical trial. *Arthritis Rheum* 2005;52:1756–65.

12 Eklund KK, Remitz A, Kautiainen H, Reitamo S, Leirisalo-Repo M. Three months treatment of active spondyloarthritis with imatinib mesylate: an open-label pilot study with six patients. *Rheumatology (Oxford)* 2006;45:1573–5.

☐ RHEUMATOLOGY SELF-ASSESSMENT QUESTIONS

New biologics for rheumatoid arthritis

1 Tumour necrosis factor alpha (TNF-α):
  (a) Is a proinflammatory cytokine found in high levels in the synovial fluid of patients with early rheumatoid arthritis
  (b) Can stimulate the secretion of other proinflammatory cytokines
  (c) Plays a key role in the body's defence against tuberculosis
  (d) Is not an important cytokine in patients with established rheumatoid arthritis

2 Regarding anti-TNF-α treatments for patients with rheumatoid arthritis:
  (a) Anti-TNF-α treatments are currently approved in the United Kingdom as a first-line antirheumatic treatment for patients with rheumatoid arthritis
  (b) Most patients go into remission after treatment with anti-TNF-α treatments
  (c) Anti-TNF-α treatments can control the symptoms of rheumatoid arthritis and slow the progression of radiographic damage
  (d) Infliximab is a soluble TNF-α receptor fusion protein

3 Regarding the safety of anti-TNF-α therapy in patients with rheumatoid arthritis:
  (a) They increase the risk of tuberculosis
  (b) They are safe to use in patients with congestive heart failure
  (c) They increase the risk of malignancy, particularly solid organ tumours
  (d) They are safe to combine with other biologics

Systemic lupus erythematosus: a problem with B cells

1 Pathological features characteristic of lupus include:
  (a) Necrosis with haematoxyphilic material
  (b) Giant cell granulomata
  (c) Complement depletion
  (d) Extensive T-cell infiltrates
  (e) Multiple autoantibodies

2 Evidence supports the following mechanisms of tissue injury in lupus:
  (a) Immune complex deposition
  (b) Immune complex-mediated cell activation
  (c) Production of cytokines by autoreactive T cells
  (d) Type II hypersensitivity (direct antibody effects on cells)
  (e) Amyloid deposition because of a prolonged acute phase response

3 Receptors on B cells that may be implicated in lupus include:
  (a) Toll-like receptor-9
  (b) Toll-like receptor-7

(c) B-cell receptor (surface immunoglobulin)
(d) Complement receptor II
(e) FcγRIIIa

4 Rituximab:
(a) Depletes B cells
(b) Targets the CD19 antigen
(c) Was developed for non-Hodgkin's lymphoma
(d) Has been shown to be effective in patients with psoriasis in controlled trials
(e) Has shown promise in open studies in lupus

New developments in spondyloarthritis

1 Concerning pathogenic factors in ankylosing spondylitis:
(a) HLA-B27 is the single most important genetic factor
(b) Susceptibility is largely genetic
(c) The IL-1 gene cluster has been excluded as a genetic risk factor
(d) HLA-B27 is a ligand of killer cell immunoglobulin-like receptors
(e) HLA-B27 is recognised only by receptors on CD4 T cells

2 In the diagnosis of ankylosing spondylitis:
(a) The mean time from onset of symptoms to diagnosis exceeds four years
(b) Awakening during the second half of the night with back pain is a feature of inflammatory back pain
(c) Spinal features in magnetic resonance images rarely precede X-ray changes
(d) HLA-B27 positivity is a useful screening test for ankylosing spondylitis
(e) Alternating buttock pain is a feature of inflammatory back pain

3 In the treatment of ankylosing spondylitis:
(a) Disease usually responds to anti-TNF treatment
(b) Adalumimab is a humanised anti-TNF monoclonal antibody
(c) Etanercept is a humanised anti-TNF monoclonal antibody
(d) Non-steroidal anti-inflammatory drugs may retard bony changes
(e) Imatinib is of proved benefit

Neurology

Ion channel disorders

Angela Vincent

□ INTRODUCTION

The neuromuscular junction (NMJ) is a prototype synapse, but one that is accessible to circulating factors, which makes it a target for neurotoxins and autoantibodies, as well as for genetic disorders. The NMJ and the targets for related genetic and autoimmune diseases are illustrated in Fig 1. The anatomy and physiology of neuromuscular transmission are reviewed in Ref 1. Autoantibodies and neurotoxins can access the NMJ from the peripheral circulation, as illustrated by the rapid onset of muscle paralysis and potentially fatal respiratory failure produced by some forms of envenomation – for example, bites of certain species of snakes, scorpions, and spiders. The toxins of these creatures bind with high affinity and specificity to different ion channels and receptors at the NMJ, which provides us with a library of tools for investigation of its disorders.

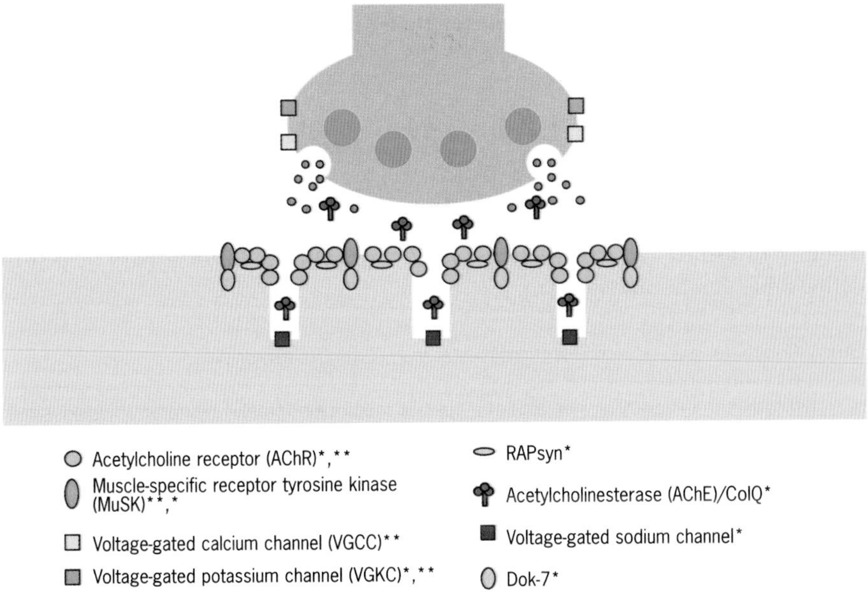

Fig 1 The neuromuscular junction (NMJ). Ion channels and related membrane receptors (for example, muscle-specific receptor tyrosine kinase (MuSK)) are shown diagrammatically and listed at the bottom. *Proteins targeted by genetic mutations in congenital myasthenic syndromes: acetylcholine receptors are the most frequent channels involved; sodium channels and MuSK have been reported in only a small number of patients. **Targets for autoantibodies in syndromes mediated by antibodies.

☐ GENETIC CHANNELOPATHIES AT THE NEUROMUSCULAR JUNCTION

Congenital myasthenic syndromes are a heterogeneous group of rare inherited disorders that result from mutations in different key proteins at the NMJ.[2] Affected patients do not have autoantibodies to ion channels in the NMJ. Congenital myasthenic syndromes probably account for about 2% of all myasthenias; a deficiency in acetylcholine receptors (AChRs) is most common, with a prevalence of around three cases per million people. Apart from 'slow channel syndrome', which is the result of a gain of function, all congenital myasthenic syndromes show recessive inheritance, and consanguinity in the family is common.

Most cases present at birth or in early childhood with ptosis, poor suck and feeding problems, and delayed motor milestones. For unknown reasons, however, some cases do not present until adolescence or young adulthood and thus may be mistaken for autoimmune seronegative myasthenia gravis. It is worth looking for distinctive features such as a history of arthrogryposis multiplex congenita at birth (caused by mutations of rapsyn), marked ophthalmoplegia (caused by mutations of the epsilon subunit of the AChR), or attacks of apnoea (caused by mutations of choline acetyltransferase (ChAT) or rapsyn), as these may point to congenital myasthenic syndromes rather than autoimmune conditions. A recently described form of limb girdle congenital myasthenic syndrome without tubular aggregates is associated with mutations in the gene for Dok-7 (see Fig 1), which is an intracellular signalling protein.[3]

☐ AUTOIMMUNE CHANNELOPATHIES AT THE NEUROMUSCULAR JUNCTION AND CENTRAL NERVOUS SYSTEM

The evidence for autoimmunity at the NMJ is overwhelming. The observations first made in myasthenia gravis (see Ref 4 for a review of the history) have helped to define other conditions (Box 1).

Box 1 Criteria for antibody-mediated diseases at the neuromuscular junction.

- Antibodies to extracellular domains of a specific membrane target – receptor or ligand-gated or voltage-gated ion channel
- Patients respond to plasma exchange and immunosuppression
- Immunoglobulin G injected into mice causes behavioural or physiological signs of disease

Myasthenia gravis

The symptoms and signs of myasthenia gravis are reviewed elsewhere.[1] Patients complain of fatigable, non-painful muscle weakness that often starts in the extraocular muscles but becomes generalised in most cases. The rest of the neurological examination produces normal findings. The diagnosis can be confirmed by detection of antibodies to the AChR or muscle-specific receptor tyrosine kinase (MuSK) in the serum, electrophysiology that shows a decrement in the compound muscle action potential on stimulation of 3Hz, increased jitter on single-fibre electromyography, or a clinical response to short-acting acetylcholinesterase inhibitors. The Tensilon test is potentially dangerous and can be misleading. Thyroid function should be tested in all patients, as this is the most common autoimmune disease associated with myasthenia gravis, and imaging of the thorax for detection of an associated thymoma should be performed in patients with anti-AChR antibodies.

Pathophysiology

About 85% of patients have anti-AChR antibodies at the NMJ, which can be measured by radioimmunoprecipitation assay (Fig 2). In patients with these antibodies, the number of AChRs at the NMJ is reduced to about 20% of normal; this results in an endplate potential that is reduced in amplitude and fails to reach threshold in a proportion of muscle fibres, which leads to muscle weakness. Failure of transmission increases with repeated effort.

The AChR is a pentameric membrane protein that exists in adult and fetal forms (Fig 3); α-bungarotoxin binds to each of the two α subunits. Anti-AChR antibodies are high affinity, polyclonal, and mainly of the immunoglobulin (Ig) G1 and IgG3 subclasses (which activate complement). Titres of anti-AChR antibodies are very

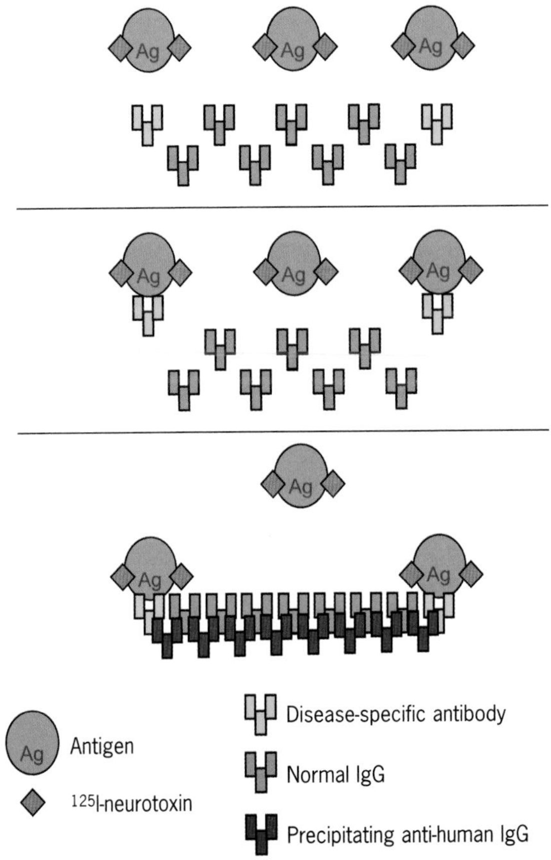

Fig 2 The radioimmunoprecipitation assay as used to test for antibodies against acetylcholine receptors, voltage-gated calcium channels, and voltage-gated potassium channels. A protein extract that contains the antigen in question is prelabelled with ^{125}I-labelled neurotoxins specific for the channel. Serum is added overnight and all of the patient's immunoglobulin (Ig) G is immunoprecipitated by a multivalent antiserum to human IgG. The precipitate is washed and counted for ^{125}I. The results are quantitative and highly specific for the condition.

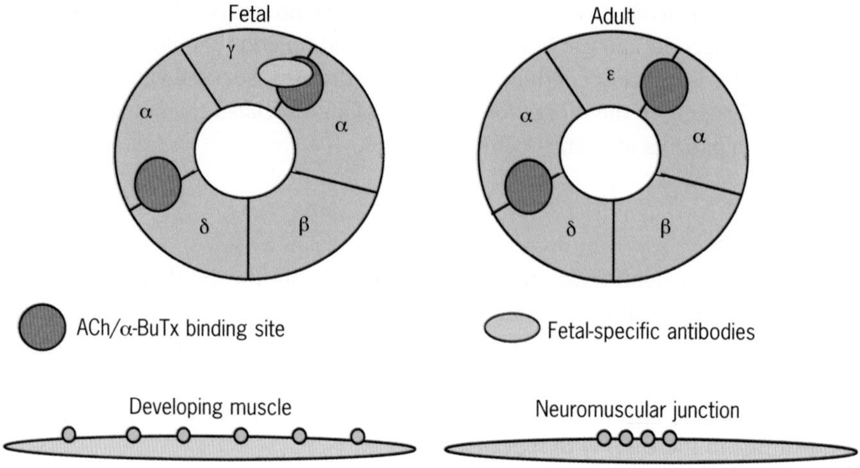

Fig 3 The adult and fetal isoforms of the acetylcholine receptor (AChR) as viewed from the nerve terminal. Acetylcholine and the snake toxin α-bungarotoxin (α-BuTx) bind to sites between each of the two α subunits and the adjacent subunits (not shown). A variable proportion of antibodies found in myasthenia gravis bind to the main immunogenic region on each of the alpha subunits. Antibodies in mothers of a few babies with arthrogryposis multiplex congenita bind strongly to a fetal epitope of the AChR and block the adjacent acetylcholine binding site, which paralyses the baby in utero.

variable between patients (ranging from 0 to >1000 nM) and overall do not correlate well with clinical severity. The levels of antibody within an individual, however, generally change in parallel with clinical scores after plasma exchange, thymectomy, or immunosuppressive treatments. Moreover, the NMJ deficits of myasthenia gravis can be transferred passively from patient to mouse (see Ref 4).

The anti-AChR antibodies cause loss of AChRs by complement-dependent lysis (which results in morphological damage), divalent cross linking of the AChR (which leads to increased internalisation and degradation), and direct inhibition of the acetylcholine binding site (which causes pharmacological blockade of function). The last mechanism seems to be uncommon in most cases.

The autoimmune attack has several knock-on effects. Firstly, the postsynaptic folds tend to be lost; this reduces the number of voltage-gated sodium channels, which increases the threshold for generation of the action potential and thus enhances the NMJ defect. There is also evidence, however, for a compensatory increase in release of acetylcholine and increased synthesis of AChRs. The final distribution and severity of muscle weakness thus must reflect not only the antibody-induced loss of AChR and secondary loss of sodium channels but also these compensatory changes.

Subgroups and prevalence

Patients with myasthenia gravis can be divided into subgroups on the basis of age at onset, human leucocyte antigen (HLA) associations, thymic involvement, and status with respect to anti-AChR antibodies (Table 1). These will not be discussed in detail here (see Ref 1). Myasthenia gravis is reported to be present in 7–15 per 100,000 of the population, but these estimates are based largely on studies from specialist centres in which most patients are young. In fact, with new evidence for presentation of myasthenia gravis in elderly people (Fig 4[5]) and probable underdiagnosis or misdiagnosis in this age group (myasthenia gravis can be mistaken for stroke or motor neurone disease, for example), the prevalence seems to be considerably higher than previously thought, at least in individuals older than 60 years. Interestingly, this is not the case in oriental countries, where childhood cases of ocular myasthenia gravis are most prevalent.

Table 1 Main types of generalised myasthenia gravis.

Type	Age at onset	Thymus	HLA	Antibody
Early onset	<40 years	Hyperplastic	B8DR3	AChR
Late onset	>40 years	Atrophic	B7DR2	AChR
Thymoma	30–60 years	Tumour	None	AChR
Myasthenia gravis with anti-MuSK antibodies	Mostly <50 years	Normal	DR14.DW5	MuSK Ab
'Seronegative'	Wide	Some hyperplasia	Not known	?AChR*

MuSK = muscle-specific receptor tyrosine tinase.
*Low affinity immunoglobulin G antibodies to acetylcholine receptors (AChRs) by an immunofluorescent staining technique are present in a subgroup of these patients.

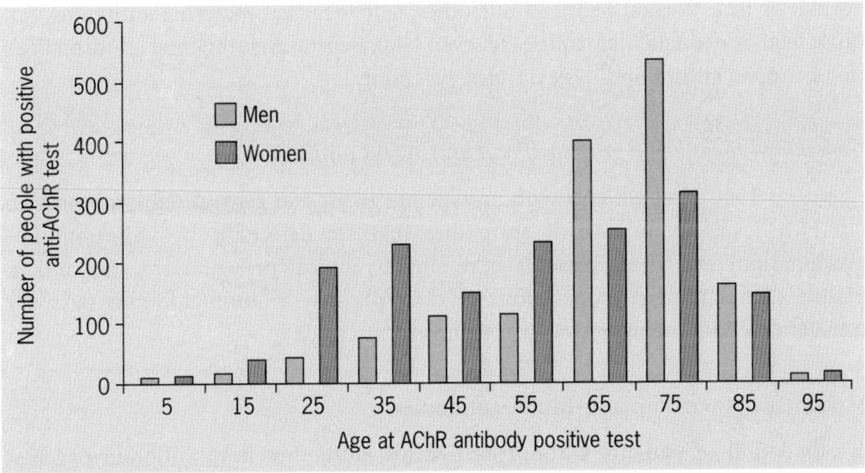

Fig 4 Age-related incidence of anti-acetylcholine receptor (AChR) antibodies in patients referred for testing in Oxford over a three-year period. As these sera represent only about 50% of patients diagnosed in the UK, the number of new patients per year is likely to be more than 1000. Although, as typically considered, women predominate in patients younger than 40 years (3:1), men predominate thereafter, and there is a striking incidence of positivity for anti-acetylcholine receptor antibodies in patients older than 75 years, with probable underdiagnosis. It should be borne in mind that the clinical status of these patients has not been determined, however, and some patients may have mild or even reversible symptoms (see Ref 5).

Paraneoplastic myasthenia gravis

Thymoma occurs in up to 10% of patients with myasthenia gravis and presents most often between the ages of 30 and 60 years. Thymoma can invade adjacent structures such as the pleura, pericardium, and great vessels and occasionally can metastasise, so it should be removed. After removal of the thymoma, however, the myasthenia rarely improves, levels of anti-AChR antibodies seldom fall, and additional immunosuppressive treatment is usually needed. The reason thymomas lead to myasthenia gravis is not clear, but the gland seems to export large numbers of mature T cells that may initiate an autoimmune response in the periphery.

Neonatal myasthenia gravis and arthrogryposis multiplex congenita

Simpson was the first to argue that passive transfer of myasthenia gravis from mother to baby supported an antibody-mediated aetiology,[4] but only a proportion of babies born to mothers with myasthenia gravis have transient respiratory and feeding difficulties.

Arthrogryposis multiplex congenita is a widely recognised condition in which the baby is born with fixed joint contractures, which usually are caused by lack of fetal movement. Inadequate development of the lungs can lead to perinatal death. This condition is relatively common and has many causes. A small number of cases have been identified in children of mothers with myasthenia gravis and in a very small number of women with anti-AChR antibodies but no clinical evidence of myasthenia gravis. These antibodies specifically block the function of the fetal isoform of the AChR (see Fig 3), which leads to fetal paralysis. Plasma exchange and intravenous immunoglobulins have been used during pregnancy in a few cases with normal or near normal neonatal outcomes. The idea that maternal antibodies can cause fetal or neonatal deformities or, even later, neurodevelopmental abnormalities (for example, autism and dyslexia) deserves study.

Generalised myasthenia gravis without anti-AChR antibodies

About 10–15% of all patients with myasthenia gravis and generalised symptoms do not have levels of anti-AChR antibodies that are detectable by radioimmuno-precipitation test. These patients have similar clinical presentations, respond to plasma exchange, and preparations of their plasma or immuglobulins passively transfer defects in neuromuscular transmission to mice.[4,6]

Myasthenia gravis with anti-MuSK antibodies

A proportion of patients without anti-AChR antibodies have antibodies against MuSK, which is a receptor tyrosine kinase restricted to the NMJ in mature muscle (see Fig 1). Interestingly, the prevalence of anti-MuSK antibodies among patients without anti-AChR antibodies is highly variable between different centres around the world,[7] which suggests a possible environmental stimulus. The antibodies are mainly of the IgG4 class and are almost never found in patients with anti-AChR antibodies or thymoma. Many of the patients are young women, but this might reflect the bias towards study of such patients in clinical practice.

The distinctive features of myasthenia gravis with MuSK are the often marked ocular, bulbar, neck, and respiratory symptoms[6] and, in contrast with myasthenia gravis with anti-AChR antibodies, patients may have normal electrophysiology in limb muscles with evidence of neuromuscular defects in facial muscles (for example, orbicularis occuli). The thymus does not show marked changes, and thymectomy is of doubtful benefit.[7] Patients respond to immunosuppression with prednisolone and azathioprine, but the response often is insufficient, and alternative immunosuppressive treatments such as mycophenolate or ciclosporin are needed. How the antibodies cause the NMJ defect is not yet clear.

Myasthenia gravis without anti-AChR and anti-MuSK antibodies

Disappointingly, some patients with typical generalised myasthenia gravis still do not have a serum antibody status defined by a laboratory test. As their clinical severity, electrophysiology, thymic pathology, and response to thymectomy tend to be similar to those in patients with myasthenia gravis with anti-AChR antibodies, we proposed that they have levels of anti-AChR antibodies undetectable by current laboratory tests. In at least a proportion of these patients, anti-AChR antibodies are detectable by a new immunofluorescent method (Leite, Willcox, and Vincent, unpublished observations).

Lambert Eaton myasthenic syndrome

Lambert Eaton myasthenic syndrome (LEMS) is a rare disorder, but it is important as the prototype paraneoplastic neurological syndrome. It is more common in men than women and usually presents with weakness that predominantly involves proximal limb muscles and a characteristic 'waddling gait'.[8] Importantly, unlike in myasthenia gravis, reflexes are absent or depressed but may increase after voluntary contraction of the relevant muscle. Autonomic symptoms (dry mouth, constipation, and impotence) are present in many patients, but need to be sought. Lambert Eaton myasthenic syndrome is diagnosed by the clinical features and improvements in strength after voluntary contraction (which reflects an increase in neurotransmitter release with repeated nerve stimulation) and confirmed by characteristic electromyographic findings and detection of antibodies to voltage-gated calcium channels (VGCCs) in the serum. Ocular symptoms are much less common than in patients with myasthenia gravis.

Small cell lung cancers (or, rarely, other tumours) are found in around 50% of patients with LEMS, but the neurological symptoms can predate the appearance of the tumour by several years. High-resolution imaging of the thorax should be performed regularly for at least five years, therefore, particularly in patients at risk (for example, smokers).

Pathophysiology

The endplate potentials in intercostal muscle biopsies are very small because the number of vesicles containing acetylcholine released per nerve impulse is decreased. During repetitive activity – such as voluntary muscle stimulation or high frequency nerve stimulation – the endplate potentials increase, which leads to an increment in compound muscle action potential and improved muscle function.

Evidence for an autoimmune pathogenesis comes from clinical and experimental observations similar to those seen for myasthenia gravis (Table 1). Patients, particularly those without a tumour, tend to have other organ-specific autoantibodies. An HLA-B8 association is seen in patients with LEMS without small cell lung cancer. Plasma exchange or treatment with intravenous immunoglobulins leads to clinical and electrophysiological improvement, and most patients also respond to immunosuppressive drugs. Moreover, passive transfer of patient's plasma or immunoglobulins into experimental animals leads to changes in the electrophysiology and morphology of the NMJ that are very similar to those seen in patients with LEMS, and IgG can be detected on the presynaptic nerve terminal.

Voltage-gated calcium channels are transmembrane proteins that comprise $\alpha1$, β, and $\alpha2/\delta$ subunits of different isoforms. The $\alpha1$ subunit contains the central ion channel and can be of a P/Q-type, N-type, or T-type in neuronal tissues. The use of neurotoxins derived from the venoms of snails and spiders has made it possible to show that the VGCCs present at the NMJ are predominantly of the P/Q-type, which is also expressed on small cell lung cancer cells. Radioimmunoprecipitation with ^{125}I-α-conotoxin labelling of mammalian brain extracts (which contain plentiful P/Q-type VGCCs) detected antibodies in more than 85% of patients with LEMS.[9]

Autonomic dysfunction is common in patients with LEMS, which suggests that IgG associated with this condition may also interfere with neurotransmission at autonomic synapses. In fact, these synapses have a much wider array of VGCC subtypes, and the P/Q-type channels are responsible for only a proportion of the nerve-induced release of neurotransmitters at the bladder or vas deferens (at least in mouse models). The situation could be different in humans, which could explain the often marked involvement of the autonomic system.

Despite the presence of P/Q-type VGCCs in the brain, particularly on the Purkinje cells of the cerebellum, most patients do not have cerebellar symptoms. Cerebellar ataxia, however, can co-occur with LEMS in rare cases. This is usually paraneoplastic cerebellar degeneration associated with small cell lung cancer, and the treatment of the peripheral symptoms (which might be unrecognised) can lead to an overall clinical improvement.

Acquired neuromyotonia and anti-voltage-gated potassium channel antibody-associated limbic encephalitis

Neuromyotonia is a syndrome of spontaneous and continuous muscle fibre contraction that results from hyperexcitability of motor nerves. It has many other names,[10] and the aetiology probably is mixed, as similar symptoms can be seen in genetic disorders and peripheral neuropathies. Neuromyotonia may be part of a spectrum of diseases that includes cramp fasciculation syndrome. Although rare, it is of particular interest because it may associate with symptoms of central nervous system disease.

A proportion of patients with this syndrome, presenting de novo, are aged 25–60 years and complain of muscle stiffness, cramps, myokymia (visible undulation of the muscle), pseudomyotonia, and weakness. Increased sweating is common and may be a significant problem. Myokymia characteristically continues during sleep and general anaesthesia (unlike muscle stiffness in stiff person syndrome). Sensory symptoms are not uncommon and usually include paraesthesia, dysaesthesia, and numbness; neuropathic pain may be a presenting symptom in rare cases. It is important to remember that neuromyotonia can also be paraneoplastic, with around 20% of cases having a thymoma or, less commonly, small cell lung cancer or another neoplastic condition.

Diagnosis is confirmed by electromyography, which shows characteristic spontaneous motor unit discharges that occur in distinctive doublets, triplets, or longer runs with high intraburst frequency (40–300 per sec). Antibodies to voltage-gated potassium channels (VGKCs) are present in about 40% of patients and more commonly in patients with associated thymoma.[10]

Pathophysiology

Neuromyotonia can be associated with other autoimmune diseases or other autoantibodies, and cerebrospinal fluid analysis may show oligoclonal bands.[10] In particular, some patients with neuromyotonia also have myasthenia gravis, or increased levels of anti-AChR antibodies – usually but not always in association with thymoma. Evidence for an antibody-mediated pathology includes the beneficial results of plasma exchange, passive transfer of disease to mice, and the effects of purified IgG on dorsal root ganglia cultures (see Refs 9 and 10). The effects of the IgG from patients with neuromyotonia were similar to those found with low concentrations of the VGKC blockers 4-aminopyridine and 3,4-diaminopyridine, which suggests that a form of VGKC is a likely target for autoantibodies.

A functional VGKC consists of four transmembrane α subunits that combine as homomultimeric and heteromultimeric tetramers. At least 10 different α subunits have been identified, and each is encoded by a different gene. Voltage-gated potassium channels of the subtypes Kv1.1 and 1.2 are highly expressed in the peripheral nervous system and also in the central nervous system. Antibodies to VGKCs can be detected in about 40% of patients with neuromyotonia by radioimmunoprecipitation of ^{125}I α dendrotoxin-labelled VGKCs extracted from the human frontal cortex. Dendrotoxin binds to the Kv1.1, 1.2, and 1.6 isoforms of VGKCs. The 60% of sera negative for these antibodies may contain antibodies to some other (as yet unidentified) peripheral nerve or motor nerve terminal ion channel or other protein.

The most exciting development in this field is the recognition that central nervous system symptoms such as insomnia, amnesia, hallucinations, delusions, and personality change may be present in patients with neuromyotonia (usually called Morvan's syndrome, see Ref 13) or in patients with very high levels of highly anti-VGKC antibodies often without neuromyotonia. About 40% of patients with Morvan's syndrome have a thymoma or other tumour. In patients without peripheral symptoms, the disease seems to represent a form of limbic encephalitis that is usually non-paraneoplastic and monophasic. This form of limbic encephalitis is increasingly being recognised, with around 40 new cases a year in the United Kingdom. Patients usually do well after sustained immunosuppression (Fig 5).[11]

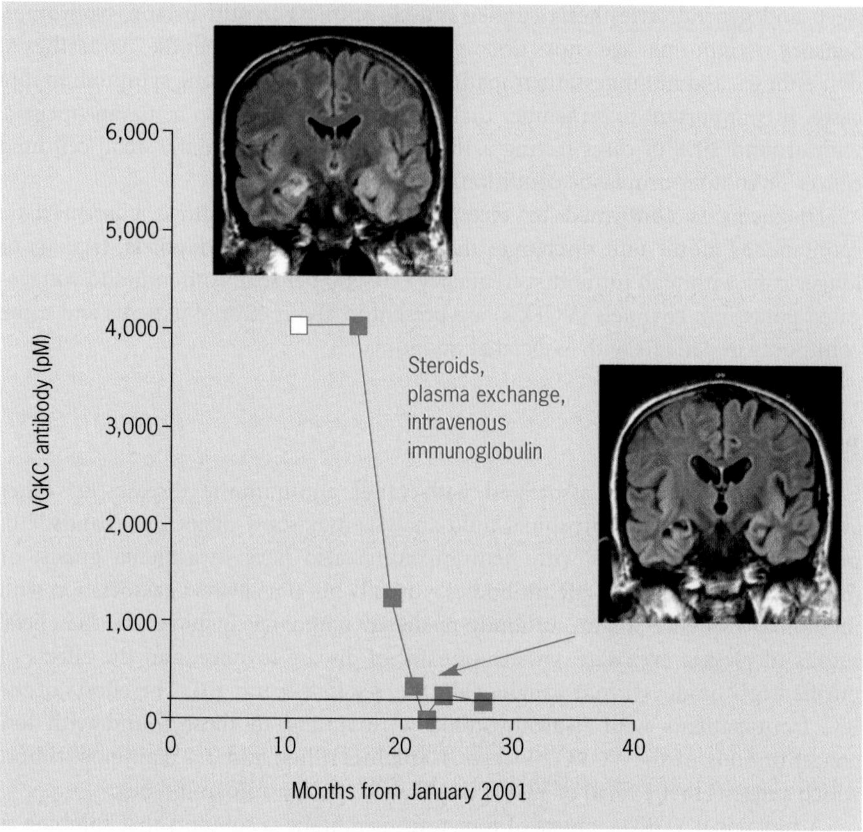

Fig 5 A case of non-paraneoplastic limbic encephalitis associated with high levels of anti-voltage-gated potassium channel (VGKC) antibodies. The patient presented with amnesia and seizures and spent five months in a district general hospital before being referred to Professor Martin Rossor at the Institute of Neurology, UCL. At this stage, levels of anti-VGKC antibodies were tested and found to be very high (normal levels up to 100 pM). The patient was treated with extensive immunotherapy and made a considerable recovery, albeit with some residual retrograde amnesia. Scans of the brain showed the typical high signal in the mesial temporal lobes at diagnosis, with sclerosed hippocampi and cerebral atrophy remaining after treatment. Data and scans courtesy of J Schott and M Rossor (see Ref 12 for more details).

☐ FINAL COMMENTS

Since the paraneoplastic disorders and now a non-paraneoplastic disorder of the central nervous system (VGKC-antibody-associated limbic encephalitis) were recognised, the search has been on for other channelopathies of the central nervous system mediated by autoantibodies. Several exciting developments are taking place (Box 2). Anti-aquaporin 4 antibodies seem to be present in up to 80% of patients with neuromyelitis optica – a condition that needs to be distinguished from multiple sclerosis. Antibodies to various N-methyl-D-aspartic acid receptors have been identified in subgroups of patients with neuropsychiatric lupus and patients with paraneoplastic limbic encephalitis related to an ovarian tumour. Glutamate receptor antibodies were identified in the 1990s in a few patients with the very rare Rasmussen's encephalitis (childhood intractable seizures) but are still not measured routinely. The discovery of further autoimmune channelopathies is likely to follow.

Box 2 Some emerging autoimmune channelopathies.

- Antibodies to aquaporin-4 in neuromyelitis optica
- Antibodies to ganglionic acetylcholine receptors in some autoimmune autonomic neuropathies
- Antibodies to N-methyl-D-aspartic acid receptors in neuropsychiatric lupus and in a rare paraneoplastic form of limbic encephalitis
- Antibodies to glutamate receptor 3 in Rasmussen's encephalitis (?)

REFERENCES

1 Vincent A, Buckley C, Burke G. Neuromuscular junction disorders. In: Schapira AHV, ed. *Neurology and clinical neuroscience.* Philadelphia, PA: Mosby Elsevier, 2007:1223–4.

2 Engel AG, Ohno K, Sine SM. Sleuthing molecular targets for neurological diseases at the neuromuscular junction. *Nat Rev Neurosci* 2003;4:339–52.

3 Beeson D, Higuchi O, Palace J *et al.* Dok-7 mutations underlie a neuromuscular junction synaptopathy. *Science* 2006;313:1975–8.

4 Vincent A. Unravelling the pathogenesis of myasthenia gravis. *Nat Rev Immunol* 2002;2:797–804.

5 Vincent A, Clover L, Buckley C, Grimley Evans J, Rothwell PM. Evidence of underdiagnosis of myasthenia gravis in older people. *J Neurol Neurosurg Psychiatry* 2003;74:1105–8.

6 Vincent A, Bowen J, Newsom-Davis J, McConville J. Seronegative generalised myasthenia gravis: clinical features, antibodies, and their targets. *Lancet Neurol* 2003;2:99–106.

7 Vincent A, Leite MI. Neuromuscular junction autoimmune disease: muscle specific kinase antibodies and treatments for myasthenia gravis. *Curr Opin Neurol* 2005;18:519–25.

8 O'Neill JH, Murray NM, Newsom-Davis J. The Lambert-Eaton myasthenic syndrome. A review of 50 cases. *Brain* 1988;111:577–96.

9 Vincent A, Lang B, Kleopa KA. Autoimmune channelopathies and related neurological disorders. *Neuron* 2006;52:123–38.

10 Hart IK, Maddison P, Newsom-Davis J, Vincent A, Mills KR. Phenotypic variants of autoimmune peripheral nerve hyperexcitability. *Brain* 2002;125:1887–95.

11 Vincent A, Buckley C, Schott JM *et al.* Potassium channel antibody-associated encephalopathy: a potentially immunotherapy-responsive form of limbic encephalitis. *Brain* 2004;127:701–12.

12 Schott JM, Harkness K, Barnes J *et al.* Amnesia, cerebral atrophy, and autoimmunity. *Lancet* 2003;361:1266.

13 Buckley C, Vincent A. Autoimmune channelopathies. *Nat Clin Pract Neurol* 2005;1:22–33.

Neurosurgery for movement disorders

Tipu Z Aziz

Surgery for movement disorders has a history that extends back more than 100 years. In the pursuit to alleviate the terrible tremors of Parkinson's disease, the nervous system was attacked at all levels.

The history of surgery for movement disorders[1] can be divided into:

- non-basal ganglia procedures
- open basal ganglia procedures
- stereotactic basal ganglia procedures.

In 1817, James Parkinson described the fact that a stroke resulted in loss of contralateral tremor. This led Sir Victor Horsley to excise the motor cortex in a dystonic patient in 1890, but he did not follow this up. In the early 20th century, many levels of the nervous system were operated on in procedures such as cervical dorsal rhizotomy, cerebellar dentatectomy, and cerebral pedunculotomy and, later on in 1939, motor cortex excision again. The aim was to induce a degree of paresis to relieve tremor.

Attention was focussed on the basal ganglia in 1940 by the work of Russell Meyer, who reported a 60% improvement in tremor and rigidity with no attendant paresis after open excision of areas of the basal ganglia. The complication rates, however, were exceedingly high. The results did point to the fact that the pallidum and its outflow pathways were the targets of choice, but open basal ganglia procedures never actually took off.

In 1953, Cooper reported a case of attempted pedunculotomy during which he damaged the anterior choroidal artery and had to ligate it. Instead of developing paresis, the patient woke up with relief of his contralateral tremor and rigidity. Anatomical studies in chimpanzees showed that the artery supplied the pallidum, and Cooper focused on targeted injections of alcohol into the pallidum with a guide attached to the patient's head. The effects were better and safer than those achieved with open anterior choroidal artery sectioning.

At the same time, the neurologist Speigel and his neurosurgical colleague Wycis considered the pallidum to be a target for Huntington's disease because carbon monoxide poisoning led to cavitating lesions in the pallidum associated with akinesia. As the condition was thought to be a hyperkinetic disorder, it seemed reasonable to lesion it to alleviate symptoms. Spiegel and Wycis did so with a human-sized stereotactic frame made to order by Sir Victor Horsley's toolmaker, who was still alive and living in London.

Horsley and Clarke devised a frame, which was reported in 1907, to lesion targets in primates' cerebella selectively without causing severe damage to structures en route. Essentially, the primate's head was fixed in a rigid frame aligned to standard landmarks. Horsley and Clarke created a cross sectional map of the primate brain, which referenced brain structures to the standard landmarks and thus allowed an electrolytic electrode to be passed directly to the target. Use of this enabled them to begin studies into the role of the cerebellum; however, neither saw a role for the frame in clinical medicine.

Speigel and Wycis saw the implications of the frame in their ambitions to perform selective orbitofrontal leucotomies and, as they had had a frame made, they made an atlas of the brain with the pineal gland as the reference point. They used this to introduce stereotaxic surgery to clinical medicine.

Over the next five years, pallidotomies were reported by many, with an overall reduction of tremor and rigidity in about 70% of patients and fairly low complication rates. To improve outcomes, the target nucleus of the pallidum – the motor thalamus – then was used. Reduction in tremor was achieved in 90% of patients operated on, and, by 1975, 75,000 patients had undergone surgery.

In 1969, at the third International Congress on Parkinson's Disease, Hoehn and Yahr described their studies in patients after thalamotomy and showed that, although 80% of patients lost their tremor, only 17% gained functional benefit because they were so akinetic. On the other hand, Cotzias showed that a new drug levodopa (L-dopa) alleviated tremor rigidity and akinesia. This heralded the end of surgery for Parkinson's disease and other movement disorders, as it was believed that drugs would become available for many and would avoid the need for the risks of surgery.

Although miraculous in the early years, L-dopa was not without complications. After five years of treatment, >70% of patients would develop crippling movement disorders called dyskinesias, which were as disabling as the untreated disease. Without an understanding of the neural mechanisms underlying the condition, however, development of better treatments was difficult.

Things changed with the case of a drug addict who injected himself with a homemade modification of pethidine called 1-methyl-4-phenyl-1,2,3,6-tetra-hydropyridine (MPTP) and was rendered severely akinetic but responsive to L-dopa. Further cases were quickly described, MPTP was administered to non-human primates, and a very accurate model of the human condition became available, with akinetic, rigid, forward flexed, and tremulous monkeys that responded to L-dopa. The use of this model led to emergence of understanding of the neural mechanisms of parkinsonism, in which loss of the nigrostriatal dopaminergic projection led to overactivity of the subthalamic nucleus (STN), which, in turn, drove the medial pallidum to excessively inhibit the motor thalamus and upper brain stem. The STN therefore seemed a target to lesion in patients with Parkinson's disease. In primates, unilateral lesions resulted in dramatic reversal of parkinsonism.

Spontaneous bleeds in the STN were known to result in intractable hemiballism, however, and an alternative to lesioning – high frequency stimulation by electrodes implanted in the nucleus – therefore was tried in primates with parkinsonism with equal effect. At such high frequencies of stimulation, the neurones essentially were suppressed. This rapidly was adopted in clinical practice, and today more than 40,000 patients have had STN stimulation for Parkinson's disease.

About 20% of patients with parkinsonism, however, have a poor response to dopaminergic treatment, and there is no medical treatment for other akinetic parkinsonian syndromes, such as progressive supranuclear palsy (PSP) and multiple system atrophy (MSA). Recent work in primates led to the finding that low frequency stimulation of a brain stem nucleus – the pedunculopontine nucleus – could relieve parkinsonian akinesia, and this has recently been confirmed in man.

The question for a neurologist is who and when to refer for surgery. Drug-resistant tremor responds well to thalamic surgery – be it thalamotomy or deep brain stimulation. In a small subgroup of patients with tremor-predominant Parkinson's disease, known as benign tremulous parkinsonism, thalamic surgery is adequate. Most patients, however, have bilateral tremor, rigidity, and bradykinesia for which thalamic surgery alone is not enough. Patients who have a good albeit brief response to L-dopa and whose disease is complicated by dyskinesias should be considered for surgery. Generally, this should be considered fairly early on, so that affected patients can resume a normal life and, if they are employed, can continue to do so. At present, deep brain stimulation of the STN is considered the best surgical treatment, although there is increasing indication that pallidal stimulation may be just as effective. Objectively, scores on the Unified Parkinson's Disease Rating Scale (UPDRS) are reduced by 50% with surgery to the STN and by 40% with pallidal surgery,[2,3] but the on drug/on stimulation improvement is the same.

A group of patients with parkinsonism are unresponsive to L-dopa, however, or become so with time (possibly as many as 20%). These patients are disabled by poor balance and gait freezing, with no hope of medical or surgical alleviation.

During the past decade, tremors in patients with other movement disorders also have been shown to be responsive to deep brain stimulation, such as the tremors of multiple sclerosis, trauma, and dystonia. Today, as knowledge of brain function increases with the help of such techniques as functional magnetic resonance imaging (fMRI), positron emission tomography (PET), and magnetoencephalography (MEG) and the results of animal studies, more conditions will become treatable.

REFERENCES

1 Gildenberg PL. Evolution of basal ganglia surgery for movement disorders. *Stereotact Funct Neurosurg* 2006;84:131–5.

2 Anderson VC, Burchiel KJ, Hogarth P, Favre J, Hammerstad JP. Pallidal vs subthalamic nucleus deep brain stimulation in Parkinson disease. *Arch Neurol* 2005;62:554–60.

3 Krack P, Poepping M, Weinert D, Schrader B, Deuschl G. Thalamic, pallidal, or subthalamic surgery for Parkinson's disease? *J Neurol* 2000;247(Suppl 2):II122–34.

☐ NEUROLOGY SELF-ASSESSMENT QUESTIONS

Ion channel disorders

1 Children with myasthenic weakness:
  (a) May have a genetic disease
  (b) Always show a recessive inheritance pattern
  (c) May have autoimmune myasthenia
  (d) Can present with apnoea

2 Myasthenia gravis:
  (a) Occurs only in young adults
  (b) Is always associated with acetylcholine receptor antibodies
  (c) Can be treated effectively by immunosuppression
  (d) Always responds to plasma exchange
  (e) Never gets better spontaneously

3 Bulbar symptoms:
  (a) Are common in patients with muscle-specific receptor tyrosine kinase (MuSK) antibodies
  (b) Do not respond to immunosuppressive treatments
  (c) May be due to muscle atrophy

4 Lambert Eaton myasthenic syndrome (LEMS):
  (a) Is only found in smokers
  (b) Is more common in men
  (c) Only gets better if the tumour is treated successfully
  (d) Affects gait more than eye movements

5 Voltage-gated potassium channel antibodies:
  (a) Are associated with limbic encephalitis
  (b) Can be found in patients without peripheral muscle hyperactivity
  (c) Are found with thymoma
  (d) Are frequent in children
  (e) Often indicate a potentially reversible disorder of the central nervous system

Neurosurgery for movement disorders

1 Surgery for movement disorders:
  (a) Is new
  (b) Is aimed to partially paralyse
  (c) Is rarely performed
  (d) Is largely ineffective

2 The most common method is:
(a) Excising the motor cortex
(b) Sectioning the spinal cord
(c) Tying the anterior choroidal artery
(d) Lesioning the thalamus
(e) Deep brain stimulation

3 Regarding deep brain stimulation:
(a) It has never been performed
(b) It is the technique most commonly used
(c) Different targets are used depending on the patient's condition
(d) It only targets the internal capsule

4 Lesional surgery:
(a) Is the most common method for treating movement disorders
(b) Has no side effects
(c) Is no longer performed
(d) Can be done bilaterally and safely
(e) Still has a role in surgery for movement disorders

Radiology

High-resolution computed tomography and diffuse lung disease – current status

Anand Devaraj and David M Hansell

☐ INTRODUCTION

It has been 25 years since the introduction of thoracic high-resolution computed tomography (HRCT). In this time, HRCT has developed from a diagnostic tool used occasionally in tertiary referral centres to an indispensable part of the investigation of diffuse lung diseases. This paper will discuss some of the recent developments in the technique and role of HRCT in the management of diffuse lung disease and will focus on its diagnostic and prognostic capabilities. It will also explore current and future areas of research, looking beyond the role of HRCT simply as a diagnostic aid. A brief description of the technological aspects of CT is provided at the outset.

☐ TECHNICAL CONSIDERATIONS

Since the first examination with CT was performed in 1971, the technology behind CT has made significant advances. The earliest machines were single-slice models by which data were acquired one row at a time. In the 1980s, the arrival of helical (or spiral) CT greatly reduced examination time.

Within this context, HRCT has been used as a way of analysing the fine anatomical detail of the lungs. The excellent spatial resolution of HRCT enables visualisation of small anatomical structures, including intralobular arteries and occasionally normal interlobular septa. High-resolution CT employs thin collimation (1 millimetre) and a sharp reconstruction algorithm and traditionally is performed as a sampling procedure with images obtained every 10 mm. This reduces the dose of radiation and examination time without affecting diagnostic ability.

In the latter part of the 1990s, manufacturers released multi-detector (or multi-slice) CT scanners (MDCT). These incorporated between four and 64 rows of detectors in the longitudinal axis, which allowed the simultaneous acquisition of multiple image slices. Thus, MDCT became capable of rapidly providing contiguous, high-resolution, sub-millimetre images of the thorax in a single breath-hold – this is referred to as volumetric HRCT.

☐ RADIATION ISSUES

The considerable increase in the number of CT examinations performed in the last 10 years has led to a corresponding increase in the dose of radiation received by the population.[1] Within this setting, the particular radiation burden from multi-detector HRCT of the thorax is worthy of discussion.

The principal reason for larger doses of radiation in thoracic MDCT is the greater volumes being scanned because of the ability to acquire contiguous slices. The effective radiation dose from a volumetric thoracic HRCT is estimated at about 7 milliSieverts (mSv), which compares less than favourably with a standard interspaced HRCT dose of 0.7 mSv (annual background radiation in the UK is 2.2 mSv). The associated risk of additional fatal cancers is estimated at 50 per million of population exposed to 1 mSv.[2]

As with all investigations that use X-rays, the radiation burden is best reduced by applying an appropriate scanning protocol to answer the clinical question being asked. Although volumetric HRCT has the potential to cover all diagnostic possibilities – and produce exquisite images in the process – in practice, most patients with interstitial lung disease can be satisfactorily assessed with conventional interspaced HRCT.

□ DIFFUSE LUNG DISEASE AND HRCT

Diagnosis and the gold standard

Many investigators have examined the diagnostic accuracy of HRCT and have attempted to characterise the imaging correlates of various diffuse lung pathologies. In this context, usual interstitial pneumonia (UIP) and non-specific interstitial pneumonia (NSIP) serve as ideal models to illustrate the diagnostic abilities of HRCT.

Histopathology is the traditional gold standard against which the diagnostic accuracy of HRCT has been judged. There are, however, a number of reasons why caution should be applied when using histology in isolation as the gold standard. The first is the obvious issue of sampling error. Flaherty *et al* showed that one quarter of patients with idiopathic interstitial pneumonia (IIP) who had surgical lung biopsy had different pathologies (NSIP or UIP) in different lobes.[3] Secondly, in contrast to estimates in the radiological literature, the degree of interobserver variation by histopathologists has been quantified only recently: studies that evaluated the histological pattern of diffuse lung disease have demonstrated only poor to fair interobserver agreement, with kappa coefficient values of 0.26 and 0.38 (values greater than 0.4 are considered to be clinically acceptable). Finally, it is important to consider the fact that biopsies are now increasingly reserved for patients with indeterminate findings from HRCT or individuals in whom there is disparity between clinical and HRCT findings, thus creating an inherent selection bias. With these caveats in mind, some of the recent research on the role of HRCT in the diagnosis of UIP and NSIP will now be reviewed.

Although many of the earlier studies examined the sensitivity of HRCT, its specificity and positive predictive value have been scrutinised only relatively recently. In various series, positive predictive values of 96% and specificities of 100% have been obtained for HRCT in the diagnosis of idiopathic pulmonary fibrosis (IPF). These results confirm that a diagnosis of UIP can be made with confidence with images from HRCT when typical features are present (Fig 1). Other studies that looked at UIP and NSIP found some variation in results. In patients with NSIP,

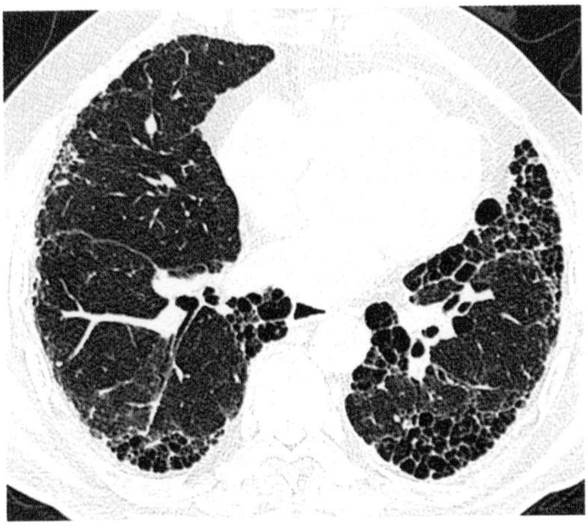

Fig 1 Characteristic appearance of usual interstitial pneumonia in an image from high-resolution computed tomography, with subpleural honeycomb change at the lung bases.

Macdonald *et al* demonstrated diagnostic sensitivity and specificity for HRCT of 70% and 63%, respectively (with corresponding sensitivity and specificity in UIP of 63% and 70%, respectively).[4] Overlap in the appearances of UIP and NSIP in images produced by CT illustrates the discordance that exists between histology and findings from HRCT, principally for the reasons alluded to earlier regarding the absence of a true gold standard. Importantly, although this issue is relevant in the setting of UIP and NSIP, it can be applied equally to the other interstitial lung diseases.

Predicting prognosis and quantifying disease

A number of investigators have examined the role of HRCT in predicting the course of disease and the ultimate endpoint, mortality, in patients with IIP. Similarly, researchers have endeavoured to correlate disease severity according to images produced by CT with the results of pulmonary function tests.

High-resolution CT can provide important prognostic information in patients with IIP. Patients with UIP confirmed on histology and radiology have higher mortality than patients with biopsy-proved UIP, and findings from HRCT that are more in keeping with NSIP. Such patients, in turn, have a worse prognosis than patients with NSIP diagnosed by both tests. Recent research has confirmed the simple concept that the presence and extent of honeycombing on HRCT (the cardinal feature of UIP in images from CT) is associated with significantly poorer mortality. For example, about one third of patients with NSIP displayed an improvement in pulmonary function at follow up compared with 14% with UIP without honeycombing and 0% with UIP and honeycombing.

The accurate quantification of disease extent in patients with IIP is a further area of interest. In this regard, CT scoring is a well-established semi-quantitative technique. Although the precise methods of scoring vary, more than one study has shown a relation between fibrosis scores according to HRCT and mortality in patients with IPF.[5] Scores of disease extent based on images from CT have also been correlated with individual pulmonary function tests, with strong relations between scores from HRCT and gas transfer as well as total lung capacity. A confounding variable in some patients with IPF, however, is the presence of coexisting emphysema. This undoubtedly complicates studies that examine such structure–function relations, with patients displaying spuriously preserved or elevated lung volumes and reduced gas transfer. In an attempt to take into account coexistent emphysema, Wells *et al* constructed the composite physiologic index, which they showed correlated strongly with the fibrosis score based on images from CT.[5] Although CT accurately illustrates the global extent of disease, scoring according to images from CT is semi-quantitative, with inherent interobserver variation, and more objective methods for assessing disease extent in CT images will be examined later.

□ THE ROLE OF HRCT IN THE MANAGEMENT OF DIFFUSE LUNG DISEASE

Conclusions about the precise role of HRCT in the management of diffuse lung disease cannot be readily drawn from the studies of diagnostic accuracy reported so far. This, in part, is because of their failure to replicate real-life circumstances. For example, in many studies, reading radiologists are provided with a fixed number of predetermined diagnostic possibilities from which to choose. Furthermore, issues that relate to the effect of HRCT on diagnostic confidence and clinical decision making have not, by and large, been addressed.

Some series, however, stand out in this regard. In a study of a wide range of diffuse lung diseases, Grenier *et al* were the first to demonstrate an incremental and substantial improvement in diagnostic accuracy and confidence with the addition of HRCT (over and above clinical and radiographic data).[6] The methods were impaired by the use of retrospective data, however, as well as the use of sensitivity as an end-point. Aziz *et al* used a radically different approach in their assessment of thin-section CT in patients with diffuse lung disease.[7] Rather than comparing the results with histology, they studied the impact of HRCT on a variety of different variables. These included diagnostic confidence, interobserver agreement, and the perceived need to perform further diagnostic tests. The authors found that assimilation of HRCT with clinical and radiographic data resulted in an increase in the level of interobserver agreement and diagnostic confidence of pulmonologists, with fewer differential diagnoses offered. Overall, the first-choice diagnosis changed in 50% of cases. Interestingly, the improvement in interobserver agreement was less impressive in cases of sarcoidosis and hypersensitivity pneumonitis than in other interstitial lung diseases. In cases of hypersensitivity pneumonitis in which there is an identifiable causative agent, it is unsurprising that CT did not change the differential diagnosis, while in sarcoidosis (in which HRCT is not performed routinely), the diagnosis is often readily made on the basis of clinical and radiographic assessment alone.

The same study looked at the impact of HRCT on the decision by clinicians to perform further investigations. Overall, requests for surgical lung biopsies fell by only 6% after findings from CT were incorporated. The reduction was more striking in the specific context of IPF, however, in which the biopsy rate decreased from 27% to 12%.[7] Biopsy was suggested to be most relevant in non-IPF cases or when radiological findings were indeterminate.

Inevitably, the influence of HRCT on the management of diffuse lung disease depends, to an extent, on the experience of the reading radiologist. Clinicians may, for example, add greater weighting to a report from an experienced radiologist. Most diagnostic series involve thoracic radiologists from referral centres, so it may be difficult to extrapolate these findings more widely.

□ CURRENT AND FUTURE AREAS OF RESEARCH

The prospect of CT serving as a sensitive and objective marker of disease severity in various diffuse lung diseases, particularly for clinical trials, is a topic that has attracted much interest recently. In particular, the phenotyping and quantitative assessment of chronic obstructive pulmonary disease (COPD), IPF, and cystic fibrosis (CF) by means of CT have been the focus of attention.

Chronic obstructive pulmonary disease

Computed tomography has been shown to characterise, with precision, both emphysema and airway disease in patients with COPD. The typical features of emphysema on HRCT are areas of low attenuation or density, which are often surrounded by normal lung parenchyma. The assessment of lung density, as determined by the number of Hounsfield Units (HU), forms the basis of simpler methods of computer-aided quantitative imaging in patients with COPD. Disease extent, for example, may be quantified by the mean lung density, the number of pixels below a certain density value, or analysis of density histograms (in which the frequency of different pixel densities is plotted). These methods have been shown to correlate well with pulmonary function testing.[8] As a significant proportion of smokers with normal lung function will show evidence of emphysema on imaging, CT is likely to represent a more sensitive marker of disease progression in clinical trials than lung function tests.

Computed tomography has also been used in the longitudinal assessment of COPD. Measurements of lung density based on images from CT can be used to document the progression of disease in patients with COPD, with a good correlation demonstrated between inflammatory markers in sputum at baseline and disease progression according to images from CT. Such applications illustrate the potential of CT for identifying prognostic indicators and patients at risk of disease progression.

Research, to date, has tended to concentrate on the assessment of lung parenchyma rather than airway remodelling in patients with COPD. The advent of multidetector CT, however, has also enabled the more precise evaluation of airway wall thickness and bronchial luminal size with computer-aided techniques. For example, investigators have shown a significant correlation between airway wall thickness and pulmonary function parameters (Fig 2).[8] Although airflow limitation and large airway wall thickness are linked, the small airways are also well known to be an important site of pathology in patients with COPD; however, precise definition, visualisation, and quantitative analysis of the 'small airways' by CT has proved more difficult.[9]

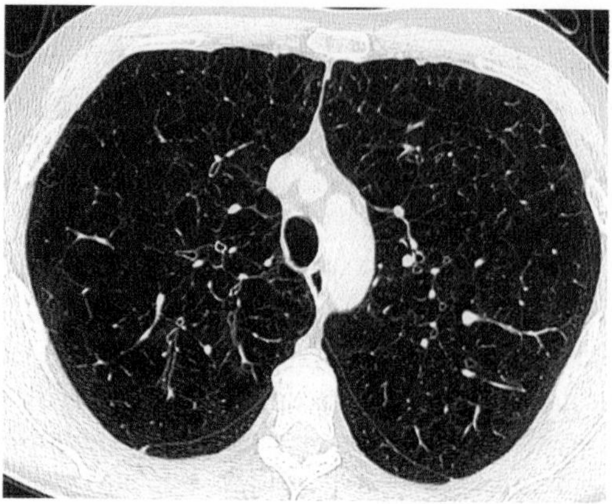

Fig 2 Image from high-resolution computed tomography of the upper lobes of an individual with chronic obstructive pulmonary disease. Both the centrilobular emphysema and the thickening of bronchial walls contribute to airflow limitation.

Areas of low attenuation in the lung are not exclusively the result of emphysema and may be the result of constrictive obliterative bronchiolitis, for example. 'Automated texture analysis' is a novel tool by which mathematical formulations are applied to MDCT to enable identification of specific subtypes of lung density. Chabat *et al* showed that texture analysis was able to discriminate between various types of obstructive lung disease with some accuracy.[10]

Finally, the pathogenesis is well recognised to differ in subgroups of patients with COPD. One phenotype is characterised by predominantly airways disease, whereas patients in another group will exhibit predominantly parenchymal destruction. Computed tomography has a crucial role to play in stratifying these groups of patients in future drug trials. For example, therapeutic interventions that target alveolar remodelling are unlikely to be successful in patients with predominantly macroscopic airway inflammation (bronchitis).

Cystic fibrosis

Visual scoring systems that use images from CT are well established in the context of CF, and it has long been postulated that CT analyses of airway dimensions could serve as an outcome marker in longitudinal studies and clinical trials. For instance, HRCT scores have been shown to be more sensitive than pulmonary function tests and chest radiographs in detecting early CF and in monitoring disease progression (Fig 3). This may be especially true in younger patients, in whom spirometry is more dependent on technique. Recently, investigators have applied more reproducible and automated software-dependent scoring systems of air trapping, airway luminal size, and wall thickness to cystic fibrosis and have used these with success in clinical trials. Despite the advantages of HRCT in the imaging of patients with CF compared with plain radiography, however, the radiation burden, as discussed earlier, cannot be ignored. The excess lifetime risk of developing radiation-induced cancer is clearly greater in the paediatric population, and it seems hard to justify the use of 'routine' HRCT in patients with CF.[11]

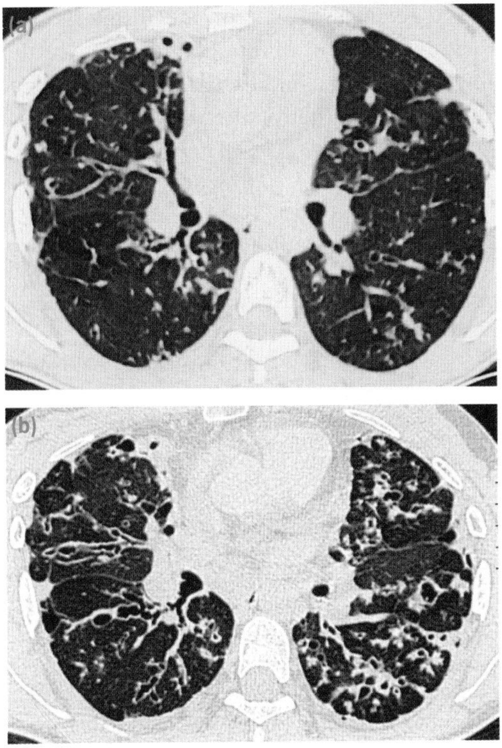

Fig 3 Serial images from computed tomography of a patient with cystic fibrosis obtained (a) at baseline and (b) 18 months later, showing marked progression of the bronchiectasis and mucous plugging. During this period, forced expiratory volume in one second (FEV_1) and forced vital capacity (FVC) decreased by less than 10%.

Idiopathic pulmonary fibrosis

The computer-derived scoring systems based on density histograms already described for COPD have also been used to analyse interstitial lung disease. Features such as mean lung attenuation, skewness, and kurtosis (that is, the sharpness and skewing of the lung density histogram peak from CT) can be analysed to produce a numerical value. The degree of correlation between these values and a range of pulmonary function parameters in patients with IPF is moderate. Interestingly, there is a significant degree of interscanner disagreement, which can be attributed to the variation in protocols used between different CT scanners.

Automated texture analysis may also have a role in the assessment of IPF. As described with COPD, this permits the identification and discrimination of different lung densities, such as ground-glass opacification or emphysema. Although such scoring systems may not yet have a place in routine clinical practice, they nevertheless have the potential to be used as a reproducible research tool in longitudinal studies of interstitial lung disease.[12]

□ CONCLUSION

Advances in CT technology have brought about the ability to produce massive volumes of high-resolution data of the thorax in a matter of seconds. Whether this new technology has resulted in improved diagnostic abilities in the purely clinical arena is questionable. Nevertheless, CT remains pivotal in the diagnosis and subsequent management of patients with a variety of diffuse lung diseases. In the future, it is also likely to have tangible benefits in clinical trials and longitudinal studies, especially in the context of automated quantitative disease evaluation.

REFERENCES

1 Dawson P. Patient dose in multislice CT: why is it increasing and does it matter? *Br J Radiol* 2004;77:S10–3.

2 Mayo JR, Aldrich J, Muller NL. Radiation exposure at chest CT: a statement of the Fleischner Society. *Radiology* 2003;228:15–21

3 Flaherty KR, Travis WD, Colby TV *et al.* Histopathologic variability in usual and nonspecific interstitial pneumonias. *Am J Respir Crit Care Med* 2001;164:1722–7.

4 MacDonald SL, Rubens MB, Hansell DM *et al.* Nonspecific interstitial pneumonia and usual interstitial pneumonia: comparative appearances at and diagnostic accuracy of thin-section CT. *Radiology* 2001;221:600–5

5 Wells AU, Desai SR, Rubens MB *et al.* Idiopathic pulmonary fibrosis: a composite physiologic index derived from disease extent observed by computed tomography. *Am J Respir Crit Care Med* 2003;167:962–9.

6 Grenier P, Chevret S, Beigelman C *et al.* Chronic diffuse infiltrative lung disease: determination of the diagnostic value of clinical data, chest radiography, and CT and Bayesian analysis. *Radiology* 1994;191:383–90.

7 Aziz ZA, Well AU, Bateman ED *et al.* Interstitial lung disease: effects of thin-section CT on clinical decision making. *Radiology* 2006;238:725–33

8 Aziz ZA, Wells AU, Desai SR *et al.* Functional impairment in emphysema: contribution of airway abnormalities and distribution of parenchymal disease. *AJR Am J Roentgenol* 2005; 185:1509–15.

9 Hansell DM. Small airways diseases: detection and insights with computed tomography. *Eur Respir J* 2001;17:1294–313

10 Chabat F, Yang GZ, Hansell DM. Obstructive lung diseases: texture classification for differentiation at CT. *Radiology* 2003;228:871–7.

11 Langton Hewer SC. Is limited computed tomography the future for imaging the lungs of children with cystic fibrosis? *Arch Dis Child* 2006;91:377–8.

12 Hoffman EA, Reinhardt JM, Sonka M *et al.* Characterization of the interstitial lung diseases via density-based and texture-based analysis of computed tomography images of lung structure and function. *Acad Radiol* 2003;10:1104–18.

Cancer imaging

Dow-Mu Koh

There is nothing permanent except change.
Heraclitus, 6th century BC

□ INTRODUCTION

The history of imaging has been characterised by rapid changes in the last century. In 1895, Wilhelm Roentgen discovered X-rays, which enabled visualisation of the bony structures within the body for the first time. The subsequent synthesis of water-soluble contrast media (1930s) and radionuclear isotopes (1940s) expanded the range of imaging tests. Ultrasound was invented in the 1960s, and this allowed soft tissue organs in the abdomen and pelvis to be explored. In 1972, Sir Godfrey Hounsfield piloted the first scanner for computed tomography (CT), which revolutionised imaging by enabling cross sectional images of the body to be acquired. A decade later, the invention of magnetic resonance imaging (MRI) provided a means of visualising the body without ionising radiation by mapping differences in the magnetic relaxivity of tissues. These techniques form the foundation of cancer imaging today and allow us to detect and stage cancer, as well as to assess the effects of treatment.

In the past decade, the field of cancer imaging has continued to expand and grow in response to new challenges posed by our increasing understanding of the molecular basis of cancer and the introduction of novel targeted treatments to clinics. Technological advancement in imaging software and hardware has enabled more rapid acquisition and processing of images, which has led to the growth of functional imaging techniques. The adoption of a multidisciplinary approach to cancer care has also placed radiologists in the heart of planning for cancer treatment and patient management.[1]

In light of recent developments, the aim of cancer imaging thus is to optimise treatment and improve outcomes by providing accurate non-invasive measurements of the morphological, pathophysiological, metabolic, and molecular properties of tumours.

□ RECENT ADVANCES IN CANCER IMAGING

A number of important imaging advances in the past decade are changing how imaging is used to assess tumours.

High-spatial resolution imaging

High-spatial resolution imaging is possible with multidetector CT and multichannel MRI technologies. Multidetector CT allows very thin (1–2 mm) axial cross sectional images of the body to be routinely acquired and reformatted to produce images in different planes (for example, the coronal and sagittal planes). Visualisation of a tumour in multiple imaging planes allows better delineation and appreciation of the relation between a tumour and adjacent structures (Fig 1).

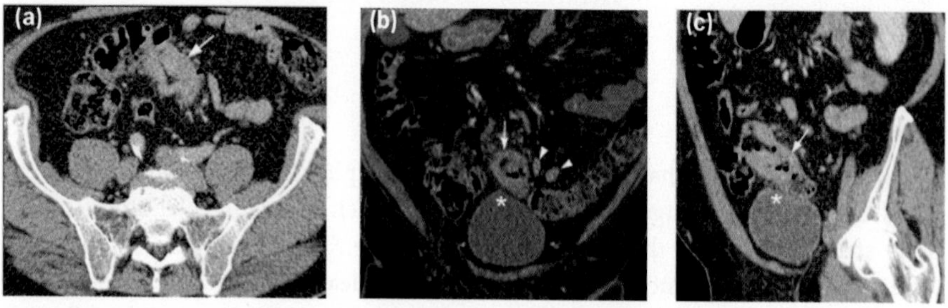

Fig 1 Images from high-spatial resolution computed tomography. **(a)** Image acquired in the axial plane shows diffuse thickening of the sigmoid colon in keeping with a carcinoma (arrow). Images reformatted in the **(b)** coronal and **(c)** sagittal planes show the relation between the tumour (arrows) and the dome of the bladder (*); no evidence of bladder involvement, which might require more radical surgery, is seen. Note also the two enlarged pericolic lymph nodes.

High-spatial resolution MRI can accurately reflect changes observed at the histopathological level. For example, MRI in patients with rectal cancer can accurately depict the morphology and stage of the primary tumour and define the relation between the tumour and important anatomical landmarks.

New contrast mechanisms

A number of new contrast mechanisms enable tumour tissues to be distinguished from normal tissues. For example, the administration of an intravenous contrast medium may highlight tumour tissues and facilitate their detection.

One recently developed contrast medium contains ultra-small particles of iron oxide (USPIO), which are used in combination with MRI to detect nodal metastases; this technique is also known as magnetic resonance lymphography. After intravenous administration, the USPIO nanoparticles escape into the interstitial spaces of tissues and are transported by lymphatic vessels into the lymph nodes. Within the lymph nodes, the USPIO are phagocytosed by nodal macrophages. Consequently, normal nodal tissues that contain macrophages appear dark on images obtained with a magnetic resonance technique sensitive to iron (T2(*)-weighted MRI). In contrast, tumour tissues that contain few macrophages appear bright in images (Fig 2).

Tumour tissues also can be distinguished from normal tissues (without the need to administer an exogenous contrast material) through differences in their intrinsic imaging properties. Diffusion-weighted MRI (DWI) derives contrast in images from

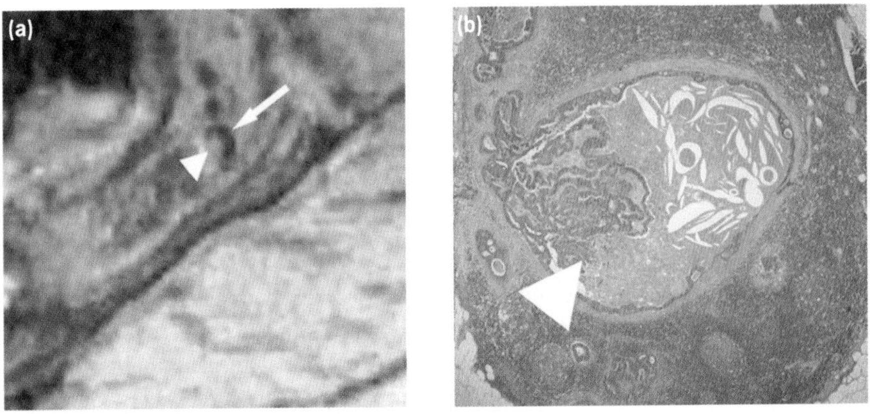

Fig 2 Images from magnetic resonance enhanced with ultra-small particles of iron oxide (USPIO). **(a)** Image obtained with T2(*)-weighted MRI after administration of USPIO shows darkening of the nodal cortex (arrow) but an eccentric bright focus (high signal intensity) remains (arrowhead). **(b)** Histopathology (haematoxylin and eosin stain, five times multiplication) confirms that the bright focus is due to metastatic disease (arrowhead) within the partially replaced node. Reproduced from Koh *et al* with permission of the Radiological Society of North America.[3]

differences in the motion of water molecules between tissues. The motion of water molecules is more restricted in tumour tissues than in normal tissues, and this difference in the mobility of water molecules can be harnessed to detect tumours through DWI (Fig 3).

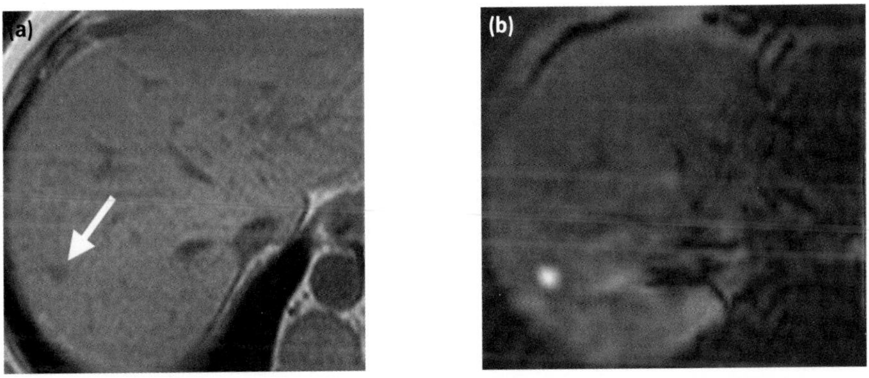

Fig 3 Diffusion-weighted magnetic resonance imaging. **(a)** Image from T1-weighted MRI shows an ill-defined metastasis in the right lobe of the liver (arrow). **(b)** The lesion is seen more clearly with diffusion-weighted magnetic resonance imaging because of the increased contrast between the metastasis and the adjacent liver, and this facilitates its detection.

Positron emission tomography (PET) relies on another contrast mechanism and detects tumours on the basis of uptake of radioactive tracers, which differs between malignant and non-malignant tissues. For example, uptake of fluorodeoxyglucose tracer reflects glucose metabolism and uptake of fluorothymidine tracer reflects cellular proliferation.

Functional imaging techniques

Functional imaging techniques probe specific aspects of tumour pathophysiology and allow quantitative measurements of these to be taken. Such methods are used increasingly to study different facets of the tumour microenvironment, such as tumour vascularity (dynamic contrast-enhanced CT and MRI), cellularity (DWI), hypoxia (PET and MRI dependent on levels of oxygenation of blood), metabolism (PET and magnetic resonance spectroscopy), cellular proliferation (PET), and tumour apoptosis (PET).

Most of these imaging techniques do not measure altered pathophysiology in tumours directly but instead measure the downstream effects of changes in the tumour's microenvironment. Imaging-derived functional measurements thus are frequently called 'surrogate imaging markers' or 'surrogate biomarkers'. Surrogate imaging markers are used increasingly in clinical studies to assess treatment responses to novel drugs, as conventional measurements of tumour size may be insensitive to the effects of such treatments.

Fusion imaging

Fusion imaging allows the diagnostic information of one imaging technique to be combined with information from another technique. This development has been facilitated by significant advances in computing capabilities and image registration techniques.

One of the most important and commonly used fusion imaging techniques is PET–CT (Fig 4). Imaging with PET yields functional information about tumour metabolism but has poor anatomical detail. In comparison, conventional CT imaging provides detailed anatomical information but no functional data. The combination of information from these two imaging methods thus can be seen as a strategy to maximise the advantages of individual techniques while minimising their disadvantages.

□ CLINICAL APPLICATIONS OF CANCER IMAGING

As a result of the recent advances, we can now use imaging for early diagnosis of cancer, to detect small volume disease, to provide roadmaps for treatment planning, and to enable novel assessment of treatment response and disease prognostication. The following section will provide illustrative examples of the evolving roles of cancer imaging.

Early diagnosis of disease

In patients with breast cancer, mammographic screening has been shown to decrease mortality. In the United Kingdom (UK), mammographic screening saves about eight lives per 1,000 women screened.

Contrast-enhanced, high-spatial resolution MRI was recently used successfully to detect cancer in women with a strong family history of breast cancer and those with a substantial genetic risk of developing breast cancer (for example, those with mutations in the *BRCA1* gene). Evidence is gathering for the use of MRI to screen for breast cancer in this select group of individuals. In one of the larger published studies (the MRI screening for breast cancer (MARIBS) trial in the UK),[2] MRI was found to be twice as sensitive as mammography for the detection of breast cancer in populations at substantial genetic risk. In patients with mutations in the *BRCA1* gene, in whom high-density normal breast tissue may obscure cancers for conventional mammography, MRI was found to be four times more sensitive than mammography. On the strength of such evidence, MRI has been advocated for screening women with an increased genetic risk of developing breast cancer.

Detection of small volume disease

The pattern of contrast enhancement achieved with MRI enhanced by USPIO can be used to identify small foci of metastatic disease in partially infiltrated lymph nodes independent of nodal size or morphology.[3] In a study of 80 patients with prostate cancer, this technique had high sensitivity (92%), specificity (93%), and negative predictive value (97%).[4] Interestingly, 71% of malignant nodes in the study did not fulfil the criteria for malignancy according to measurements of their size. A recent meta-analysis of several published series showed that MRI enhanced by USPIO resulted in 88% (95% confidence interval 85% to 91%) sensitivity and 96% (95% to 97%) specificity for the detection of malignant nodes.[5]

Imaging with 2-deoxy-2-^{18}F-D-glucose (^{18}FDG) PET can be used to identify and localise unusual sites of disease dissemination. In patients with colorectal cancer, PET has high sensitivity and specificity for detecting extrahepatic disease, which can result in significant changes to management in up to 33% of patients (see Fig 4).[6]

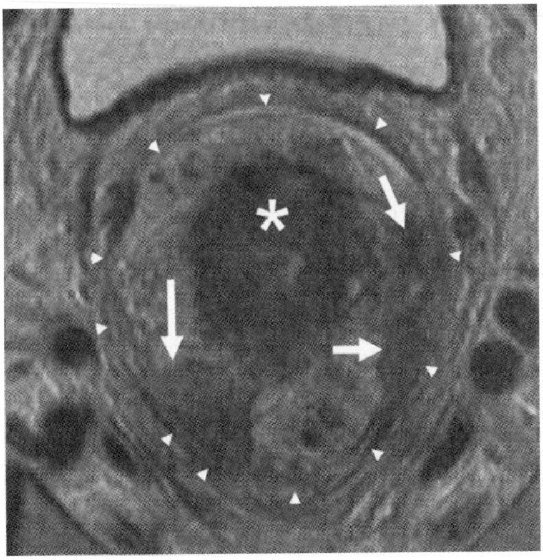

Fig 4 Magnetic resonance imaging predicts involvement of the circumferential resection margin at surgery. Image obtained with T2-weighted magnetic resonance in the axial plane shows an irregular rectal tumour (*) with disease extension into the mesorectum (arrows) (perirectal fat). Note that the local extension of the tumour is encroaching on the plane of total mesorectal excision surgery (arrowhead). Preoperative chemoradiation may be administered to downsize and downstage the tumour before surgery.

Roadmap for treatment planning

Imaging is now used routinely to plan treatment with surgery or radiotherapy. In patients with rectal cancer, curative surgery by total mesorectal excision surgery is achieved by sharp instrumental dissection along the mesorectal fascia, which forms the circumferential resection margin (CRM). Such surgery allows the tumour, surrounding mesorectal fat, and lymph nodes to be removed as an en bloc surgical specimen to minimise spillage of tumour cells.

Magnetic resonance imaging can accurately assess the relation between the tumour and the potential CRM. If the tumour is shown to reside within 1 mm of the CRM, this predicts involvement of the circumferential surgical margin.[7] Long term survival in patients with tumour involvement of the CRM is substantially worse than when the CRM is not involved.[8] The preoperative use of MRI to predict involvement of the CRM thus means that patients with tumour extension to the CRM can be offered neoadjuvant chemoradiation to downsize and downstage the disease before surgery (Fig 5).

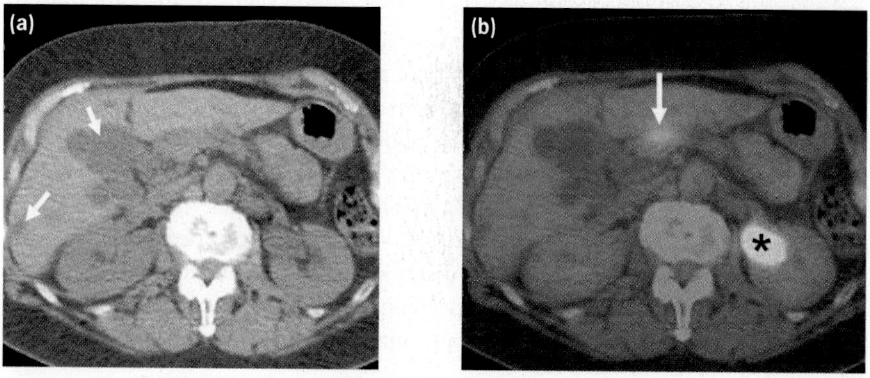

Fig 5 Positron emission tomography–computed tomography in a man aged 54 years with potentially curable colorectal cancer. **(a)** Image obtained with computed tomography shows a few hepatic cysts (arrows) but no other significant abnormality in the upper abdomen. **(b)** Fusion imaging with 2-deoxy-2-^{18}F-D-glucose positron emission tomography–computed tomography shows a hypermetabolic focus in the pancreas (arrow), which was proved to be malignant. Note also the increased tracer activity (*) within the left renal pelvis due to renal excretion of the tracer.

Novel assessment of treatment response

Tumour cells secrete proangiogenic factors, and these result in the transcription and translation of proteins that stimulate growth of endothelial cells. A number of drugs inhibit this pathway – for example, through direct effects on endothelial cells (eg combrestatin) or inhibition of activators of angiogenesis (eg bevacizumab). Other drugs act via other pathways, such as preventing matrix breakdown or other cell signalling pathways.

Conventional assessment of treatment response relies on serial measurements of tumour size as a surrogate response marker. Such measurements are insensitive, however, especially to the early effects of treatment. The use of functional imaging techniques allows quantitative parameters that reflect tumour vasculature – such as tumour blood volume, blood flow, and vascular permeability – to be derived through dynamic, contrast-enhanced CT or MRI studies. Such techniques are now employed widely in clinical trials to provide surrogate measurements of the effects of drugs (Fig 6).[9] Although direct imaging of drug activity at the site of drug interaction is now possible in animal models, such imaging is still limited in humans.

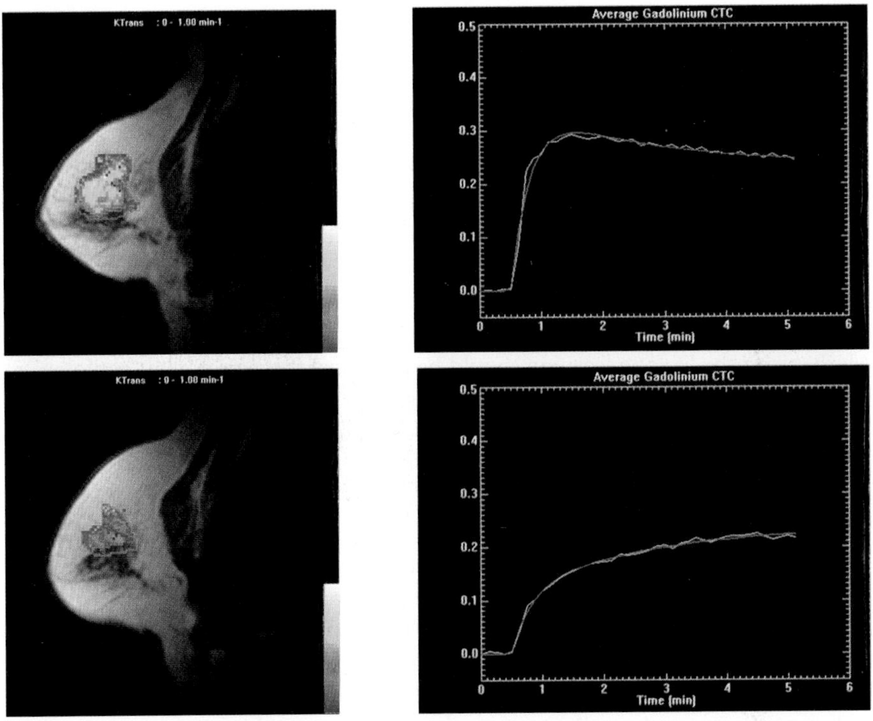

Fig 6 Quantitative maps of K^{trans} (an imaging-derived index that reflects blood flow and vascular permeability) and accompanying curves obtained from a woman with breast cancer through dynamic-enhanced magnetic resonance imaging show the rate of contrast uptake in the tumour during assessment of tumour vascularity. Before treatment, the tumour had high K^{trans} values and rapid contrast enhancement followed by early contrast washout typical of malignant tissue. After chemotherapy was complete, K^{trans} reduced within the tumour and the enhancement curve normalised. Reproduced courtesy of James D'Arcy.

Disease prognostication

Measurements of function through imaging can provide novel prognostic information. For example, DWI allows determination of a quantitative parameter – the apparent diffusion coefficient (ADC) of tissues, which reflects tissue cellularity and the integrity of cell membranes. This coefficient is low in highly cellular tissues with intact cellular membranes (such as tumour tissue); in contrast, necrotic tissues have high ADCs.

Diffusion-weighted MRI has shown that a low ADC before treatment can predict better responses to chemotherapy and radiotherapy. This effect has been shown in patients with primary rectal cancers[10] and, more recently, in those with colorectal cancer and metastases in the liver. The biological basis for this observation is not entirely clear, but it may relate to the fact that tumours with high ADC values are more likely to be necrotic. Necrotic tumours are more frequently hypoxic and poorly perfused, which diminishes their sensitivity to chemotherapy and radiotherapy. In the future, such prognostic information may help to individualise treatment strategies for patients with cancer.

☐ ISSUES AND CHALLENGES

Despite significant advancements in cancer imaging, there clearly are challenges ahead. As imaging becomes more sophisticated, new technologies are often expensive and not widely available. Healthcare providers thus must rationalise their use of such new techniques. Cost effective analysis can assess the cost to benefit ratio of these techniques for clinical use and healthcare delivery.

Imaging technologies are changing and progressing at a rapid pace. New imaging techniques are increasingly complex, and doctors involved in imaging have to keep abreast of new developments in the field of radiology, as well as molecular medicine. Mechanisms for lifelong learning should be enhanced through existing radiological communities and meetings, as well as through new e-learning initiatives, which can harness the power of the world wide web and digital media for education and delivery of information.

The past decade has seen a significant decrease in mortality from cancer in the UK, largely as a result of earlier diagnosis and improved treatment of cancer. Although new imaging techniques are transforming our ability to visualise cancers, the ultimate impact of these technologies on patient survival and outcome currently is unclear. As such, long term studies on the health impact of imaging techniques are needed, although such studies may not be easy to conduct, as imaging technology is changing at such a phenomenal pace. Indeed, new techniques may supersede existing techniques before such studies are completed, and it would be difficult to deter the introduction of new and promising technologies into the healthcare market.

☐ CONCLUSIONS

Imaging is central to the management of patients with cancer. Recent advances in cancer imaging have had a major impact on the diagnosis, staging, treatment planning, and monitoring of treatment in patients with cancer. Functional imaging techniques are increasingly used to assess response to new treatments and can provide unique prognostic information that may help in the development of individualised management strategies in the future.

REFERENCES

1 Koh DM, Cook GJ, Husband JE. New horizons in oncologic imaging. *N Engl J Med* 2003; 348:2487–8.

2 Leach MO, Boggis CR, Dixon AK *et al.* Screening with magnetic resonance imaging and mammography of a UK population at high familial risk of breast cancer: a prospective multicentre cohort study (MARIBS). *Lancet* 2005;365:1769–78.

3 Koh DM, Brown G, Temple L *et al.* Rectal cancer: mesorectal lymph nodes at MR imaging with USPIO versus histopathologic findings – initial observations. *Radiology* 2004;231:91–9.

4 Harisinghani MG, Barentsz J, Hahn PF *et al.* Noninvasive detection of clinically occult lymph-node metastases in prostate cancer. *N Engl J Med* 2003;348:2491–9.

5 Will O, Purkayastha S, Chan C *et al.* Diagnostic precision of nanoparticle-enhanced MRI for lymph-node metastases: a meta-analysis. *Lancet Oncol* 2006;7:52–60.

6 Vogel WV, Wiering B, Corstens FH, Ruers TJ, Oyen WJ. Colorectal cancer: the role of PET/CT in recurrence. *Cancer Imaging* 2005;5 (Spec No A):S143–9.

7 MERCURY Study Group. Extramural depth of tumor invasion at thin-section MR in patients with rectal cancer: results of the MERCURY study. *Radiology* 2007;243:132–9.

8 Adam IJ, Mohamdee MO, Martin IG *et al.* Role of circumferential margin involvement in the local recurrence of rectal cancer. *Lancet* 1994;344:707–11.

9 Workman P, Aboagye EO, Chung YL *et al.* Minimally invasive pharmacokinetic and pharmacodynamic technologies in hypothesis-testing clinical trials of innovative therapies. *J Natl Cancer Inst* 2006;98:580–98.

10 Dzik-Jurasz A, Domenig C, George M *et al.* Diffusion MRI for prediction of response of rectal cancer to chemoradiation. *Lancet* 2002;360:307–8.

Endocrine imaging

Nicola Hilary Strickland

□ INTRODUCTION

This article concentrates on some specific areas of endocrine imaging, in particular:

- pancreatic neuroendocrine tumours
- carcinoid tumours
- pituitary tumours
- adrenal lesions.

Some varied pathology is demonstrated, and the clinical applications of the various imaging techniques and their pitfalls are discussed.

□ PANCREATIC NEUROENDOCRINE TUMOURS

Pancreatic neuroendocrine tumours may be sporadic or may occur in association with multiple endocrine neoplasia 1 (MEN1) – an autosomal dominant adenomatous hyperplasia (Table 1).

Table 1 Approximate incidence of tumours in patients with multiple endocrine neoplasia type 1 (MEN1).

Tumour type	Approximate incidence (%)
Pancreatic islet cell tumours	70
Gastrinoma (Zollinger–Ellison syndrome)	60
Insulinoma	30
VIPoma	
Parathyroid (mainly hyperplasia)	>95
Pituitary adenomata	40
With or without carcinoid, adrenal nodular hyperplasia, thymoma, lipoma, etc	About 10

Pancreatic islet cell tumours characteristically enhance avidly in the arterial phase of contrast enhancement (about 25 seconds after peripheral intravenous injection), and this vascular blush persists well into the venous phase of contrast enhancement (about 60 seconds, and longer after injection) (Fig 1). Both the primary islet cell tumour and its metastases show vascular enhancement well into the portal venous phase of contrast enhancement (Fig 2).

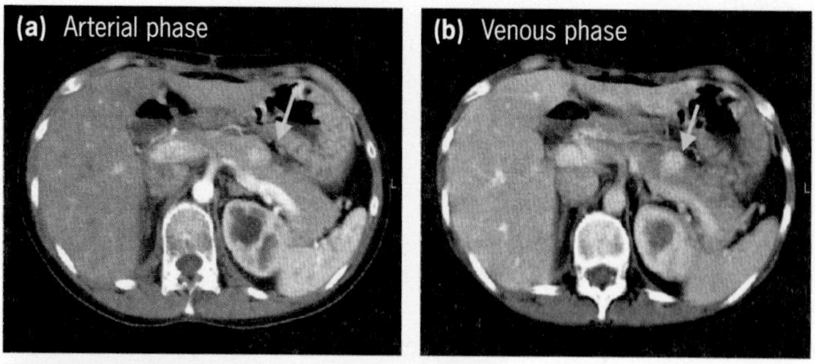

Fig 1 **(a)** Insulinoma in pancreatic body in arterial phase of contrast enhancement; and **(b)** the same lesion showing enhancement persisting into venous phase.

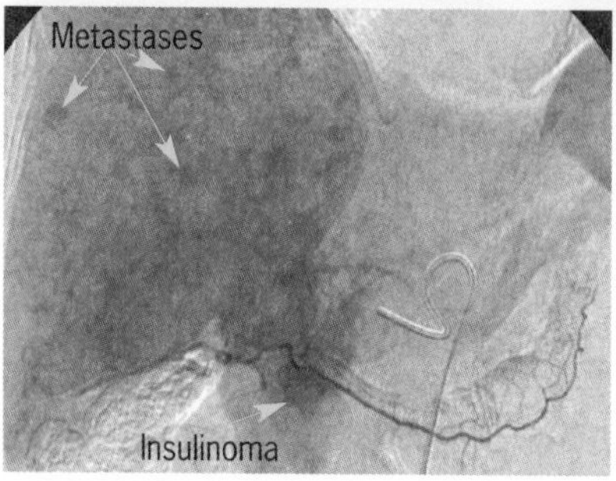

Fig 2 Metastases in liver on venous phase of a digital subtraction angiogram, with the primary insulinoma in the neck of pancreas, all showing persistent enhancement.

Gastrinomata may be tiny and multiple in the wall of the duodenum or stomach, or both. Their detection is facilitated by distending the stomach and upper small bowel with water (which the patient drinks before scanning takes place) and by giving intravenous hyoscine butylbromide to induce gastrointestinal stasis and better distend the upper gastrointestinal tract during computed tomography (CT). Hypersecretion of gastrin from a gastrinoma frequently induces gastric rugal hyperplasia (Fig 3). (Rugal hyperplasia cannot be assessed in a collapsed stomach, which may give the spurious impression of prominent rugae.)

Pancreatic islet cell tumours are often small, and their avid enhancement by contrast agents easily can be mistaken for a vessel if careful analysis of the normal anatomy is not made. Review of CT scans on monitors in cine or stack mode

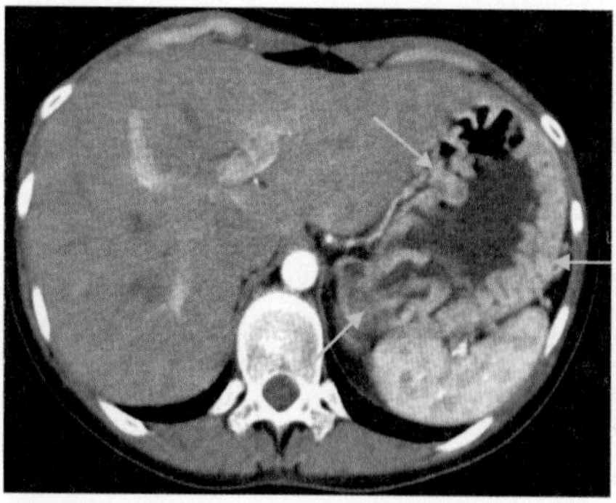

Fig 3 Rugal hyperplasia in a patient with duodenal and pancreatic gastrinomata (not shown).

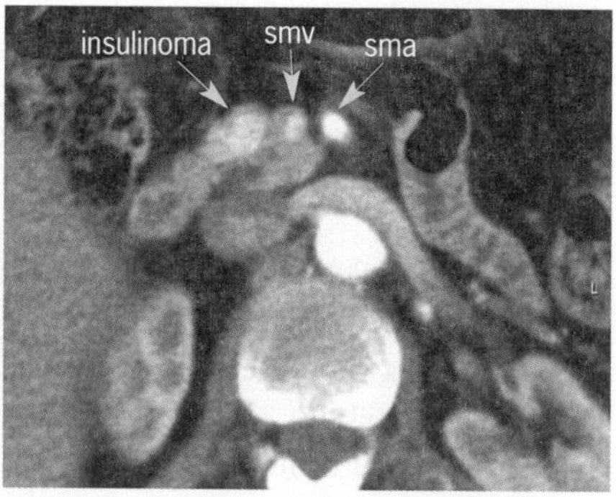

Fig 4 Small insulinoma lying just lateral to normal superior mesenteric vein (smv) and superior mesenteric artery (sma), and medial to water-filled second part of duodemum.

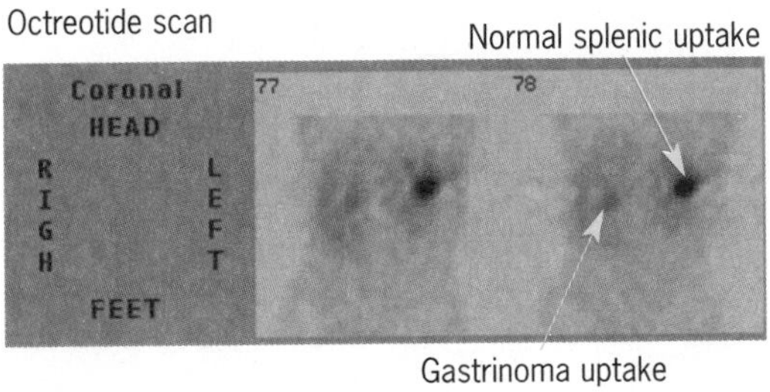

Fig 5 Octreotide-avid small gastrinoma in the right of the abdomen.

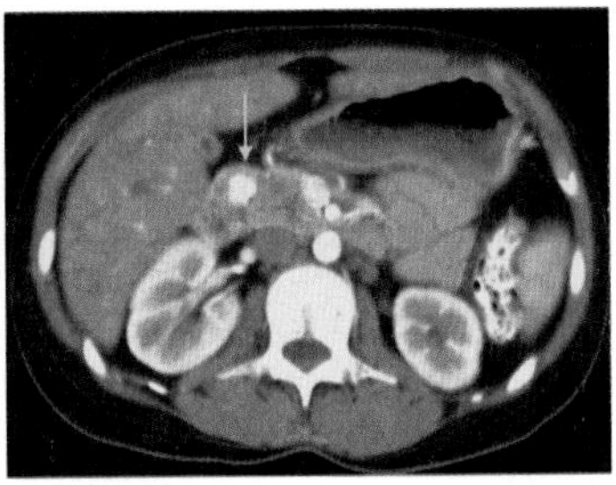

Fig 6 Gastrinoma (arrow) located by CT scan to lie in medial wall of second part of the duodenum, just lateral to the pancreatic head (same patient as Fig 5).

facilitates tracing the vascular anatomy from slice to slice by delineating the cranial and caudal extent of the small pancreatic tumours and thus distinguishing them from continuous vessels (Fig 4)

A nuclear medicine scan with radiolabelled octreotide is used to identify pancreatic islet cell tumours. Octreotide is a somatostatin analogue of eight amino acids, which binds to somatostatin receptors. Somatostatin receptors are expressed in almost 100% of gastrinomas, glucagonomas, VIPomas (vasoactive intestinal peptide-secreting tumours), and carcinoid tumours, but in only about half of insulinomas. It is important to use single-photon emission computed tomography (SPECT) for a three-dimensional acquisition effect when scanning with octreotide in order to avoid the problem of avid splenic uptake of octreotide, which obscures small pancreatic islet cell tumours in the pancreatic tail that would otherwise be masked on planar imaging alone. As with all nuclear medicine imaging, octreotide scanning is a functional imaging modality that is sensitive to the presence of a pancreatic islet cell tumour but poor at anatomical localisation, as illustrated in Fig 5. The dedicated CT scan in Fig 6 allows precise anatomical localisation of the tumour.

Most centres nowadays report all cross-sectional imaging from soft copy (on monitors) and therefore can exploit the numerous soft-copy imaging tools to manipulate the image – for example, magnification and alteration of the width and level of greyscale contrast windows. Fig 7 illustrates the angiogram of a patient who had had a gastrinoma resected many years earlier and presented with markedly increased levels of gastrin, which indicated a recurrence. On first examination of the CT scan, the recurrence was not spotted, but the lesion is more evident when the width and level settings of the greyscale contrast window are narrowed (Fig 8). Imaging for endocrine tumours, particularly pancreatic islet cell tumours, should be carried out only after evidence for the presence of such a biochemically active lesion has been established from laboratory results.

A powerful tool for the localisation of small pancreatic islet cell tumours is invasive intra-arterial stimulation of the tumour with selective injection of calcium gluconate followed by venous sampling. Selective catheterisation of the superior mesenteric, gastroduodenal, splenic, right hepatic, and various subselective arteries

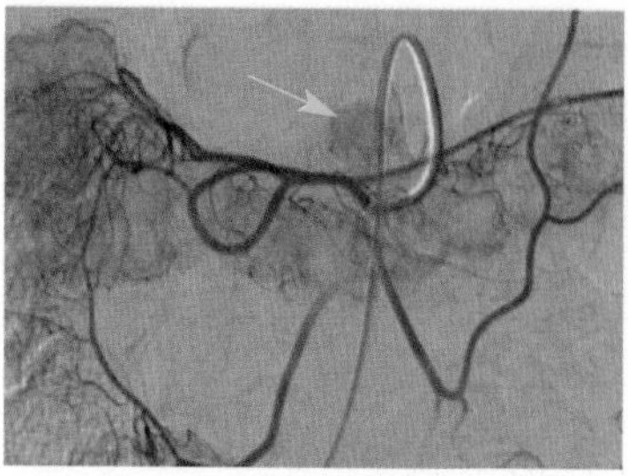

Fig 7 Gastrinoma recurrence seen as a vascular nodule, lying centrally superior to the transverse colon, on late arterial phase of a digital subtraction angiogram.

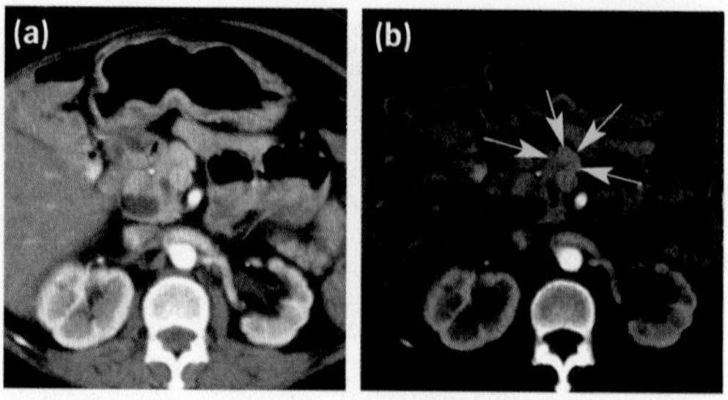

Fig 8 Gastrinoma recurrence (same patient as Fig 7) lying just anterior to the superior mesenteric vein, barely visible in **(a)** but much more conspicuous (arrowed) in **(b)**, where the greyscale contrast settings have been narrowed.

is performed, samples from the right hepatic vein are collected after injection of calcium gluconate, and a battery of hormonal assays are performed. Rigorous protocol, with meticulous recording of the injection sites in correct chronological order and obsessive labelling of the collected samples, is essential to the success of this technique. It generally is best to delegate this responsibility to a member of the clinical team so that the angiographer can concentrate on the imaging procedure.

Pancreatic islet cell tumours generally can also be well demonstrated with magnetic resonance imaging, which has the advantage of not using ionising irradiation. Magnetic resonance images take longer to acquire than CT scans and often require a variety of different sequences in order to show the lesion. Fig 9 shows a small insulinoma that, in this particular case, was only shown on one sequence of the magnetic resonance scan and had not been detected by CT. On careful retrospective review of this patient's CT scan (Fig 10), however, the lesion could be identified but was extremely subtle. When the width of the greyscale contrast window was narrowed, the lesion could be accentuated (Fig 10b).

The characteristic vascular enhancement of pancreatic islet cell tumours well into the late venous phase of angiographic imaging and CT can be a helpful diagnostic clue for aetiology. This is illustrated by a case (Fig 11), in which a woman presented with a history of both renal cell and breast carcinomata but now had new enhancing pancreatic lesions that, on CT-guided fine needle biopsy, were shown to be secondary metastatic deposits from her previous renal cell carcinoma rather than

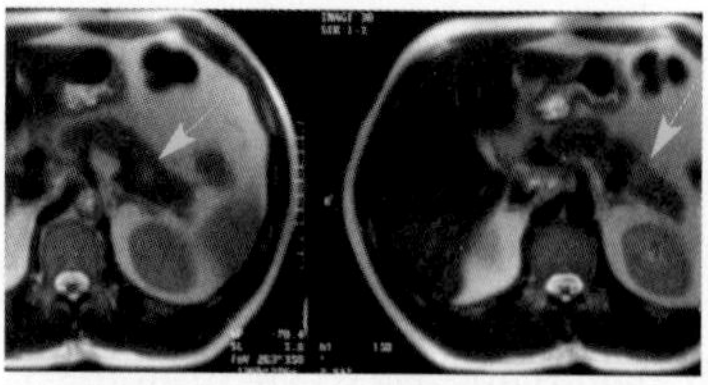

Fig 9 Contiguous sections of an MR scan showing small insulinoma in the pancreatic body.

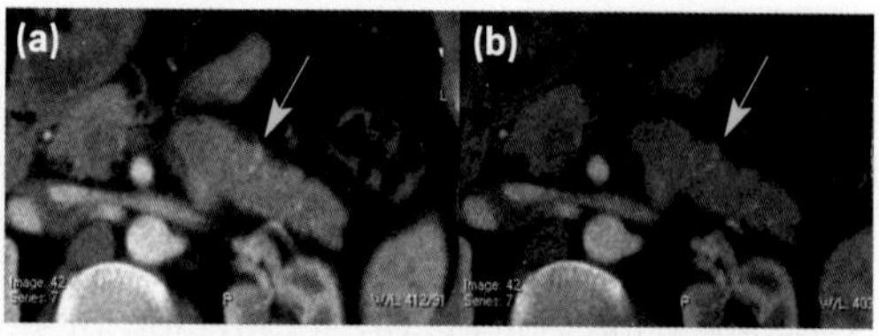

Fig 10 (a) CT scan of the same patient as in Fig 9. This insulinoma atypically shows only a minor vascular blush, which is more conspicuous on narrowing the greyscale window setting **(b)**.

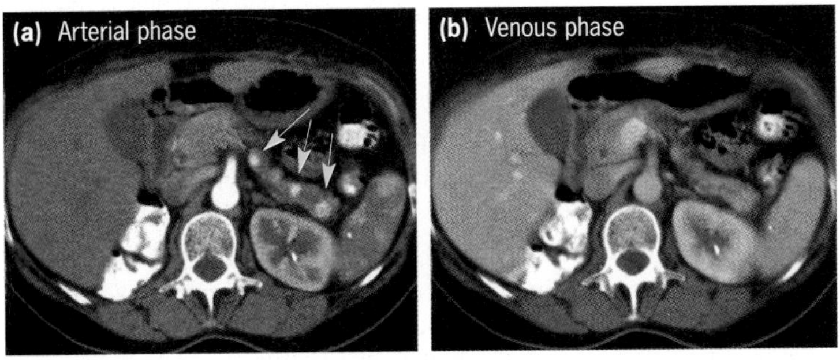

Fig 11 Renal carcinoma metastases in body and tail of pancreas that enhances in the arterial phase **(a)** but not in the venous phase **(b)**, unlike endocrine tumours.

the differential diagnostic possibility of new, non-secreting, pancreatic islet cell tumours. This result was suspected from the lack of persistent enhancement of these lesions on the venous phase of the scan, as expected for non-endocrine metastases.

It is worth noting, incidentally, that the differential diagnosis for huge tumours of the pancreas includes non-secreting endocrine lesions, as well as non-Hodgkin's lymphoma. Adenocarcinoma of the pancreas rarely reaches massive proportions before becoming symptomatic.

Ultrasound examination is a useful rapid initial investigation when looking for neuroendocrine pancreatic tumours and does not use ionising radiation, but it often is hampered by technical difficulty due to gas in the small bowel obscuring the pancreas, or due to patient obesity: both factors limit the resolution of the study. Endoscopic ultrasound is very sensitive for identifying lesions in the pancreatic head, uncinate process, and neck and proximal body, but it is less successful at showing lesions more distant from the endoscopic probe in the tail of the pancreas and for identifying metastatic lymphadenopathy. Computed tomography thus remains the mainstay of neuroendocrine pancreatic imaging, being quick and easily accessible in all centres. It is essential that multi-modality imaging (for example, endoscopic ultrasound) is tailored to the clinical problem and to local expertise.

□ CARCINOID TUMOURS

Pancreatic carcinoid and other gastrointestinal primary tumours sometimes can calcify, which gives a clue as to their possible aetiology (Fig 12). Calcified lesions are

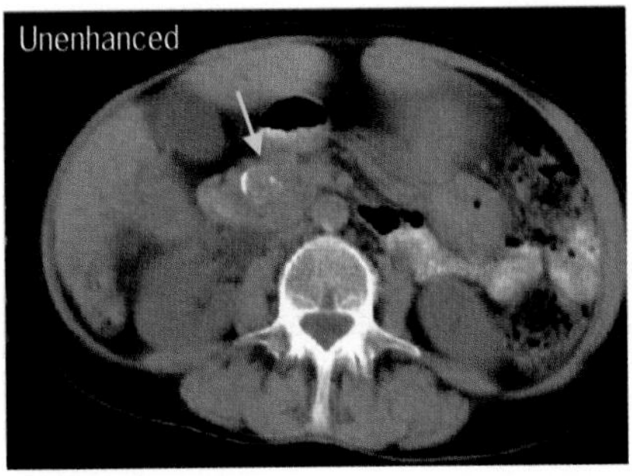

Fig 12 Calcified carcinoid tumour in head of pancreas (arrow) on an unenhanced CT scan.

well seen on CT, particularly on bone window settings. Most hepatic carcinoid metastases are best shown in the venous phase of CT. On first scanning a patient with hepatic carcinoid metastases, it is advisable to perform a triple-phase CT scan of the liver (unenhanced, arterial, and venous phase of contrast enhancement) to identify which phase renders the hepatic metastases most conspicuous. This phase of imaging then can be chosen for follow-up studies to maximise the accuracy of sequential lesion measurement (see Fig 13). Fig 14 shows an example of a nuclear medicine scan of hepatic carcinoid with radiolabelled octreotide. Carcinoid tumours are relatively slow growing compared with 'conventional' cancers such as colonic metastases, and patients are often followed for many years on medical treatment.

Symptoms in carcinoid hepatic metastatic disease are controlled by medical treatment, and only when the burden of tumour is such that symptoms can no longer be controlled medically, or there is pain from stretching of the hepatic capsule due to hepatomegaly would more aggressive therapeutic options be considered. These include arterial embolisation of the lesions by interventional radiology (Fig 15) or the administration of radiolabelled octreotide or lanreotide. It is important to remember that no treatment alters the course of disease in patients with metastatic hepatic carcinoid. Arterial hepatic artery embolisation is effective in selectively necrosing carcinoid metastases; metastases derive their blood supply entirely from the hepatic artery, whereas the normal hepatic parenchyma is supplied by the portal vein.

Carcinoid bone metastases are characteristically sclerotic, and the CT scan should be checked on a bone a window setting to render any bone metastases more conspicuous. Octreotide scans may also demonstrate bony metastases (see Fig 16).

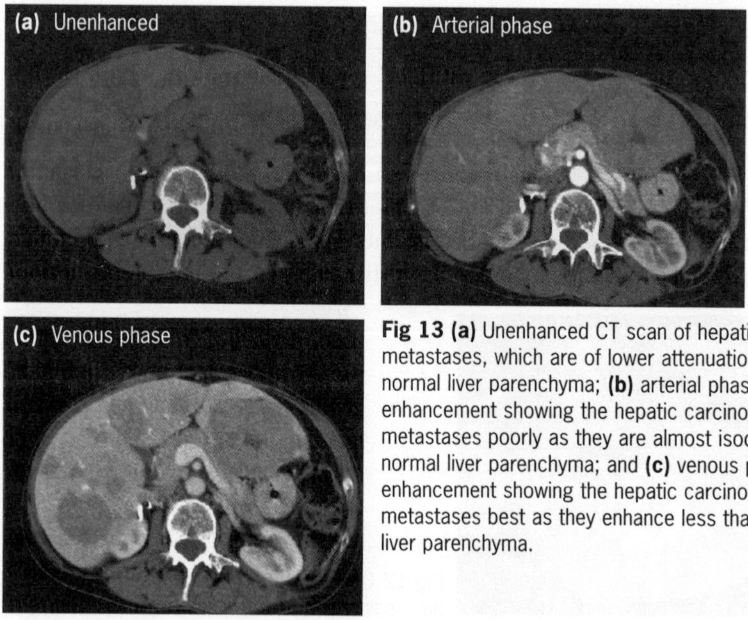

Fig 13 (a) Unenhanced CT scan of hepatic carcinoid metastases, which are of lower attenuation than normal liver parenchyma; **(b)** arterial phase enhancement showing the hepatic carcinoid metastases poorly as they are almost isodense with normal liver parenchyma; and **(c)** venous phase enhancement showing the hepatic carcinoid metastases best as they enhance less than normal liver parenchyma.

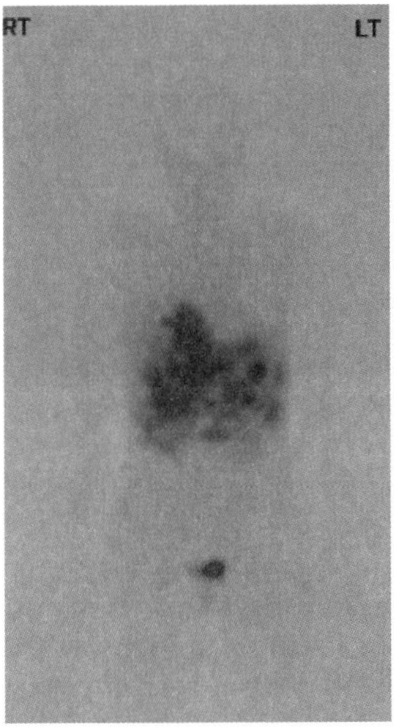

Fig 14 Octreotide scan showing avid uptake of isotope in carcinoid metastases in an enlarged liver. (The hotspot over the bladder is excreted radiolabel).

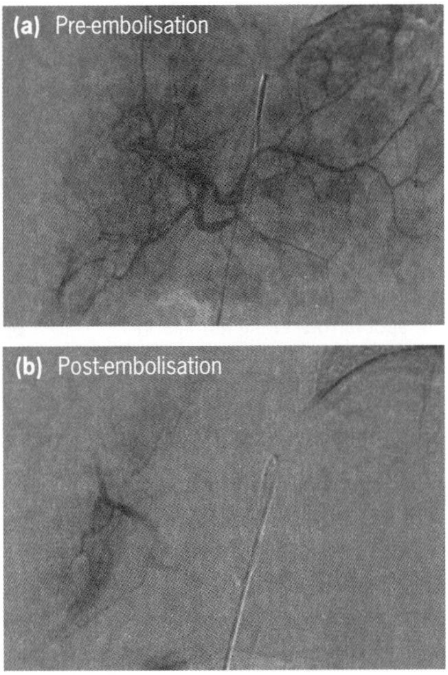

Fig 15 (a) Multiple vascular hepatic carcinoid metastases seen on a digital subtraction angiogram selectively injecting contrast into the hepatic artery (pre-embolisation) and **(b)** marked reduction in the number of carcinoid metastases visualised after their hepatic artery supply has been embolised (post-embolisation).

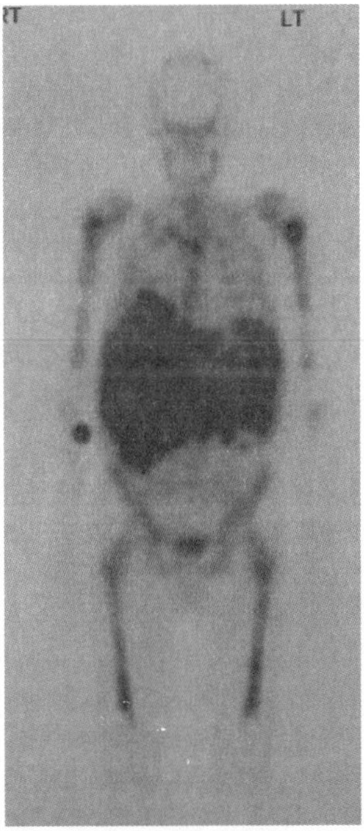

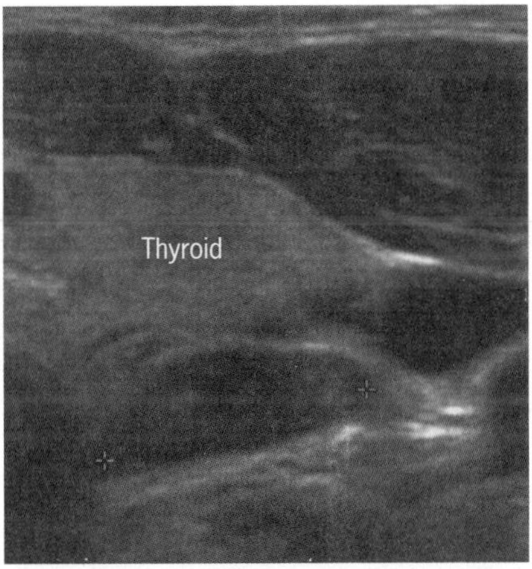

Fig 17 Longitudinal section through the thyroid, with an ovoid, low echogenicity parathyroid adenoma (marked by cursors) lying posterior to its left inferior pole.

Fig 16 Octreotide scan showing radioisotope uptake into multiple bony metastases throughout the skeleton, as well as in the hepatic metastases. (The hot spot over the right wrist is the injection site and that in the pelvis is radiotracer excreted into urine in the bladder.)

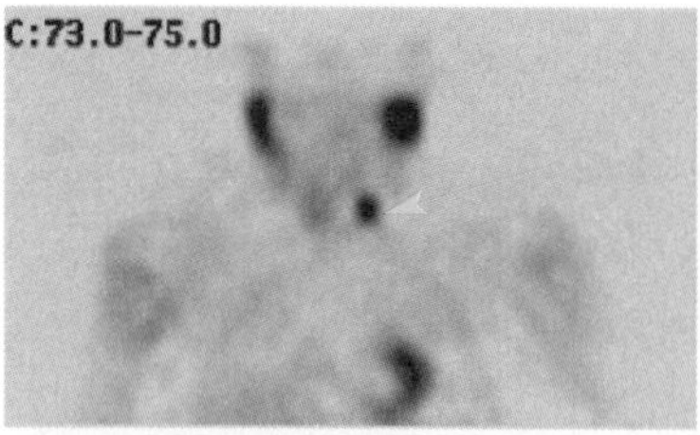

Fig 18 Same patient as Fig 17: parathyroid adenoma seen as persistent hot spot (arrow) in the left inferior parathyroid gland on coronal views (normal uptake in the parotid glands and in the myocardium is also visible).

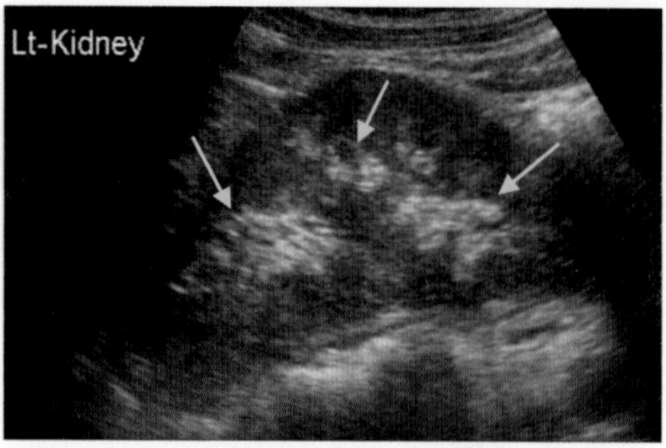

Fig 19 Nephrocalcinosis seen as hyperechoic renal medulla on ultrasound.

☐ PARATHYROID LESIONS

Parathyroid lesions are composed largely of adenomata, hyperplasia, or, rarely, carcinoma. Ultrasound is a very sensitive, non-invasive, method for imaging the parathyroid glands. In the neck it is unaffected by obesity of the patient and is readily reproducible. Normal-sized parathyroid glands are not usually seen on ultrasound. Fig 17 shows a low echogenicity parathyroid adenoma. This correlates well with the technetium-99m methoxyisobutyl isonitrile (MIBI) scan in Fig 18. The same patient incidentally had nephrocalcinosis associated with the hyperparathyroidism (Fig 19).

☐ PITUITARY TUMOURS

Pituitary tumours are classified broadly as microadenomata when <10 mm in craniocaudal dimension or macroadenomata when larger. Other lesions, such as pituitary metastases (for example, from breast carcinoma) or hypothalamic lesions that extend down into the pituitary gland, are seen occasionally. Fig 20 shows a coronal magnetic resonance scan of the normal pituitary gland. Fig 21 demonstrates

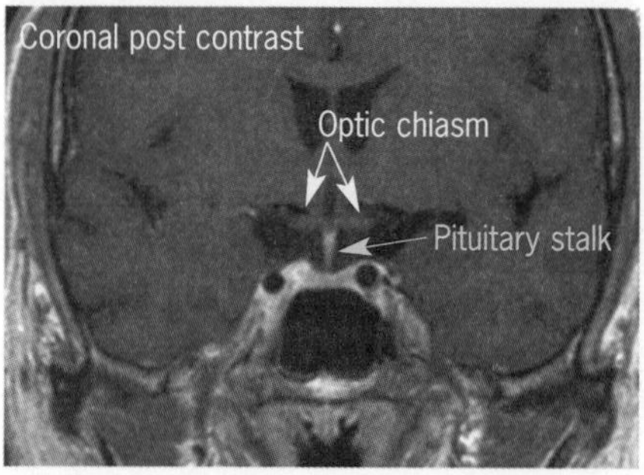

Fig 20 Normal pituitary coronal magnetic resonance imaging scan after gadolinium contrast: the pituitary stalk inserts centrally into the concave-upwards margin of the gland.

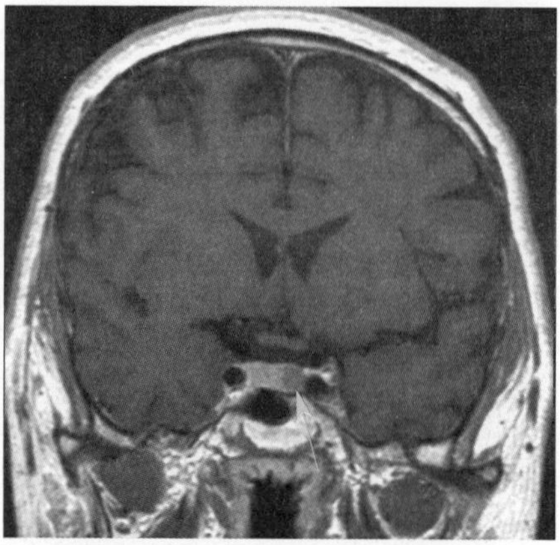

Fig 21 Microadenoma (arrow) shows reduced enhancement compared with normal pituitary gland after intravenous contrast.

a microadenoma in the left of the pituitary. Petrosal vein sampling (Fig 22) is a useful (although specialised and invasive) technique for identifying laterality of a secreting microadenoma. These lesions may secrete prolactin, and simultaneous sampling from the two petrosal vein catheters will reveal a higher level of hormone on the side of a functioning tumour. As non-functional microadenomata are quite commonly found incidentally, it can be important to confirm the position and activity of a microadenoma identified on magnetic resonance imaging. Sampling of the petrosal veins also can be useful for identifying the presence of a secreting microadenoma that has not been visualised on magnetic resonance scanning.

Fig 23 shows a typical large macroadenoma in the coronal plane. Fig 24 shows an example of an unusual lesion involving only the pituitary stalk and the posterior pituitary, which was a case of Wegner's granulomatosis.

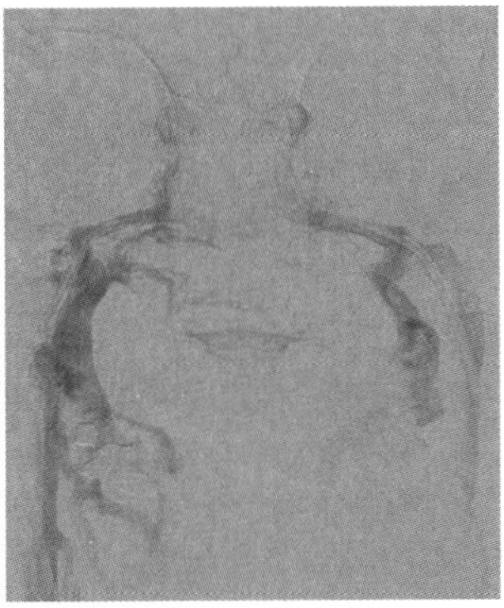

Fig 22 Digital subtraction venogram showing catheters in both petrosal veins for simultaneous sampling.

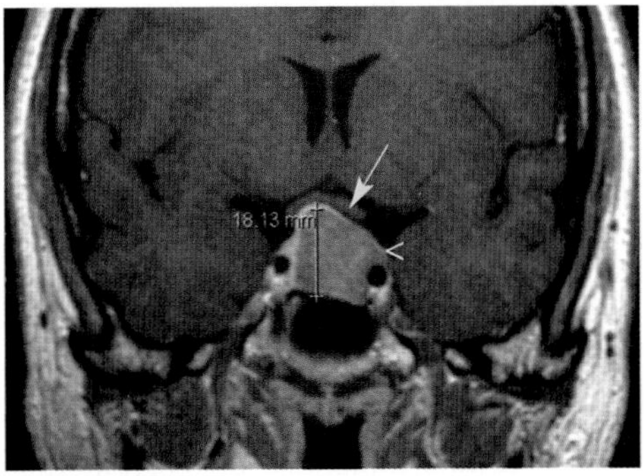

Fig 23 Macroadenoma that has expanded out of the pituitary fossa cranially and is elevating and stretching the optic chiasm above it (arrow) and invading into the left (<) but not into the right cavernous sinus.

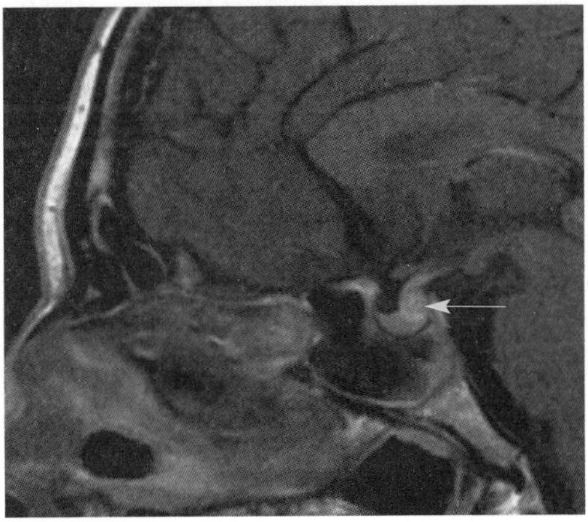

Fig 24 Wegner's granulomatosis of pituitary stalk and posterior pituitary: contrast-enhanced sagittal magnetic resonance section, with the infiltration markedly thickening the pituitary stalk and invading the posterior pituitary (arrow), leaving a normal anterior pituitary. The optic chiasm is not affected.

☐ ADRENAL IMAGING

It is important to establish convincing evidence of a secretory adrenal lesion before embarking upon imaging, as the imaging method and protocol must be tailored carefully to the type of adrenal lesion suspected. Benign, non-secreting adrenal adenomata are common in the adult population (4–6%) and lesions <4 cm in diameter can be safely dismissed as benign adenomata if they are shown to have a high content of fat. These adenomata have a density ≤10 Hounsfield units on unenhanced CT scans. Unfortunately, a minority of benign adenomata are relatively lipid-poor and have a pre-contrast density ≤10 Hounsfield units. These lesions can also be shown to have a relatively high lipid content by in-phase and out-of-phase magnetic resonance imaging. Fat-containing lesions (adenomata) show signal loss on the out-of-phase scanning, in which the signal from fat is nulled. This is shown in Fig 25. Lipid-poor lesions, which are most unlikely to be adenomata, do not show such signal dropout. Computed tomography also can be useful to distinguish benign adenomata from metastases. The adrenals are scanned pre-contrast, 60 seconds after intravenous injection of 100 ml of iodinated contrast material, and again after a delay of 15 minutes. A region of interest is drawn over the enlarged adrenal for each of the scans, a quantitative Hounsfield unit density value is measured, and the formulae for iodinated contrast washout shown in Box 1 are applied.

No consensus has been reached on whether, or how often, follow-up scanning of benign adrenal adenomata should be performed. Practice in the United States favours follow-up scans at 6, 12, and 24 months.[3]

The magnetic resonance image in Fig 26 shows an example of a large left adrenal phaeochromocytoma, and the corresponding anterior nuclear medicine scan with iodine-131-meta-iodobenzylguanidine (MIBG) (Fig 27) shows corresponding increased activity. The MIBG localises in storage granules in adrenergic tissue and therefore shows hyperactivity of the adrenal medulla and sympathetic nervous tissue. It generally is labelled with radioactive iodine (iodine-123 or -131).

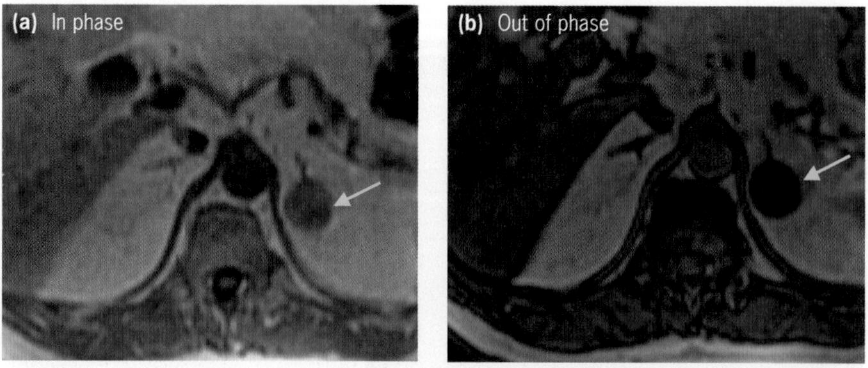

Fig 25 (a) In-phase magnetic resonance scan of adrenals showing intermediate signal of adrenal mass (adenoma) in posterior aspect of a limb of the left adrenal and **(b)** out-of-phase magnetic resonance scan showing the left adrenal mass in Fig 25(a) changes to a much lower signal because of its fat content. Right adrenal is normal.

Box 1 Adrenal mass characterisation on computed tomography (CT): adenoma.

HU = Hounsfield unit value of tissue density on CT.
Dynamic = 60 seconds after injection of intravenous contrast agent.
Delayed = 15 minutes after injection of intravenous contrast agent.

Pre-contrast density
If pre-contrast density is ≤10 HU, adrenal mass is a benign adenoma.

Absolute percentage washout

$$\text{Absolute percentage washout} = \frac{\text{dynamic HU} - \text{delayed HU}}{\text{dynamic HU} - \text{Pre HU}} \times 100$$

If absolute percentage washout is >60%, adrenal mass is a benign adenoma.

Relative percentage washout

$$\text{Relative percentage washout} = \frac{\text{dynamic HU} - \text{delayed HU}}{\text{dynamic HU}} \times 100$$

If relative percentage washout is >40%, adrenal mass is a benign adenoma.

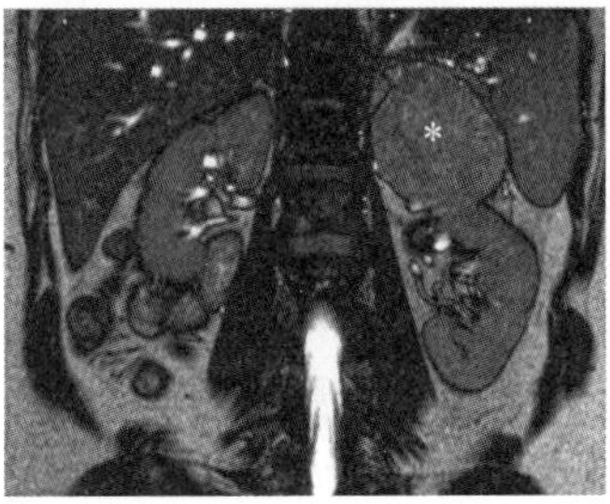

Fig 26 Coronal magnetic resonance scan showing large left adrenal phaeochromocytoma (*).

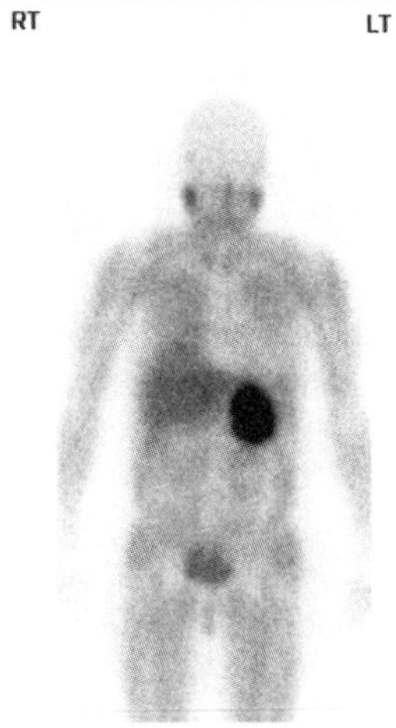

Fig 27 Iodine-131-meta-iodobenzyl-guanidine (MIBG) scan of same left adrenal phaemochromocytoma as in Fig 26.

Conn's tumours may be difficult to identify because they are often small. As they contain fat, they should also show signal dropout on the out-of-phase magnetic resonance image. The invasive technique of adrenal vein sampling may be used to measure the ratio of levels of aldosterone between the two adrenal glands. If the ratio is >10:1, it is highly suggestive of a unilateral Conn's tumour. This technique is very useful for differentiating a solitary hyperactive Conn's tumour from adrenal hyperplasia, which may be nodular, as shown in Fig 28. Adrenal vein sampling in this case showed levels of aldosterone of 151,000 pmol/l on the left and 57,000 pmol/l on the right; this gives a ratio of only about 3:1, which is indicative of bilateral adrenal hyperplasia (and not Conn's syndrome due to a dominant hypersecreting nodule). Nuclear medicine scanning with 131-iodonorcholesterol can be performed, with images obtained on days 4, 7, and 11 after administration of the contrast agent. Iodonorcholesterol is taken up by the renal cortex when it is hyperactive and can also

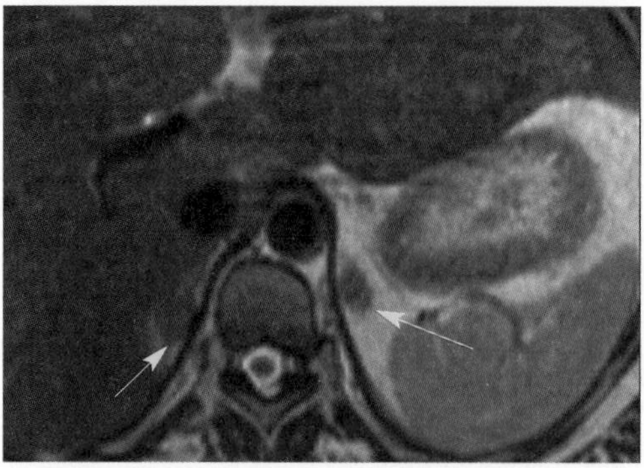

Fig 28 Nodular adrenal hyperplasia: two of the nodules, one in each adrenal gland, are seen on this section of the magnetic resonance image.

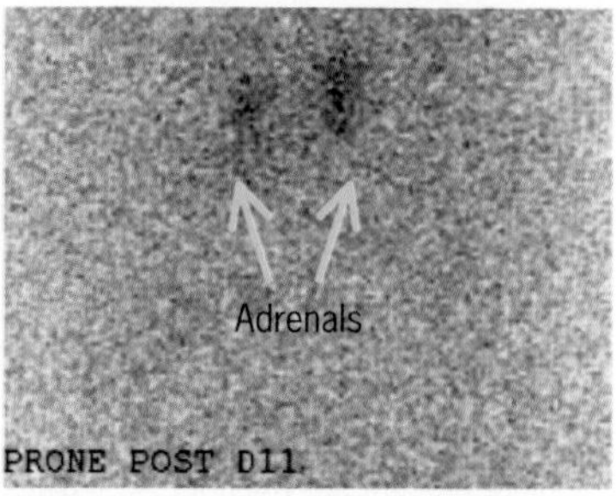

Fig 29 131-iodonorcholesterol nuclear medicine scan of bilateral adrenal hyperplasia with radiolabel uptake in both adrenal glands.

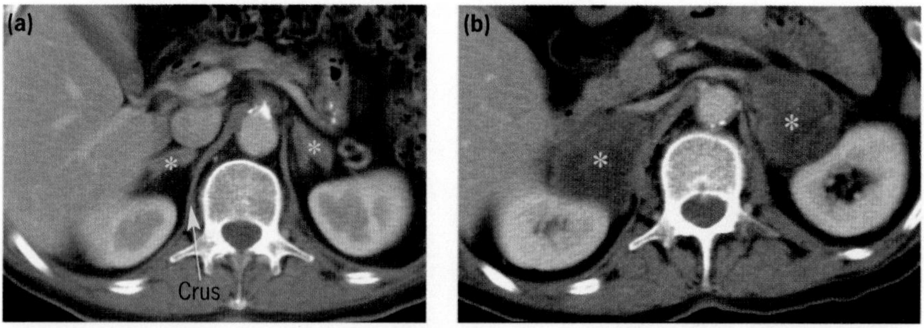

Fig 30 (a) Non-Hodgkin's lymphoma of the adrenals, with marked hyperplasia of the adrenals (*). As a rough guide, the limbs of a normal adrenal gland should not be larger than the adjacent crura of the diaphragm. **(b)** 10 months later.

be useful in differentiating a solitary hypersecreting Conn's nodule from bilateral adrenal hyperplasia (Fig 29).

Fig 30 illustrates a rare case of apparent adrenal hyperplasia, which shows sequential CT scans from September 2005 (a) and July 2006 (b); however, there was no biochemical evidence of Conn's syndrome or other abnormality. Non-Hodgkin's lymphoma was diagnosed on biopsy.

□ CONCLUSION

It is essential that endocrine imaging should be guided by the clinical problem and that the results of all biochemical tests should be known before imaging. This guides the location and type of imaging to be performed – for example, if adrenocorticotropic hormone (ACTH) is suppressed in a patient with Cushing's syndrome, there is no point imaging the pituitary as the pathology clearly must lie within the adrenals or in an extra-adrenal ectopic location. Very close cooperative investigation by physicians and radiologists – carried out via regular, well-documented, multidisciplinary team meetings – is indispensable.

REFERENCES

1 Turner HE, Wass JAH, eds. *Oxford handbook of endocrinology and diabetes.* Oxford: Oxford University Press, 2002.

2 Rockall AG, Britton KE, Grossman AB, Resnek RH. *Neuroendocrine tumours in imaging and oncology.* Abingdon: Taylor and Francis, 2004:789–817.

3 Young WF. The incidentally discovered adrenal mass. *N Engl J Med* 2007;356:601–10.

☐ RADIOLOGY SELF-ASSESSMENT QUESTIONS

High-resolution computed tomography and diffuse lung disease – current status

1 The addition of findings from high-resolution computed tomography (HRCT) to clinical and radiographic information in patients with diffuse lung disease has been shown to:
(a) Improve diagnostic confidence
(b) Change the first-choice diagnosis in 50% of cases
(c) Significantly improve interobserver diagnostic agreement for patients with sarcoidosis
(d) Improve interobserver diagnostic agreement for patients with idiopathic pulmonary fibrosis (IPF)
(e) Reduce the rate of biopsies in patients with IPF by 6%

2 Concerning the radiological and pathological diagnosis of usual interstitial pneumonia (UIP) and non-specific interstitial pneumonia (NSIP):
(a) Histology is the final arbiter for differentiating between UIP and NSIP
(b) Studies evaluating histopathological interobserver variation have shown kappa coefficient values >0.4
(c) Histological interlobar concordance in patients with UIP and NSIP is estimated at 75%
(d) HRCT has a positive predictive value for UIP of 96%
(e) HRCT is more sensitive than specific for the diagnosis of UIP

3 With respect to the imaging of airways disease:
(a) Lung parenchymal density is measured in Hounsfield Units
(b) Multidetector computed tomography (CT) can accurately show the indirect signs of small airway diseases
(c) Automated texture analysis is used routinely to discriminate between small and large airway diseases
(d) Correlation between the thickness of the airway wall according to CT and lung function tests in patients with chronic obstructive pulmonary disease (COPD) is poor
(e) The distinction between panacinar emphysema and obliterative bronchiolitis can be readily made with HRCT

Cancer imaging

1 Magnetic resonance lymphography
(a) Is performed after administration of ultra-small nanoparticles of manganese oxide
(b) Can be used to identify partially infiltrated malignant lymph nodes
(c) Does not affect overall nodal staging accuracy compared with size criteria for nodal assessment
(d) Contrast nanoparticles are phagocytosed by lymphocytes in lymph nodes
(e) Malignant nodes appear dark on imaging sequences that detect presence of the contrast nanoparticles

2 The following are functional imaging techniques that may be useful for assessment of tumours:
 (a) Magnetic resonance spectroscopy
 (b) Magnetic resonance imaging (MRI) dependent on levels of oxygenation of blood
 (c) Diffusion-weighted MRI
 (d) Positron emission tomography (PET) with 18-fluorothymidine
 (e) High spatial resolution multidetector CT

3 Regarding the application of imaging for tumour assessment:
 (a) MRI has a recognised role for the screening of women who are genetically predisposed to develop ovarian cancer
 (b) MRI can accurately predict the relation of rectal cancer to the potential circumferential resection margin
 (c) Imaging with 2-deoxy-2-^{18}F-D-glucose (^{18}FDG) PET is unhelpful for demonstrating sites of extrahepatic disease in patients with colorectal cancer
 (d) Dynamic contrast-enhanced CT imaging may be used to evaluate the effects of antiangiogenic drug treatment
 (e) Diffusion-weighted MRI provides information related to tissue cellularity

Endocrine imaging

1 Pancreatic islet cell tumours:
 (a) Enhance avidly in the arterial phase of CT
 (b) Show enhancement in the portal venous phase of CT
 (c) Very rarely metastasise to liver
 (d) Can be asymptomatic
 (e) Are usually vascular on angiography

2 Octreotide scanning:
 (a) Uses octreotide because it binds to somatostatin receptors
 (b) Can be used effectively only for large tumours
 (c) Shows up almost 100% of insulinomas
 (d) Shows up almost 100% of gastrinomas
 (e) Gives very accurate anatomical localisation of tumours

3 Regarding carcinoid tumours:
 (a) Primary tumours can calcify
 (b) Liver metastases may be difficult to see on unenhanced CT scans
 (c) They usually give lytic bone metastases
 (d) Liver metastases can be embolised for symptomatic relief
 (e) Liver metastases are supplied by the hepatic artery

Endocrinology

New therapies in the management of type 2 diabetes

Ebaa Al-Ozairi and Philip Home

□ BACKGROUND

Diabetes mellitus has become a major focus of attention in the last 10 years, largely because its health impact in terms of complications, particularly cardiovascular complications, has been generally recognised. Furthermore, decreasing levels of physical activity and increasing levels of calorie consumption are increasing the incidence of type 2 diabetes at ever younger ages. An additional factor in the increased prevalence is longer life expectancy, because lifespan with diabetes is longer with earlier onset and because of advances in the prevention and management of cardiovascular disease.

New treatments for the management of diabetes are not limited just to glucose-lowering drugs. The statins, for example, are particularly important in people with diabetes: although the relative risk reduction is the same as for other groups, the background risk is much higher than in the general population (2–3 times higher), even in those with declared cardiovascular disease (about 2.5 times higher). Statins and other drugs are thus much more cost effective in people with diabetes. Other examples of newer non-glucose-lowering drugs that have had considerable evidence-based impact in the management of diabetes are the renin–angiotensin system blockers, antiplatelet drugs such as clopidogrel, and new lipid-lowering drugs. Meanwhile there have been some disappointments, such as the failure of new microvascular complication inhibitors to progress into clinical care and the failure of thiazolidinediones to show cardiovascular protection beyond that predicted from conventional risk factors (glucose, triglycerides, high-density lipoprotein (HDL) cholesterol, and blood pressure).[1]

It is the glucose-lowering drugs that are providing excitement in 2006–7 (Table 1), however, and this review is confined to those launched or due to be launched 12 months before and after the date of writing. Peroxisome proliferator-activated receptor (PPAR) γ agonists (including the thiazolidinediones) have been covered in a previous volume of *Horizons in Medicine*.[2] A major disappointment has been the failure of newer, more potent, PPAR agonists to complete the clinical development process.

The new drugs are of interest in coming from classic pharmacological approaches to drug development, and in marking a return of endocrinology to the management of type 2 diabetes. Rimonabant acts through blockade of cannabinoid receptors in the central nervous system and peripherally, modulating synaptic transmission. Exenatide

Table 1 New treatments introduced since 1995 and future treatments with glucose-lowering properties.

Period	Development
1995–2005	• Rapid-acting insulin analogues • Extended-acting insulin analogues • Thiazolidinediones • Inhaled insulin
2006–2007	• Cannabinoid receptor blockers (rimonabant) • GLP-1 mimetics (exenatide) • Dipeptidyl peptidase IV (DPP-4) inhibitors (sitagliptin, vildagliptin)
2010–2020	• Further examples of the above • Glucokinase activators • Glycogenolysis inhibitors • Peroxisome proliferator-activated receptor (PPAR) δ and pan-PPAR agonists • Gluconeogenesis inhibitors

is a distant analogue of GLP-1 – a hormone that enhances insulin secretion, is normally released by the gut after feeding, and acts through physiological GLP-1 receptors (the full name of this peptide is misleading and best forgotten). The two dipeptidyl peptidase IV (DPP-4) inhibitors, sitagliptin and vildagliptin, inhibit an enzyme that degrades physiological GLP-1, thus enhancing its action in people with type 2 diabetes, in whom secretion of GLP-1 is abnormally low.

□ RIMONABANT (CANNABINOID RECEPTOR BLOCKER)

Background

Preparations from the plant *Cannabis sativa* have been known since ancient times because of their pleasantly intoxifying effects as well as their medicinal uses. The active principle in the plants has in recent decades been identified as D9-tetrahydrocannabinol. The concept of pharmacologically active plant extracts that bind to receptors responsible for normal brain functions (such as opioids – morphine and derivatives) is long established; for the cannabinoids this is known as the endocannabinoid system.

At least in part the endocannabinoid system seems to be a modulatory system affecting behavioural drive, the mesolimbic dopaminergic system, and is particularly involved in feeding behaviour. Recent work has suggested that the endocannabinoids are synthesised in postsynaptic cells from lipid precursors but that they act presynaptically on cannabinoid CB1 receptors, thus acting as retrograde messengers to inhibit neurotransmitter release and thus modulate synaptic activity. A major part of the function of this system seems to be regulation of systems of energy balance, and indeed there seem to be peripheral effects involving the endocannabinoid system in adipose tissue particularly, but also in liver and skeletal muscle.[3]

In rodents, hypothalamic levels of endocannabinoids increase when they are deprived of food and reduce when they are fed. Knockout of the CB1 receptor or the use of CB1 receptor blockers (such as rimonabant) blunts feeding behaviour in fasted animals. Jamshidi and colleagues injected the endocannabinoid anandamide directly into the hypothalamus of satiated rats and showed that this caused resumption of feeding, which could be blocked by rimonabant.[4] In normal mice, high-fat diets result in an excess in body weight of about 25%; this can be stopped by deletion of the CB1 receptors, and even normal weight mice lacking such receptors gain weight more slowly than usual.

Clinical studies

Five studies have been published or presented in which rimonabant was used in people with obesity, with glucose intolerance, and with type 2 diabetes. In general, the results are consistent with the findings of the study published on its use in people with diabetes. In this population, which had a mean body weight of 96 kg, weight loss over 12 months was 3.9 kg more with 20 mg/day rimonabant than with placebo.[5] In studies in people without diabetes, absolute changes were greater because the people with diabetes had had considerable lifestyle advice in the years before the study. The weight loss was accompanied by improvements in glycated haemoglobin (HbA_{1c}) and fasting plasma glucose concentrations; the reduction in HbA_{1c} was in the order of –0.7% (standard deviation 0.1%) HbA_{1c} – a useful improvement from the relatively low baseline levels. Weight loss, which is assumed to result from a decrease in the level of calorie intake, would be expected to improve glucose control in itself, but calculations using data on changes in weight and HbA_{1c} with placebo (which must be entirely the result of advice on calorie restriction) show that about 50% of the reduction in glucose levels is secondary to changes in food intake; the other 50% is presumably the result of direct metabolic effects on the endocannabinoid system.[5]

This is consistent with observations from the other studies in which improvements are seen in a variety of features of the metabolic syndrome, such as insulin insensitivity and serum levels of HDL cholesterol and triglycerides. A core feature of the metabolic syndrome is abdominal adiposity, and waist circumference consistently decreased in studies in which rimonabant was used at the 20 mg dose now licensed.

The downside of a cannabinoid blocker might be expected from the positive mood effects of cannabis. Indeed, people with a history of depression were excluded from the studies. Marked discontinuation rates were found in the studies; apart from nausea, which was a minor but significant problem, the most notable side-effects were mood-related changes of depression and anxiety. The relatively small numbers exposed in the trials (about 2,500) cannot provide information on whether more serious or irreversible psychological changes may rarely occur, and it is not clear from the publications whether larger proportions of people might have suffered some loss of well being.

The possible clinical role of rimonabant is discussed below.

☐ GLP-1 MIMETICS – EXENATIDE

Background

'Incretin' is a term used to describe enhancement of insulin secretion, and Nauck and colleagues provided the key demonstration of the incretin effect in 1986. Their pertinent observation was that matching the increased arterial concentrations of glucose found after a meal by intravenously infusing glucose in the same people in a separate study resulted in much lower levels of insulin secretion. In other words, feeding stimulated insulin secretion by mechanisms additional to those of increased concentrations of glucose. The effect was shown in people with and without diabetes. Subsequent work found that two peptides produced by the gut were of significance, namely GLP-1 and GIP (as with GLP-1, the full name of this peptide is misleading and best forgotten). In people with type 2 diabetes, production of GLP-1 is decreased but its action is normal, which makes it a suitable candidate for replacement treatment; the opposite is true of GIP.[6]

Nauck and colleagues subsequently showed that intravenous infusion of GLP-1 into fasted people with type 2 diabetes led to a steady normalisation of plasma levels of glucose over about four hours. This was associated with an increase in plasma concentrations of insulin and a decrease in plasma concentrations of the hormone glucagon. Glucagon is responsible for maintaining plasma concentrations of glucose by stimulating output of glucose from the liver in the fasting state, and is secreted in excessive amounts in people with type 2 diabetes. Studies of longer duration subsequently showed that both the basal and prandial hyperglycaemia of type 2 diabetes could be reversed by infusion of GLP-1, but the very need for intravenous infusion means that GLP-1 itself is not a therapeutic candidate.[6]

There are two reasons for this. Firstly, GLP-1 is a peptide, which means it cannot be taken by mouth and must be injected. Secondly, GLP-1 is degraded in the circulation even more quickly than insulin; unlike insulin, however, this is not because of removal through its effector receptors but rather through the enzyme DPP-4, which is expressed by endothelial cells. The physiological significance of this remains a mystery. This enzyme acts on a peptide bond located near the end of the peptide chain of GLP-1, however, so a change in the sequence of amino acids at this point, which does not affect the peptide's activity, thus protects against rapid degradation. This approach is being used by Novo Nordisk: a fatty acid residue is also attached to the peptide, which further prolongs the peptide's residence in the circulation because of binding to the fatty acid binding sites of albumin. Novo Nordisk's derivative peptide liraglutide shows promise in clinical trials but is not licensed at present.

Exenatide, the preparation currently on the market, is a synthetic version of exendin-4, which is a peptide found among a myriad of others in the saliva of the Gila monster of the American south-west – one of the two known venomous lizards. Exenatide is not only resistant to degradation by DPP-4 but is also some 10 times more potent in binding to GLP-1 receptors; this is a useful property, as the peptide has only 50% homology with human GLP-1 and might be expected to be quite antigenic were it not for the very small doses (up to 10 μg twice daily) needed.

Clinical studies

Exenatide has been the subject of a number of clinical trials that have been directed largely at establishing the size of its efficacy and have therefore been comparisons against placebo. As a new and therefore relatively expensive injectable is unlikely to become the first-line choice for glucose lowering, the most clinically relevant studies are those in which exenatide was used on a background of metformin or a sulphonylurea, or both. The findings can be summarised as suggesting that exenatide has useful glucose-lowering effects that seem to be about the same size as those obtained with the other non-insulin drugs already available.[7]

What was exceptional (at least until rimonabant was licensed) was an accompanying weight loss in the order of 2 kg over 30 weeks in people who had a starting weight of about 98 kg and who should have gained about 2 kg from amelioration of glycosuria and reduction of glucose metabolism driven by hyperglycaemia.[8] Probably more importantly, this weight loss seems to continue for quite long periods (it is not yet known how long), and anecdotal reports of very large amounts of weight loss (>10 kg) in some people are easily found among physicians in the United States, who have had access to exenatide since May 2005.

Exenatide has been compared to insulin in two studies. Both were of poor quality, however, with doses of insulin inadequately titrated so that the comparator arm was invalid.[9]

Mimetics of GLP-1 (and thus also the DPP-4 inhibitors discussed below) have become the subject of other interesting studies on durability of glucose-lowering effects. These stem from observations of islet B-cell regeneration and death in rodents and the potential of GLP-1 to enhance islet B-cell neogenesis and decrease the rate of apoptosis. Direct extrapolation to man is difficult, however, because it is clear that the rate of islet turnover in humans is much lower than in rodents and may not occur at all. If the inexorable decline in islet B-cell function in people with diabetes could be stopped, however, the need for more and more glucose-lowering drugs with time could be ameliorated, which would result in considerable savings in health and costs. The studies will focus on durability of blood glucose control over three years or more; similar studies are planned for the DPP-4 inhibitors.

The possible clinical role of exenatide is discussed below.

□ DPP-4 INHIBITORS (GLIPTINS)

Background

As discussed above, plasma levels of the incretin hormone GLP-1 are low in people with type 2 diabetes, and the islet B-cells responsible for insulin secretion function inadequately. As GLP-1 is degraded rapidly by the endothelial enzyme DPP-4, a logical approach to glucose-lowering therapy is to enhance endogenous GLP-1 levels by preventing its degradation and therefore to enhance insulin secretion and normalise secretion of glucagon (Fig 1). It is relatively easy to identify substances that inhibit this enzyme – up to 18 different compounds have been in clinical development – but a key issue is enzyme specificity, notably with respect to the related peptidases DPP-8 and DPP-9. Two compounds are currently leading candidates in this area: sitagliptin is already licensed in the United States, while vildagliptin has been approved subject to some further studies. European licences were being granted in spring and summer of 2007.

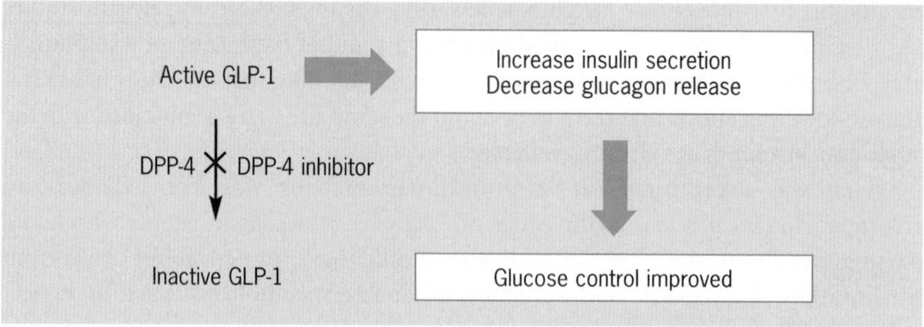

Fig 1 The concept that underlies the dipeptidyl peptidase IV (DPP-4) inhibitors. Endogenous GLP-1 is normally degraded rapidly by the enzyme DPP-4, which is expressed on endothelial cells. By inhibiting the enzyme pharmacologically, plasma levels of GLP-1 can be enhanced in people with type 2 diabetes, which increases insulin secretion and corrects glucagon hypersecretion. As a result, control of blood glucose levels is improved.

Sitagliptin and vildagliptin seem to have the appropriate enzyme specificity to be considered for human use. Both are highly potent and seem suitable for once-daily dosing, although suitability is clearer for sitagliptin, with which 70% inhibition seems to be maintained to 24 hours. Sitagliptin is excreted renally, so the dose needs downward adjustment in patients whose estimated glomerular filtration rate is severely impaired; vildagliptin is probably not so affected. The safety profiles are discussed below, but the only notable problem of this class of drugs in animals is skin problems in monkeys – a side-effect that, as yet, does not seem to have a clinical correlate in man. In addition, there is no embryotoxicity in animal studies, but there is also no experience of use during human pregnancy.

Clinical studies

In studies of 28 days' duration in people with type 2 diabetes, Mari and colleagues were able to show that vildagliptin enhanced levels of GLP-1 and GIP in the basal and postprandial states throughout the day. Levels of GLP-1 increased about threefold. In the same studies, concentrations of insulin in plasma were also increased at all time points and concentrations of glucagon in plasma were reduced by about 25%. In other studies, vildagliptin restored the blunted 'first-phase' insulin response to an intravenous glucose challenge by 12 weeks.[10]

A number of clinical studies have been performed, most of which are available from detailed copies of meeting posters distributed freely for both drugs. Studies generally have been 6–12 months in duration (with extensions now to 24 months) and have included monotherapy and combination use, and active or placebo comparators. Studies have even been performed in combination with other drugs that act to enhance insulin secretion from the islet B-cells – namely the sulphonylureas.

The conclusion from these studies can be summarised as follows: glucose lowering is similar to, or in some circumstances slightly less than, that achieved with traditional glucose-lowering drugs, hypoglycaemia is not a problem (although in combination with sulphonylureas or insulin, better glucose control will inevitably give a higher incidence of hypoglycaemia), and there is no weight gain.[11] Note that the last of these should be regarded as a positive effect. If glucose control is improved by any means, glycosuria is reduced and glucose metabolism driven by glucose concentration is reduced; both of these conserve carbohydrate, which ultimately can be stored only as fat. The mechanism of the effect of DPP-4 inhibitors on body weight is unclear but presumably is a lesser manifestation of the effects seen with GLP-1 mimetics. Indeed DPP-4 inhibitors have a smaller effect on levels of GLP-1 than when giving a GLP-1 mimetic, which has led to speculation that another mechanism may be at work.

Other important aspects of preventative care in people with type 2 diabetes are control of dyslipidaemia and blood pressure. The effect of DPP-4 inhibitors on the blood lipid profile is neutral. They may have some beneficial effect on blood pressure, but this is small and may be of the order of that seen with the thiazolidinediones.

The other feature of sitagliptin and vildagliptin is their adverse event profile – or rather the lack of it. The glucose-lowering drug market is filled by drugs with significant side-effects that occur with a relatively high prevalence, or with contraindications (risk of serious adverse events) (Table 2). Inhibition of DPP-4, a non-specific peptidase, was expected to result in enhancement of levels of other peptides, perhaps in times of metabolic or immunological stress. This concern as yet has come to nothing; the explanation is perhaps that although DPP-4 is non-specific, GLP-1 and GIP are the only peptides wholly 'dependent' on it for degradation.

Table 2 Common causes of intolerance to and contraindications of glucose-lowering drugs. This table includes only more common adverse events and contraindications and is not intended as prescribing advice.

Drug or drug class	Intolerance	Contraindication
Metformin	Diarrhoea Nausea +	Renal impairment
Sulphonylureas	Hypoglycaemia Weight gain +	–
Thiazolidinediones	Fluid retention Weight gain ++	Heart failure
Rimonabant	Mood change Nausea +	History of depression
DPP-4 inhibitors (gliptins)	–	–
Exenatide	Nausea ++	–
Insulin	Hypoglycaemia Weight gain +/++	–

☐ ROLE OF THE NEW GLUCOSE-LOWERING DRUGS

Considerable consensus exists over the use of current glucose-lowering drugs; this may be summarised as follows: metformin is the first-line drug after lifestyle measures alone fail to achieve glucose targets, sulphonylureas generally are added when metformin alone is inadequate, thiazolidinediones are used in triple therapy (or sometimes added directly to metformin), and insulin is started only later in the evolution of islet B-cell deficiency in an individual person.[12] Where then do rimonabant, exenatide and the gliptins fit in? An important point here is that all these new drugs are expensive, particularly compared with generic metformin and sulphonylureas, which means they must show distinct advantages in health (quality of life) to be cost effective.

Nothing at present will displace metformin from first-line use, as long as it is tolerated and not contraindicated. The good adverse event profile of the gliptins, however, might mean that they would displace sulphonylureas as second-line treatment (added to metformin) in richer societies. Evidence currently suggests that they can be used together with the sulphonylureas, so they may also be used where the alternative choice would be one of the thiazolidinediones, which paradoxically remain a good choice in obese, insulin-resistant patients, in whom they seem to be particularly effective.

Rimonabant and exenatide would seem to be useful alternatives, or perhaps additions, to the treatment armamentarium in people in whom body weight is, or is perceived to be, a special problem. This is not a small market. Again, where it can be afforded, rimonabant might be used instead of a sulphonylurea, although the alternative would often be a thiazolidinedione. Exenatide is an injectable drug, but it requires much less in the way of self-monitoring or dose titration than insulin, and so is likely to find its main use in people who would otherwise be starting insulin.

☐ CONCLUSION

The endocannabinoid blocker rimonabant, the DPP-4 inhibitors, and the GLP-1 mimetic exenatide are all useful additions to the limited range of glucose-lowering drugs available to date. All have unique profiles, and together they clearly tackle the problem of weight gain that is associated with most of the currently available drugs. The exact clinical role of all of these new drugs remains to be determined, and cost effectiveness will be a significant part of the necessary decision making in that respect.

Duality of interest: PH, on behalf of Newcastle University, has advised or provided educational activities for the manufacturers of rimonabant, the gliptins, and other glucose-lowering drugs. All the companies involved have supported organisations and initiatives with which he is associated.

REFERENCES

1 Dormandy JA, Charbonnel B, Eckland DJ *et al.* Secondary prevention of macrovascular events in patients with type 2 diabetes in the PROactive Study (PROspective pioglitAzone Clinical Trial In macroVascular Events): a randomised controlled trial. *Lancet* 2005;366:1279–89.

2 Home PD. Thiazolidinediones: increasing insulin sensitivity. In: Amiel S. *Horizons in Medicine, volume 13*. London: Royal College of Physicians, 2002:185–94.

3 Di Marzo V, Goparaju SK, Wang L *et al.* Leptin-regulated endocannabinoids are involved in maintaining food intake. *Nature* 2001;410:822–5.

4 Jamshidi N, Taylor DA. Anandamide administration into the ventromedial hypothalamus stimulates appetite in rats. *Br J Pharmacol* 2001;134:1151–4.

5 Scheen AJ, Finer N, Hollander P *et al.* Efficacy and tolerability of rimonabant in overweight or obese patients with type 2 diabetes: a randomised controlled study. *Lancet* 2006;368: 1660–72.

6 Meier JJ, Nauck MA. Glucagon-like peptide 1 (GLP-1) in biology and pathology. *Diabetes Metab Res Rev* 2005;21:91–117.

7 Kendall DM, Riddle MC, Rosenstock J *et al.* Effects of exenatide (exendin-4) on glycemic control over 30 weeks in patients with type 2 diabetes treated with metformin and a sulfonylurea. *Diabetes Care* 2005;28:1083–91.

8 Ratner RE, Maggs D, Nielsen LL *et al.* Long-term effects of exenatide therapy over 82 weeks on glycaemic control and weight in over-weight metformin-treated patients with type 2 diabetes mellitus. *Diabetes Obes Metab* 2006;8:419–28.

9 Nauck MA, Duran S, Kim D *et al.* A comparison of twice-daily exenatide and biphasic insulin aspart in patients with type 2 diabetes who were suboptimally controlled with sulfonylurea and metformin: a non-inferiority study. *Diabetologia* 2007;50:259–67.

10 Mari A, Sallas WM, He YL *et al.* Vildagliptin, a dipeptidyl peptidase-IV inhibitor, improves model-assessed β-cell function in patients with type 2 diabetes. *J Clin Endocrinol Metab* 2005;90:4888–94.

11 Rosenstock J, Baron MA, Dejager S, Mills D, Schweizer A. Comparison of vildagliptin and rosiglitazone monotherapy in patients with type 2 diabetes: a 24-week, double-blind, randomized trial. *Diabetes Care* 2007;30:217–23.

12 Clinical Guidelines Task Force. *Global guideline for type 2 diabetes.* Brussels: International Diabetes Federation, 2005. Available at: www.idf.org (last accessed 16 May 2007).

Management of adrenal insufficiency in severe stress and surgery

Wiebke Arlt and Christopher J Mowatt

'While on a visit to London in the fall of 1947, Congressman Kennedy became so seriously ill with weakness, nausea, vomiting, and low blood pressure that he was given the last rites of the Roman Catholic Church. The physician who examined him diagnosed his condition as Addison's disease and told one of Kennedy's friends that "he hasn't got a year to live".'[1]

Fortunately, John F Kennedy was diagnosed with Addison's disease as great advances were being made in the study of steroid function, with an ultimate breakthrough due to the synthesis of cortisone, which led to the award of the Nobel Prize to Edward Kendall, Tadeusz Reichstein, and Philipp Hench in 1950.

After John F Kennedy's illness was diagnosed in London, its course was not always smooth, and he suffered several adrenal crises related to stress during his election campaigns. He was also forced to undergo surgery while a senator, when surgery on patients with Addison's disease was fraught with danger. Luckily, he narrowly survived the stress of major surgery (a lumbosacral and sacroiliac fusion) after perioperative infusion of hydrocortisone; this was an absolute novelty at the time and led to the publication of his case in an article in the American Medical Association's Archives of Surgery *in 1955.*[2]

☐ INTRODUCTION

More than a century ago, the French physiologist Bernard speculated that the 'milieu interne' must be preserved to maintain life. His theory that the body responds to external influence to maintain a constant internal environment remains one of the central tenets of medicine. Thomas Addison first made the connection between 'disease of the suprarenal capsules' and the clinical signs and symptoms of adrenal insufficiency. At this time, however, no specific treatment was available, and diagnosis was followed imminently by death. An increase in levels of corticosteroids in tissues during acute stress is an important protective response. The hypothalamic–pituitary–adrenal (HPA) axis has a central role in the body's ability to respond to stress, which may be generated by almost any threat to homeostasis, such as infection, trauma, and surgery. The importance of corticosteroids for survival was illustrated clearly by Dunlop in a survey that examined the outcomes in patients treated for adrenal insufficiency from 1928 to 1962.[3] Until 1939, most patients died within two years of diagnosis. When deoxycortisone acetate became available in

1939, survival increased significantly, and since the advent of cortisone (a purified glucocorticoid preparation) in 1949, patients with Addison's disease have been able to lead nearly normal lives.

☐ PHYSIOLOGY OF STEROIDS

Glucocorticoids are cholesterol derivatives produced in the zona fasiculata of the adrenal cortex. In a healthy unstressed person, cortisol is secreted according to a diurnal pattern under the influence of corticotrophin released from the pituitary gland, with peak levels between 4 am and 8 am. Secretion of corticotrophin, in turn, is under the influence of hypothalamic corticotrophin-releasing hormone, and both hormones are subject to negative feedback control by cortisol itself. Cortisol circulates in bound and unbound forms – the bound form is primarily carried on cortisol-binding globulin (90%), and it is the unbound form that is active physiologically and regulated homeostatically. Current routine clinical assays measure total levels of cortisol because of technical difficulties associated with measurement of the free fraction, which usually requires equilibrium dialysis followed by tandem mass spectrometry and thus an effort that is difficult to justify routinely. Recent data, however, highlighted the potential significance of free levels of cortisol in the context of acute inflammation, such as severe sepsis and states associated with shifts in circulating albumin and other binding proteins.

Glucocorticoids exert their effects by binding to an intracellular glucocorticoid receptor (GR) protein. This receptor – a member of the nuclear receptor superfamily – is ubiquitous in the cytoplasm of nucleated cells, which reflects the vital role it plays in homeostasis. When GR is activated by a ligand, it translocates to the nucleus and binds as a homodimer to glucocorticoid response elements (GREs) in the DNA sequence, which elicits transcription of glucorticoid target genes.

☐ CAUSES OF ADRENOCORTICAL FAILURE

Primary adrenal failure

Adrenal insufficiency may be of primary or secondary origin.[3] Primary adrenal failure results from destruction of the adrenal cortex itself and has a prevalence of 39–60 per million population. The mean age at diagnosis is 40 (range 17–72) years. In Thomas Addison's time, the most frequent cause was tuberculous adrenalitis, and this still predominates in the developing world, with 5% of patients with active tuberculosis being affected. This is likely to become a more frequent manifestation in the United Kingdom as the increase in cases of tuberculosis continues. Autoimmune adrenal disease accounts for 80–90% of cases of primary adrenal insufficiency, and involves slow destruction of the adrenal cortex by cytotoxic lymphocytes. It may arise as an isolated phenomenon (40%; with a slight male preponderance) or in the context of a polyglandular deficiency syndrome. Autoimmune polyendocrinopathy syndrome type 1 (APS1) is a rare autosomal-recessive disorder that affects up to 15% of patients with autoimmune adrenalitis. The first manifestation is neonatal-onset muco-cutaneous candidiasis, with subsequent development of hypoparathyroidism and adrenal failure. The gene responsible for APS1 has been identified as the autoimmune regulator gene *AIRE*, which drives the expression of self-antigens in the thymic medulla and plays an essential role in 'central' tolerance in humans and mice.

Autoimmune polyendocrinopathy syndrome type 2 (APS2) is more common than APS1 and occurs in an autosomal dominant pattern with variable penetrance. The major features of this polyendocrinopathy are adrenal failure, autoimmune thyroid disease, and type 1 diabetes mellitus. As is the case in APS1, there is often gonadal failure. Other components that are seen in patients with APS1 may also be present (alopecia, vitiligo, and pernicious anaemia) but are much less commonly associated with APS2. No single gene is responsible, but a strong association exists with the genes for major histocompatibility complex, class II, DR beta 3 (*HLA-DR3*) and cytotoxic T lymphocyte antigen 4 (*CTLA-4*).

Adrenomyeloneuropathy and adrenoleukodystrophy (ALD) are increasingly recognised as causes of adrenal insufficiency in young men. These X-linked recessive disorders are caused by a mutation in the *ABCD1* gene, which encodes a peroxisomal membrane protein. The defect results in impaired metabolism of very long chain fatty acids (VLCFAs), which accumulate in the white matter of the nervous system and result in demyelination. The clinical picture comprises adrenal insufficiency and neurological impairment. Adrenal insufficiency can precede the onset of neurological symptoms and is the sole manifestation of the disease in 15% of cases.

Fungal infection remains an important cause of adrenal insufficiency, particularly in immunocompromised people, in whom cryptococcosis is the most frequent cause. Human immunodeficiency virus (HIV) adrenalitis and adrenal insufficiency are increasingly recognised as causes of primary adrenal insufficiency without superadded infection. Adrenal haemorrhage that results in destruction of the adrenal cortex can occur as a result of sepsis and associated coagulopathy. Waterhouse–Friderichsen syndrome (WFS) is massive, usually bilateral haemorrhage into the adrenal glands caused by fulminant meningococcaemia. It is characterised by overwhelming bacterial infection, rapidly progressive hypotension that leads to shock, and disseminated intravascular coagulation (DIC) with widespread purpura.

Adrenal production of cortisol can become impaired by the administration of pharmacological agents. The anaesthetic agent etomidate inhibits the mitochondrial 11β-hydroxylase enzyme (CYP11B1) of the adrenal steroid synthesis pathway. Prolonged infusions have been related to marked increases in mortality,[5] and it is likely that single-dose adrenal suppression is an under-recognised clinical problem.[6,7]

Secondary adrenal failure

Adrenal insufficiency most frequently occurs as a result of pharmacological treatment with glucocorticoids. Treatment with exogenous glucocorticoids suppresses the production of corticotrophin-releasing hormone and corticotrophin and can induce adrenal atrophy. This effect may persist for months after treatment with corticosteroids is stopped and depends on the dose and duration of treatment, but it should be anticipated in any patient who has been receiving >7.5 mg/day prednisolone (30 mg/day hydrocortisone or 0.75 mg/day dexamethasone) for more than three weeks. Patients are particularly at risk of hypoadrenalism if treatment with glucocorticoids is withdrawn abruptly. Patients on low-dose glucocorticoid treatment or within two months of stopping may have normal basal production of cortisol but still be unable to mount a full response if confronted with a physiologically stressful event. Case reports that appeared shortly after the introduction of chronic treatment with glucocorticoids described life-threatening adrenal crises in patients subjected to medical or surgical stresses who were not receiving adequate corticosteroid supplementation.

If exogenous glucocorticoid treatment is excluded as a cause of secondary adrenal insufficiency, the next most frequent cause is a tumour of the hypothalamic–pituitary region, with secondary adrenal insufficiency presenting as a consequence of tumour growth or treatment of the tumour with surgery or irradiation. Few patients have isolated adrenal insufficiency, and the involvement of other hormonal axes or the development of neurological or ophthalmological conditions may precede the development of adrenal insufficiency. Of note, production of mineralocorticoids is preserved in patients with secondary adrenal insufficiency, as it is under the regulatory control of the renin–angiotensin–aldosterone (RAA) system, which is driven by the juxtaglomerular cells in the kidney and the zona glomerulosa of the adrenal cortex.

☐ CORTICOSTEROIDS AND STRESS

Stress from many sources stimulates the HPA axis and increases the secretion of cortisol. The pathways through which the HPA axis is activated are diverse, which reflects the wide variation in forms of stress. The stressor may be emotional, so-called 'social' stress, or physical in response to a multitude of challenges to homeostasis, including pain, tissue injury, sepsis, and hypoxia. By the 1930s, the extreme sensitivity of adrenal-deficient animals to stress was evident; the adrenocortical function of conferring resistance to stress eventually was ascribed to the glucocorticoids. The anti-inflammatory action of corticosteroids was not predicted in the early work on steroids, however – in fact, quite the reverse was the case. Hans Selye, the renowned physiologist, postulated that diffuse rheumatic diseases were caused by excessive secretion of steroids in response to stress. This was dismissed, of course, with the discovery of the dramatic and near-miraculous relief from the symptoms of rheumatoid arthritis provided by treatment with cortisone or adrenocorticotropic hormone (ACTH), which yielded the Nobel Prize for Hench, Kendall, and Reichstein in 1950. To quote one author of the time, 'the most unusual thing about this discovery was its unexpectedness'.

Activation of the HPA axis is facilitated by anatomical connections with the amygdala and hippocampus through which sensory pathways project. The hypothalamus integrates these responses with the monoamine neurotransmitters dopamine, norepinephrine, and serotonin, which are important in regulation of the response.

Glucocorticoids have numerous physiological actions relevant to the adaptation to stress.[8] These will be discussed in turn below.

Metabolic actions of glucocorticoids

Glucocorticoids increase levels of glucose in the blood, which increases the rate of hepatic gluconeogenesis by increasing the activity of phosphoenolpyruvate carboxykinase and glucose-6-phosphatase. There is also stimulation of release of free fatty acids from adipose tissue and liberation of amino acids from body proteins. These processes act to supply energy and substrate to cells for the response to stress and repair of injury.

Effects of glucocorticoids on the cardiovascular system

Adrenal insufficiency predisposes individuals to hypovolaemia and subsequent low blood pressure, and it may lead to circulatory shock in cases of severe stress; these responses can be prevented by replacement doses of corticosteroids. This reflects the role of not only mineralocorticoids but also glucocorticoids in the maintenance of vascular tone, endothelial integrity, and vascular permeability and the distribution of total body water. Glucocorticoids are required for normal cardiovascular reactivity to angiotensin II, epinephrine, and norepinephrine, partly mediated through the increased transcription and expression of receptors for these hormones. Production of nitric oxide, which is important in the modulation of vascular permeability, is reduced in response to glucocorticoids.

Chronic adrenal insufficiency is characterised by decreased systemic vascular resistance and decreased cardiac contractility. Hypotension in patients with acute adrenal insufficiency may mimic the 'shutdown' picture of hypovolaemic shock or the vasodilated pattern typical of hyperdynamic 'septic' shock, depending on whether or not secretion of mineralocorticoids is preserved and fluid resuscitation has been attempted. The possibility of the diagnosis of adrenal insufficiency should be considered in both these circumstances, particularly in patients who fail to respond to fluid challenges and vasopressor drugs.

Anti-inflammatory and immunosuppressive actions of glucocorticoids

Glucocorticoids possess anti-inflammatory and immunosuppressive actions that are mediated through specific receptor mechanisms. Most of the effects of glucocorticoids on the pathways involved in immune and inflammatory reactions are the result of modulation or activity of cytokines, complement activation, and other inflammatory mediators. The effects of glucocorticoids on production of mediators tend to result in an increase in anti-inflammatory factors (for example interleukin (IL) 10, soluble tumour necrosis factor (TNF) receptor, and IL-1 receptor antagonist) and inhibition of the transcription of genes that encode pro-inflammatory mediators. Glucocorticoids decrease the accumulation and function of cells that participate in the immune and inflammatory reactions at sites of tissue injury.

The feedback effect of cytokines on the HPA axis is complicated, with the proinflammatory cytokines IL-1α, IL-1β, and IL-6 increasing activity of the HPA axis, which increases levels of ACTH, corticotropin-releasing hormone (CRH), and glucocorticoids. Cytokines may also suppress activity of the HPA axis, with excessive secretion of inflammatory cytokines leading to systemic or tissue-specific-induced resistance to corticosteroids.

The integration of these mechanisms, as part of the more generalised stress response, serves to protect an individual from threats to homeostasis. Excessive amounts of glucocorticoids can prove harmful, however: immunosuppression, impaired wound healing, and glucocorticoid-induced metabolic abnormalities may be life threatening in certain circumstances. Debate over the years has surrounded the relative importance of the physiological effects of glucocorticoids and the pharmacological effects seen when glucocorticoids are administered in higher doses. The physiological function of stress-induced increases in levels of glucocorticoids has been proposed to protect against an 'overshoot' of host defences that, left unchecked, might itself threaten homeostasis.

Adrenal androgens in stress

Whereas levels of cortisol derived from the adrenal zona fasciculata increase in the serum in response to stress, circulating levels of dehydroepiandrosterone sulphate (DHEAS) – the major product of the adrenal zona reticularis and the most abundant adrenal steroid in the human circulation – decrease.[9] This has been interpreted as a stress-induced shift from adrenal production of androgens towards biosynthesis of glucocorticoids. Such a shift may have a negative effect on the immune response by disrupting the balance between cortisol- and DHEA-induced immune effects. Administration of DHEA in models of sepsis in rodents has been shown to be beneficial for survival; however, rodent adrenals do not usually synthesise DHEA in large amounts, which illustrates the importance of the human model in investigating, in particular, the physiological significance of adrenal androgens.

The adrenal glands secrete DHEA and DHEAS, but only DHEA is considered to be biologically active. A recent study showed that despite low circulating levels of DHEAS, levels of DHEA actually were increased significantly in patients with sepsis – a finding that detracts from the previous concept of DHEA deficiency in patients with septic shock.[10] This response to sepsis is proposed to maintain the physiological ratio of cortisol to DHEA and thereby stabilise the balance between glucocorticoid- and DHEA-mediated effects, which may be favourable for an effective endocrine response to septic shock.

□ TREATMENT WITH CORTICOSTEROIDS IN STRESS

Patients with adrenal insufficiency are unable to mount a normal glucocorticoid response to stress. Intercurrent stressful events may result in adrenal crises, with hypotension and resultant organ hypoperfusion that is potentially life threatening. It is important to recognise situations in which a patient's supply of glucocorticoid may not meet the demands placed on physiological systems by external stress and to treat this appropriately. The conventional recommendations for corticosteroid supplementation in patients with known or suspected adrenal insufficiency are empirical and based on advice from case reports in the early 1950s that described cardiovascular collapse and death during surgery in young patients who received treatment with exogenous corticosteroids. These reports are considered the initial clinical recognition of iatrogenic adrenal insufficiency. Since recommendations for perioperative steroid cover were made in light of these case reports, clinical practice has often involved the administration of large doses of steroids to 'cover' stressful events.

Advances in our knowledge of glucocorticoid physiology have led to attempts to develop a more rational individualised approach for patients with adrenal insufficiency who face stressful events. The key questions in determining appropriate levels of steroid replacement are:

- Who should it be given to?
- Is it necessary?
- How much should be given?
- How should it be given?

The increase in circulating levels of cortisol in response to surgical trauma is one component of the 'stress response'. Acutely stressful events such as surgery result in rapid increases in levels of corticotrophin and cortisol in serum, and the magnitude of the postoperative increase in levels of cortisol in serum is thought to correlate positively with the extent of surgery; however, detailed data on this are still lacking.

The widespread practice of administering large doses of corticosteroids (200–300 mg hydrocortisone) to patients at risk of adrenal crises during induction ofanaesthesia before surgery should be discouraged. The use of supplemental corticosteroids should be individualised to the degree of challenge, and extended durations of dosing should be avoided.

During stress, the normal diurnal variation in secretion of cortisol is lost. Continuous infusions in these circumstances provide more physiological levels of glucocorticoids and limit the rapid clearance and peak levels associated with bolus administration. Intramuscular injection or continuous intravenous infusion may provide a better pharmacokinetic profile than intravenous bolus dosing, although the significance of this is unclear.

Some doctors suggest the use of longer acting glucocorticoid preparations, such as dexamethasone and methylprednisolone, for similar reasons. Synthetic corticosteroids show high variability with regard to their mineralocorticoid activity, however, while hydrocortisone binds the mineralocorticoid receptor with an affinity similar to that of aldosterone. Replacement with the physiological substance cortisol (i.e. hydrocortisone) is, therefore, certainly the preferred option.

Patients with adrenal insufficiency

Patients who receive steroid replacement for adrenal insufficiency should be given supplemental treatment with corticosteroids during any severe illness or surgery. Patients are advised to double their usual daily dose of oral replacement in case of intercurrent illness. In case of prolonged vomiting or diarrhoea, they need parenteral administration of hydrocortisone, and prescription of an emergency injection kit with an ampoule of 100 mg hydrocortisone (eg SoluCortef) for intramuscular self-injection has proved useful. Minor procedures (like routine dental checks) and psychosocial stresses (such as exams) do not require routine adjustment of the dose of glucocorticoid, although this may be necessary before prolonged physical exercise (for example, an additional 5 mg of hydrocortisone 1–2 hours before exercise). All patients with chronic adrenal insufficiency should carry a steroid emergency card and should be trained regularly with regard to procedures for the adjustment of doses of glucocorticoids during stress or illness.

When a person presents to hospital with a full-blown adrenal crisis, 100 mg hydrocortisone should be administered intramuscularly or intravenously as a bolus, followed by 200 mg hydrocortisone every 24 hours as a continuous infusion in 5% glucose or by intramuscular injection (50 mg four times daily). Importantly, hypovalaemia has to be tackled by concurrent infusion of saline – initially at a rate of 1 litre per hour, which requires close cardiac monitoring.

Minor surgical stress – for example, a tooth extraction or the removal of a skin lesion under local anaesthesia – should be covered by doubling the oral dose on the day of surgical intervention. Moderate-to-major surgical stress should be covered by administration of 100 mg hydrocortisone as a continuous infusion in 5% glucose or by intramuscular administration (50 mg four times daily). It should be appreciated, however, that these are empirical recommendations and that no single publication has comprehensively addressed the comparability of the pharmacokinetics of cortisol after intravenous bolus, intravenous infusion, and intramuscular injection of hydrocortisone.

The dose of hydrocortisone usually can be tapered rapidly alongside clinical recovery. Assessment of the adequacy of replacement of steroid should be based on clinical features.

Patients with glucocorticoid-induced suppression of the adrenal axis

Evaluation of the HPA axis and adrenal reserve is not informative in patients who are currently receiving exogenous glucocorticoids for the pharmacological treatment of diseases other than adrenal insufficiency – for example, prednisolone for the treatment of rheumatoid arthritis. Generally, adrenal suppression can be assumed if a patient is receiving the equivalent of >7.5 mg prednisolone for more than four weeks. In patients who are receiving doses equivalent to 5–10 mg prednisolone, no further adjustment is necessary during routine surgery, as these doses yield glucocorticoid activity equivalent to the levels of cortisol observed during moderate and major surgical stress. During emergency surgical procedures and in case of a prolonged stay in the intensive care unit (ICU) for treatment of infectious complications, hydrocortisone may be administered at the usual dose for stress of 100 mg per 24 hours.

Patients with critical illness

The role of the HPA axis in critical illness has been the subject of much debate. Adrenal insufficiency has been implicated as an important contributing factor to the poor outcomes in patients with severe sepsis and septic shock.[11] Clinical signs of adrenal insufficiency may be difficult to detect in patients with critical illness, and a high index of suspicion is required. The debate is complicated by uncertainty as to how best to assess the activity of the HPA axis during critical illness: the changes in cortisol-binding globulin that occur in the critically ill,[12] the influence of tissue-specific resistance to glucocorticoids, and how to determine appropriate pass or fail criteria are a few of the problems that confuse the issue.[13]

Evidence supports the use of supplemental corticosteroids in patients with established septic shock, and some have suggested that the response to hydrocortisone depends on the response of the adrenal gland to stimulation by ACTH, as per the short synacthen test.[14] It may well be possible, however, that we are looking at a cytokine-induced phenomenon that is a bystander and not a causative factor in severe sepsis and septic shock, and more research is needed into the recovery of parameters for the adrenal axis after treatment in the ICU. High-dose glucocorticoids have been shown to adversely affect outcome in patients with septic shock,[15] and whether the current approach recommended by Annane[14] – 50 mg by intravenous bolus every six hours – really represents a 'low-dose' approach or whether this kind of treatment aims at pharmacological effects rather than replacement is questionable.

Current practice in ICUs is to arrange for a short synacthen test on diagnosis of septic shock followed by initiation of hydrocortisone treatment (50 mg four times a day). This practice may have to be scrutinised, however, depending on the results reported in the imminent publication of the Corticosteroid Therapy of Septic Shock (CORTICUS) trial – a multinational effort to assess the efficacy of treatment with hydrocortisone in the context of septic shock.

In 2007, 60 years after John F Kennedy was diagnosed with Addison's disease, we have considerably more detailed knowledge on glucocorticoid physiology and pharmacology, but many questions remain to be answered with regard to management of glucocorticoid deficiency in stress. We hope that future studies will enable us to give precise answers that will enhance our clinical practice, which, in this specific area, currently is based more on pragmatic experience than scientific evidence.

REFERENCES

1 Gilbert RE. *JFK and Addison's*. Boston, MA: John F Kennedy Presidential Library and Museum, 1992. Available at: www.jfklibrary.org/Historical+Resources/Archives/Reference+Desk/JFK+and+Addisons+ Disease.htm (last accessed 13 Dec 2007).

2 Nicholas JA, Burstein CL, Umberger CJ, Wilson PD. Management of adrenocortical insufficiency during surgery. *AMA Arch Surg* 1955;71:737–42.

3 Dunlop DM. The diagnosis and treatment of Addison's disease. *Proc R Soc Med* 1953;46:565–6.

4 Arlt W, Allolio B. Adrenal insufficiency. *Lancet* 2003;361:1881–93.

5 Allolio B, Stuttmann R, Fischer H, Leonhard W, Winkelmann W. Long-term etomidate and adrenocortical suppression. *Lancet* 1983;2:626.

6 Allolio B, Stuttmann R, Leonhard U, Fischer H, Winkelmann W. Adrenocortical suppression by a single induction dose of etomidate. *Klin Wochenschr* 1984;62:1014–7.

7 Annane D. ICU physicians should abandon the use of etomidate! *Intensive Care Med* 2005;31:325–6.

8 Arlt W, Stewart PM. Adrenal corticosteroid biosynthesis, metabolism, and action. *Endocrinol Metab Clin North Am* 2005;34:293–313, viii.

9 Beishuizen A, Thijs LG, Vermes I. Decreased levels of dehydroepiandrosterone sulphate in severe critical illness: a sign of exhausted adrenal reserve? *Crit Care* 2002;6:434–8.

10 Arlt W, Hammer F, Sanning P *et al.* Dissociation of serum dehydroepiandrosterone and dehydroepiandrosterone sulfate in septic shock. *J Clin Endocrinol Metab* 2006;91:2548–54.

11 Annane D, Sébille V, Troché G *et al.* A 3-level prognostic classification in septic shock based on cortisol levels and cortisol response to corticotropin. *JAMA* 2000;283:1038–45.

12 Hamrahian AH, Oseni TS, Arafah BM. Measurements of serum free cortisol in critically ill patients. *N Engl J Med* 2004;350:1629–38.

13 Cooper MS, Stewart PM. Corticosteroid insufficiency in acutely ill patients. *N Engl J Med* 2003;348:727–34.

14 Annane D, Sébille V, Charpentier C *et al.* Effect of treatment with low doses of hydrocortisone and fludrocortisone on mortality in patients with septic shock. *JAMA* 2002; 288:862–71.

15 Sprung CL, Caralis PV, Marcial EH *et al.* The effects of high-dose corticosteroids in patients with septic shock. A prospective, controlled study. *N Engl J Med* 1984;311:1137–43.

Making sense of 'funny thyroid function tests'

Mark Gurnell

□ INTRODUCTION

Disorders of thyroid function (for example, hyperthyroidism and hypothyroidism) are common causes of morbidity in the general population. In some instances, the presence of thyroid disease is not immediately obvious, and a diagnosis is made only when thyroid function tests are requested on the basis of an associated complication such as atrial fibrillation (AF). Most doctors are all too aware of the importance of not missing a diagnosis of underlying thyroid dysfunction in this and other clinical settings, and thyroid function testing accordingly has become one of the most common investigations in patients admitted through the acute medical route. Similarly, general practitioners frequently request thyroid function tests in patients who complain of a variety of non-specific symptoms, including tiredness, lethargy, and weight gain or loss. The average clinical biochemistry department therefore faces a significant challenge to provide rapid and accurate measurement of levels of thyroid-stimulating hormone (TSH) and, where necessary, thyroid hormones (thyroxine (T4) and triiodothyronine (T3)). Fortunately, the introduction of sensitive assays, coupled with high-throughput platforms, ensures that most laboratories provide a high-quality service in a timely manner.

Interpretation of the results of most thyroid function tests is straightforward, and more than 90% of patients investigated ultimately are deemed to have normal function of the thyroid gland. In the remaining patients, combined measurement of TSH with T4 or T3, or both, usually enables a simple diagnosis of hyperthyroidism or hypothyroidism. However, a small but important number of situations in which the results of assays of TSH, T4 and T3 seem to point in different directions, remain, thereby producing clinical confusion. Although some of these cases represent an increasingly recognised, albeit rare, group of genetic disorders of the hypothalamic–pituitary–thyroid axis, most of these 'funny thyroid function tests' ultimately can be attributed to concomitant illness, drug treatment, poor compliance with thyroid medication, or interference in one or other of the laboratory assays. These atypical patterns of thyroid function tests are easily misdiagnosed by unwary clinicians, which may lead to inappropriate recommendations for treatment. In this article, I provide guidance to the general physician on how to avoid these pitfalls, thus ensuring the correct interpretation and management of patients with 'funny thyroid function tests'.

☐ THYROID FUNCTION TESTS

Thyroid hormones regulate a diverse array of biological processes (including reproduction, metabolism, and neurological development and function). Hypothalamic thyrotropin-releasing hormone (TRH) stimulates the secretion of TSH from anterior pituitary thyrotrophs, which in turn directs production and release of T4 and T3. The predominant hormone secreted by the thyroid gland is T4, and this is converted to T3, the biologically active hormone, by the actions of a family of deiodinase enzymes. Throughout life, circulating levels of T3 and T4 are maintained within a fairly narrow range in any given individual. In people with an intact hypothalamic–pituitary–thyroid axis, small changes in thyroid status are reflected initially by compensatory changes in hypothalamic TRH and pituitary TSH secretion. Measurement of TSH thus is the most sensitive indicator of thyroid status in those with normal hypothalamic–pituitary function. Accordingly, most laboratories offer a highly sensitive (second- or third-generation) assay for TSH, with a limit of detection <0.1 mU/l, as the initial screening test for thyroid dysfunction. An estimate of T3 or T4 alone is not recommended for routine screening, as small changes in levels of T3 or T4 may yield results that still lie within the reference range, thereby allowing so-called 'subclinical' disease to go undetected. Where TSH is used as the initial screening test, the level of T4 (with or without T3) should be checked after an abnormal level of TSH is detected. In some cases, a combination of all three tests (TSH, T4, and T3) will be needed.

It is worth noting that a small number of laboratories still offer total thyroid hormone assays (total T4 (TT4) and total T3 (TT3)), and it is important to remember that alterations in thyroid hormone binding carrier proteins (for example, thyroxine-binding globulin (TBG), prealbumin and albumin) may affect these measurements and suggest the presence of thyroid dysfunction in an otherwise euthyroid individual. Pregnancy, oestrogens (for example, from oral contraceptive preparations and hormone replacement therapy), and hepatic disorders can cause increases in levels of TBG. Accordingly, whenever possible, assays of free hormones (free T4 (FT4) and free T3 (FT3)) should be used; for the remainder of this article, all references to levels of T4 and T3 will relate to measurements of the free hormones unless stated otherwise.

Where TSH alone is used as the first-line screening test, it is important to remember that a small number of diagnoses may be missed (Table 1). If any of these conditions are clinically suspected, therefore, it is important to check the level of FT4 (with or without FT3) together with the level of TSH.

In practice, seven different patterns of the three main thyroid function tests (TSH, FT4, and FT3) may be encountered (Fig 1).

Convergent thyroid function tests

Normal levels of TSH, FT4, and FT3

In general, if all three parameters fall within their respective laboratory reference ranges, thyroid disease can confidently be excluded in the vast majority of patients. Interestingly, some patient advocacy groups and a small number of clinicians have

Table 1 Conditions and situations in which measurement of thyroid-stimulating hormone (TSH) levels alone may be misleading.

Common	Rare
• Non-thyroidal illness • Recent treatment for hyperthyroidism • Central hypothyroidism (hypothalamic and/or pituitary disease)	• TSH-secreting pituitary adenoma • Resistance to thyroid hormone (RTH)

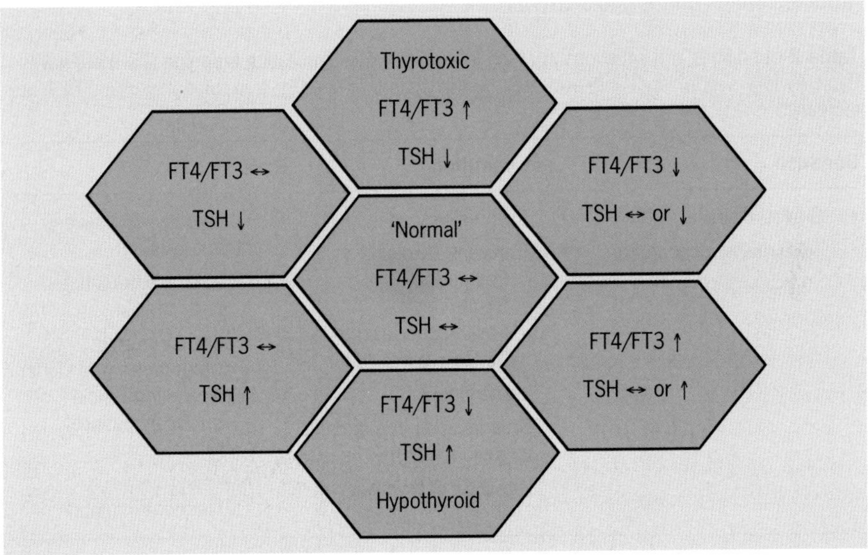

Fig 1 Patterns of thyroid function tests.

argued that it is possible to have symptoms genuinely attributable to hypothyroidism despite entirely normal thyroid function tests. Indeed, many endocrinologists are aware of euthyroid patients who have been treated with thyroid hormones by private practitioners even though this treatment is based on no serious scientific data or physiologically plausible hypothesis. Moreover, where data that has been subject to appropriate scientific scrutiny exists, it has failed to support this approach. For example, in the simple but well-conducted study of Pollock and colleagues, thyroxine was found to be no more effective than placebo in improving cognitive function and psychological well being in patients with symptoms of hypothyroidism but normal thyroid function tests.[1] For now, therefore, if the levels of TSH, FT4, and FT3 all lie within the normal range, patients should be advised that there is no evidence to support the use of T4 or T3 to treat 'hypothyroid symptoms'. Only one exception to this rule should be considered; in individuals who are receiving thyroxine replacement for existing hypothyroidism, restoring TSH levels to the normal range occasionally does not fully alleviate the patient's symptoms – in this setting, the levels of FT4 and FT3 typically are 'low normal' and the level of TSH is 'high normal', which suggests that the patient's intrinsic axis operated with higher levels of FT4 or FT3, or both, before the development of hypothyroidism. In these circumstances, it may be appropriate to make a small increment to the thyroxine dose so as to push the level of TSH down to the lower part of the reference range (for example, between 0.4 mU/l and 2 mU/l).

Low levels of TSH and increased levels of FT4 and/or FT3

This pattern of thyroid function tests indicates primary hyperthyroidism, the causes of which are shown in Table 2. In this context, the level of TSH should be 'undetectable' (that is, <0.1 mU/l).

Table 2 Conditions and situations in which levels of thyroid-stimulating hormone (TSH) are low (typically fully suppressed) and levels of free thyroxine (FT4) and/or free triiodothyronine (FT3) are increased.

Common	Less common	Rare
• Graves' disease • Toxic multinodular goitre	• Toxic solitary adenoma • Transient thyroiditis – Postpartum – Silent – Postviral (for example, De Quervain's) • Iodine induced • Drug induced (for example, by amiodarone) • Ingestion of thyroxine	• Ectopic thyroid tissue or struma ovarii • Metastatic differentiated follicular thyroid carcinoma • Pregnancy related – Hyperemesis gravidarum – Hydatidiform mole – Familial gestational thyrotoxicosis • Activating germline TSH-receptor mutation

Increased levels of TSH and low levels of FT4 and FT3

This pattern of thyroid function tests indicates primary hypothyroidism, the causes of which are shown in Table 3.

Table 3 Conditions and situations in which levels of thyroid-stimulating hormone (TSH) are increased and levels of free thyroxine (FT4) and/or free triiodothyronine (FT3) are low.

Common	Less common	Rare
• Autoimmune thyroiditis – Hashimoto's thyroiditis – Atrophic thyroiditis • Previous treatment for thyrotoxicosis – Thyroidectomy – Treatment with radioiodine	• Hypothyroid phase of thyroiditis • Drug induced (for example, by antithyroid agents, amiodarone, or lithium) • Deficiency or excess of iodine • After external beam irradiation of neck	• Riedel's thyroiditis • Infiltration – Tumour – Amyloid • Congenital – Thyroid agenesis or hypoplasia – Defects in hormonogenesis – Resistance to thyroid-stimulating hormone (TSH)

Divergent ('funny') thyroid function tests

Low levels of TSH and normal levels of FT4 and FT3

Clinical vignette 1

A 67-year-old woman with a past history of hypercholesterolaemia and hypertension was admitted to the emergency assessment unit with a three-week history of progressive shortness of breath. This had been associated with intermittent palpitations but no chest pain. She had no known history of ischaemic heart disease. Her medications included bendroflumethiazide (2.5 mg/day) and simvastatin (40 mg/day).

Physical examination revealed a resting tremor and small goitre. Her pulse was 130–140 beats per minute and she was in AF, but there was no evidence of cardiac failure and the remainder of the physical examination was unremarkable.

The initial electrocardiogram confirmed AF but without ischaemic changes. Her chest X-ray did not show any evidence of pulmonary oedema or cardiomegaly. Thyroid function tests requested by the admitting doctor showed that her level of TSH was <0.1 mU/l (reference range 0.4–4.0 mU/l) and her level of FT4 was 18.0 pmol/l (reference range 9.0–20.0 pmol/l). A FT3 test also was requested, and her level was found to be normal (7.3 pmol/l; reference range 3.0–7.5 pmol/l). Thyroid autoantibodies were not detected.

What is the most likely explanation for this pattern of thyroid function tests?

Low levels of TSH with normal levels of FT4 and FT3 may be seen in several conditions (Table 4). In the case described above, the patient had no history of thyroid disease and was not taking any drugs known to alter hypothalamic– pituitary–thyroid status. Further investigation included thyroid scintigraphy, which showed the appearances of a multinodular goitre. A diagnosis of subclinical hyperthyroidism was made, therefore, although it could reasonably be argued that the condition was not truly 'subclinical', as the patient's presentation with AF was likely to be a direct manifestation of her thyroid dysfunction. In subclinical hyperthyroidism, pituitary thyrotrophs respond to minor increments in levels of thyroid hormones, which remain within the normal range, by switching off production and secretion of TSH. Although an absence of symptoms was once considered an important criterion for diagnosing this condition, it is now well recognised that subtle symptoms or signs of thyrotoxicosis often are present.[2] The very nature of the condition makes it difficult to predict accurately the rate of progression from subclinical to overt hyperthyroidism, although it has been estimated that this approaches 5% per year in patients with a demonstrable multinodular goitre.[2] Even in the absence of progression, several studies have reported that people with persistently suppressed levels of TSH are at increased risk of developing AF[3,4] and osteopenia or osteoporosis.[5] Considerable debate remains among endocrinologists, however, as to the merits of recommending antithyroid treatment (for example, antithyroid drugs or radioiodine) in this setting; many advocate a patient-tailored approach – for example, although it would be reasonable to adopt a surveillance policy in younger asymptomatic patients without evidence of a nodular goitre, antithyroid treatment may be indicated in older patients with AF or

Table 4 Conditions and situations in which levels of thyroid-stimulating hormone (TSH) are low and levels of free thyroxine (FT4) and free triiodothyronine (FT3) are normal.

Common	Less common
• Subclinical hyperthyroidism • Recent treatment for hyperthyroidism	• Drug induced (for example, by glucocorticoids or dopamine) • Non-thyroidal illness

osteoporosis that could have been caused or exacerbated by mild excess of thyroid hormones.

Among patients who have been admitted to hospital, treatment with high-dose glucocorticoids or dopamine can directly suppress pituitary release of TSH. This pattern of blood tests is also seen occasionally with non-thyroidal illness (see below). Accordingly, unless there is an urgent need to institute treatment, repeat thyroid function tests after recovery should help to identify those with true thyroid pathology who need further evaluation or intervention.

Low or normal levels of TSH and low levels of FT4 and/or FT3

Clinical vignette 2

A previously fit and well 58-year-old woman was referred to hospital with increasing respiratory distress on a background of a seven-day history of productive cough, pleuritic chest pain, and fluctuating pyrexia. Her past medical history was notable only for a laparoscopic cholecystectomy, and she was on no regular medication.

On examination, she was pyrexial (temperature 38.5°C), in fast AF (140 beats per minute), and had a blood pressure of 95/65 mmHg. Examination of the chest showed coarse crepitations and bronchial breath sounds at the right base. The admitting doctor noted the patient to have a small goitre but no other features of thyroid dysfunction.

Her level of TSH measured on admission was subnormal at 0.27 mU/l (reference range 0.4–4.0 mU/l), and her level of FT4 was 9.8 pmol/l (reference range 9.0–20.0 pmol/l). An FT3 level was requested and found to be low at 2.6 pmol/l (reference range 3.0–7.5 pmol/l). A test for thyroid peroxidase antibodies was mildly positive (155 U/l; reference range <100 U/l).

What is the most likely explanation for this lady's thyroid function test results?

Low or normal levels of TSH together with low levels of FT3 (with or without low levels of FT4) are a commonly encountered pattern of thyroid function tests in patients who are systemically unwell, indicating the presence of so-called non-thyroidal illness (NTI; sometimes referred to as 'sick euthyroid syndrome'). A summary of the key features of this disorder is shown in Box 1.

In people without obvious concomitant illness, central hypothyroidism must be considered in the differential diagnosis of this pattern of thyroid function tests. In this context, the level of TSH frequently falls within the normal range but clearly is inappropriate for the ambient levels of thyroid hormones. Bearing this in mind, it is

Box 1 Non-thyroidal illness (NTI).

Definition

- A condition characterised by abnormal thyroid function tests that are not a consequence of primary hypothalamic–pituitary–thyroid disease

Patterns of thyroid function tests in NTI

Test		**Result**
TSH		Reduced or normal
T4	• Total T4	Normal, reduced or (elevated)
	• Free T4	Normal, reduced or (elevated)
T3	• Total T3	Reduced or (normal)
	• Free T3	Reduced or (normal)

TSH = thyroid-stimulating hormone; T4 = thyroxine; T3 = triiodothyronine.

Aetiology and pathogenesis

- Contentious but may include:
  - alterations in serum thyroid hormone-binding capacity
  - reduced cellular uptake of T4
  - decreased peripheral conversion of T4 to T3
  - reduced hypothalamic secretion (of TRH) and pituitary secretion (of TSH) (role of interleukin (IL) 1, IL-6, leptin, glucose, and availability of oxygen)
  - other factors, such as cortisol, exogenous glucocorticoids, and dopamine

Adaptive or maladaptive?

- Induced hypothyroidism – a 'beneficial' response

or

- Central hypothyroidism – a potentially 'disadvantageous' response?

Table 5 Conditions and situations in which levels of thyroid-stimulating hormone (TSH) are low or normal and levels of free thyroxine (FT4) and/or free triiodothyronine (FT3) are low.

Common	**Less common**	**Rare**
• Non-thyroidal illness	• Central hypothyroidism (for example, pituitary disease)	• Isolated deficiency of TSH

vital to request measurements of FT4 or FT3, or both, together with TSH, in any patient in whom this diagnosis is suspected. Failure to recognise hypopituitarism could have dire consequences for vision if compression of the optic chiasm by a pituitary macroadenoma goes unrecognised and may even be life threatening in the presence of coexistent hypoadrenalism. Other rarer causes of this pattern of thyroid function tests are shown in Table 5.

Increased levels of TSH with normal levels of FT4 and FT3

Clinical vignette 3

A 46-year-old woman presented to her general practitioner complaining of weight gain of 8 kg over the preceding six months, which had occurred despite her attempts to 'diet'. On direct questioning, she also admitted to tiredness and lethargy. Her past medical history was notable for hyperthyroidism, which had been treated with a subtotal thyroidectomy at the age of 20 years. Thereafter, she had been taking thyroxine replacement treatment (150 µg/day).

Physical examination showed that she was obese (body mass index 32.5 kg/m^2). No thyroid remnant was palpable, and, although her skin was dry to touch, there were no other overt features of hypothyroidism and her resting pulse was 72 beats per minute in sinus rhythm. The remainder of the physical examination was unremarkable.

Thyroid function tests showed a normal level of FT4 (14.0 pmol/l; reference range 9.0–20.0 pmol/l) but a significantly increased level of TSH (42 mU/l; reference range 0.4–4.0 mU/l). In light of these findings, the duty biochemist had also requested a FT3 test, which showed normal levels (4.8 pmol/l; reference range 3.0–7.5 pmol/l).

What is the most likely explanation for this lady's presentation and abnormal thyroid function tests?

Increased levels of TSH with normal levels of FT4 and FT3 are commonly an indicator of mild thyroid failure (so-called subclinical hypothyroidism). Population studies have suggested that 5–10% of all women may be affected by this condition at some time during their life (typically with positive tests for antithyroid peroxidase antibodies).[6] The level of TSH, however, is usually only slightly increased. If the level of TSH is increased to a value that is usually associated with a frankly low level of FT4 or FT3 (that is, >20 mU/l) or does not show appropriate suppression with the introduction or titration of thyroxine replacement treatment, the possibility of interference with laboratory assays should be considered. It is beyond the scope of this article to describe the various mechanisms through which assays for TSH and free thyroid hormones may be rendered unreliable, but most clinical biochemistry laboratories are equipped to help screen for these possibilities once clinical concern has arisen. Accurate assessment of the patient's clinical thyroid status can provide an important pointer as to the likely artefactual result. If assay interference is detected, the patient should be informed for future reference, as the phenomenon may persist for several years.

In the case presented in Clinical vignette 3, interference with assays was considered and subsequently excluded. It was noted that although the patient had previously been clinically and biochemically euthyroid on the same dose of thyroxine, she was now reporting symptoms consistent with hypothyroidism. In this context, it is important to consider two possibilities: firstly, if the patient has developed malabsorption (for example, due to coeliac disease), she may have diminished absorption of thyroxine and reappearance of hypothyroid features. This diagnosis was considered unlikely, however, given that the patient had gained weight (arguing against significant malabsorption), and, moreover, the increased level of TSH was markedly disproportionate to the ambient levels of FT4 and FT3. The question of erratic compliance with thyroxine replacement treatment therefore was raised. Omission of thyroxine over several days can be associated with a marked rebound increase in levels of TSH; however, if the patient takes one or two doses of thyroxine just prior to a blood test, this can result in normal circulating levels of T4 and T3 but is insufficient to fully restore the level of TSH to the normal range. This possibility should be considered in cases where there is a significant discordance between the magnitude of the increase in levels of TSH and the circulating levels of free thyroid hormones. In this particular case, the patient subsequently admitted to poor compliance with her thyroxine treatment. Other causes of increased levels of TSH and normal levels of FT4 and FT3 are shown in Table 6.

Table 6 Conditions and situations in which levels of thyroid-stimulating hormone (TSH) are increased and levels of free thyroxine (FT4) and free triiodothyronine (FT3) are normal.

Common	Less common	Rare
• Subclinical hypothyroidism – Autoimmune – Post-thyroid ablation treatment	• Poor compliance with thyroxine replacement treatment • Malabsorption of thyroxine • Assay interference • Drugs (for example, amiodarone – especially during the early stages of treatment) • Non-thyroidal illness recovery phase	• TSH resistance (for example, inactivating germline TSH-receptor mutation)

Normal or increased levels of TSH with increased levels of FT4 ± FT3

Clinical vignette 4

A 67-year-old woman was admitted under the care of the orthopaedic team after a fall in which she sustained a fracture of the right neck of the femur. Her past medical history included mild hypertension, which was well controlled on amlodipine 10 mg/day, and she had undergone a hysterectomy at the age of 40 years for menorrhagia.

During the early postoperative period, she developed fast AF (130 beats per minute) but without cardiovascular compromise. The remainder of the physical examination was unremarkable; specifically, she was euthyroid with no palpable goitre.

In the absence of any obvious primary cardiac or respiratory pathology, the medical registrar, who was called to see the patient the next day, requested thyroid function tests. The level of TSH was mildly increased at 4.6 mU/l (reference range 0.4–4.0 mU/l) and her level of FT4 was 45.2 pmol/l (reference range 9.0–20.0 pmol/l). The level of FT3 also was increased at 14.5 pmol/l (reference range 3.0–7.5 pmol/l). A test for thyroid peroxidase antibodies was mildly positive (160 U/l; reference range <100 U/l).

What is the most likely explanation for this pattern of thyroid function tests?

A normal or increased level of TSH with increased levels of free thyroid hormones is an unusual finding that is most commonly artefactual or drug related, but it can also be found in two rare but clinically important conditions. In this case, as in all other instances, the results of thyroid function tests must be interpreted in the clinical context – is the patient hypothyroid, euthyroid or hyperthyroid? In the case presented here, the presence of AF triggered the request for a TSH test, with the anticipation of diagnosing possible subclinical or mild overt hyperthyroidism, so the finding of an increased level of TSH was unexpected. Similarly, the magnitude of increase in the level of FT4 (and FT3) was disproportionate to the clinical context. In this situation, the validity of the laboratory results must be questioned. For example, the presence of antiiodothyronine antibodies (anti-T4 antibodies or anti-T3 antibodies, or both) in the patient's serum may interfere with assays of free thyroid hormone, thus yielding artificially increased levels of hormones. As indicated above, most laboratories should be able to advise on how best to screen for assay interference.

If assay interference is excluded, a number of other possibilities should be considered (Table 7). In a patient who is taking thyroxine replacement, this pattern of results may indicate poor compliance, with the ingestion of a large dose of thyroxine just prior to the blood test. Alternatively, it is well recognised that a small number of patients who are taking thyroxine replacement treatment need to run a level of FT4 that is mildly above the upper limit of the reference range in order to maintain a satisfactory level of TSH and clinical euthyroidism. In this setting, the level of FT3 almost invariably is normal. Treatment with amiodarone, because it inhibits conversion of T4 to T3, can yield similar results. Most doctors are well versed in the possible consequences for thyroid function of treatment with amiodarone, but surprisingly few are aware of the effects of the much more commonly prescribed agent heparin. Administration of fractionated and unfractionated heparin can produce an artefactual increase in measured levels of free thyroid hormones.[7,8] The mechanism that underlies these abnormalities is not fully understood but seems to involve displacement of T4 and T3 from their carrier protein binding sites in response to an increase in free fatty acids (FFAs). Heparin activates endothelial lipoprotein lipase (LPL), which produces an increase in circulating levels of FFAs (Fig 2). The extent to which FFAs rise is variable, which may explain why abnormal levels of free thyroid hormones are not

Table 7 Conditions and situations in which levels of thyroid-stimulating hormone (TSH) are normal or increased and levels of free thyroxine (FT4) ± free triiodothyronine (FT3) are increased.

Common	Less common	Rare
• Interference with assays (for example, antiiodothyronine (T3 or T4) antibodies; TSH interference)	• Thyroxine replacement treatment (including poor compliance) • Drugs (for, example, amiodarone or heparin) • Non-thyroidal illness – Acute psychiatric illness	• TSH-secreting pituitary tumour (TSHoma) • Resistance to thyroid hormone (RTH)

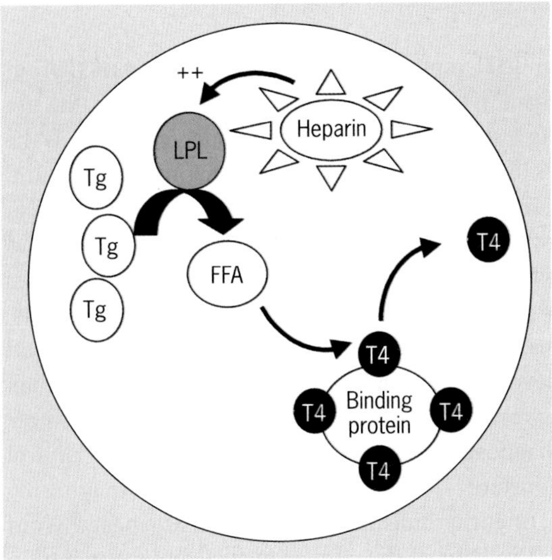

Fig 2 Proposed model of heparin-induced displacement of thyroid hormones from their binding proteins. FFA = free fatty acids; LPL = lipoprotein lipase; T4 = thyroxine; Tg = triglyceride.

seen in all patients treated with heparin. As the displacement continues *in vitro*, pre-analytical delay can compound the situation. Ideally, therefore, when thyroid dysfunction is suspected, samples should be collected before administration of heparin. Alternatively, as the artefact is secondary to hormone displacement, measurements of the levels of total T4 or T3 usually remain normal and assaying these can circumvent the problem. In the case presented here, the surgical team had started heparin before the patient was reviewed by the medical registrar, and when tests of TSH, FT4, and FT3 were repeated on a preoperative blood sample, the TSH was confirmed to be slightly increased (which in the presence of positive thyroid antibodies was likely to reflect latent autoimmune hypothyroidism), but levels of free thyroid hormones were normal.

If assay interference, drug effects, and non-thyroidal illness have been excluded, two rare but important conditions must be considered:

- TSH-secreting pituitary adenoma (TSHoma)[9]
- resistance to thyroid hormone (RTH).

Resistance to thyroid hormone is a genetic disorder in which loss-of-function mutations in the thyroid receptor β (TRβ) isoform are associated with variable tissue refractoriness to thyroid hormone action,[10] which leads to an altered set-point of the hypothalamic–pituitary–thyroid axis. Features that favour a diagnosis of TSHoma include an increased α-subunit:TSH molar ratio, the presence of a pituitary adenoma on magnetic resonance imaging or computed tomography, an attenuated TSH response to exogenous TRH administration and lack of inhibition of TSH secretion by exogenous T3 (reflecting autonomous tumour function), and an increased level of sex-hormone binding globulin (SHBG) (hepatic production of SHBG is strongly dependent on thyroid hormones).[9] In contrast, a family history of similarly affected individuals strongly favours the diagnosis of RTH.[10]

□ SUMMARY/CONCLUSION

As changes in circulating levels of TSH represent the earliest indicator of thyroid dysfunction in patients with an intact hypothalamic–pituitary–thyroid axis, the use of TSH alone as the initial screening test of thyroid status is reasonable, as long as the requesting doctor is aware of its limitations, with central hypothyroidism and pituitary failure the most important potential 'missed diagnoses'. Interpretation of the results of thyroid function tests in most patients with primary thyroid dysfunction is straightforward, with levels of TSH and free thyroid hormones typically showing a pattern that is classic for the underlying disorder (for example, suppressed levels of TSH and increased levels of FT4 or FT3 in hyperthyroidism and increased levels of TSH and low levels of FT4 or FT3 in hypothyroidism). A small number of situations in which the results of thyroid function tests seem to diverge or fail to support the clinical diagnosis remain. In these cases, careful clinical reappraisal of the patient is important – what is the evidence for diagnosing hypothyroidism, hyperthyroidism, or euthyroidism? Interpretation of repeat thyroid function tests (TSH, FT4, and FT3) in light of the clinical history and examination findings should help to determine which of the results is discordant or unexpected. Knowledge of the various conditions that can be associated with each of the patterns of 'funny TFTs' (see Tables 4–7) should allow a correct diagnosis in most cases, thereby ensuring that inappropriate further investigation and treatment are avoided.

REFERENCES

1 Pollock MA, Sturrock A, Marshall K *et al.* Thyroxine treatment in patients with symptoms of hypothyroidism but thyroid function tests within the reference range: randomised double blind placebo controlled crossover trial. *BMJ* 2001;323:891–5.

2 Toft AD. Clinical practice. Subclinical hyperthyroidism. *N Engl J Med* 2001;345:512–6.

3 Sawin CT, Geller A, Wolf PA *et al.* Low serum thyrotropin concentrations as a risk factor for atrial fibrillation in older persons. *N Engl J Med* 1994;331:1249–52.

4 Biondi B, Palmieri EA, Lombardi G, Fazio S. Effects of subclinical thyroid dysfunction on the heart. *Ann Intern Med* 2002;137:904–14.

5 Faber J, Jensen IW, Petersen L *et al.* Normalization of serum thyrotrophin by means of radioiodine treatment in subclinical hyperthyroidism: effect on bone loss in postmenopausal women. *Clin Endocrinol (Oxf)* 1998;48:285–90.

6 Vanderpump MPJ, Tunbridge WMG, French JM *et al.* The incidence of thyroid disorders in the community: a twenty-year follow-up of the Whickham Survey. *Clin Endocrinol (Oxf)* 1995;43:55–68.

7 Laji K, Rhidha B, John R, Lazarus J, Davies JS. Abnormal serum free thyroid hormone levels due to heparin administration. *QJM* 2001;94:471–3.

8 Stevenson HP, Archbold GP, Johnston P, Young IS, Sheridan B. Misleading serum free thyroxine results during low molecular weight heparin treatment. *Clin Chem* 1998;44: 1002–7.

9 Beck-Peccoz P, Brucker-Davis F, Persani L, Smallridge RC, Weintraub BD. Thyrotropin-secreting pituitary tumors. *Endocr Rev* 1996;17:610–38.

10 Gurnell M, Beck-Peccoz P, Chatterjee VKK. Resistance to thyroid hormone. In: DeGroot LJ, Jameson JL, eds. *Endocrinology*. Philadelphia: Elsevier Saunders, 2005:2227–37.

☐ ENDOCRINOLOGY SELF-ASSESSMENT QUESTIONS

New therapies in the management of type 2 diabetes

1 Comparing the background risk of cardiovascular disease in people with diabetes and the general population:
   (a) It is 2–3 times higher in people with diabetes
   (b) It is 1.5 times higher in people with diabetes
   (c) It is four times higher in people with diabetes
   (d) There is no difference
   (e) None of the above

2 The following drugs are contraindicated in people with heart failure:
   (a) Insulin
   (b) Thiazolidinediones
   (c) Dipeptidyl peptidase IV (DPP-4) inhibitors
   (d) Metformin
   (e) Exenatide

3 Regarding treatment:
   (a) Exenatide can be used without special caution in people with diabetes who are taking antidepressant drugs
   (b) Gliptins should be discontinued in patients with mild renal impairment
   (c) Rimonabant is currently recommended as first-line treatment for obese people with diabetes and metabolic syndrome
   (d) Thiazolidinediones offer specific cardiovascular protection through reductions in conventional risk factors

4 The following are associated with weight loss in clinical trials:
   (a) Metformin
   (b) Gliptins
   (c) Inhaled insulin
   (d) Exenatide
   (e) Rimonabant

Management of adrenal insufficiency in severe stress and surgery

1 Concerning adrenocortical failure:
   (a) Primary adrenal failure is a common condition with a prevalence of 200 per million population
   (b) It most frequently affects those aged 25–30 years
   (c) The most frequent cause of adrenal insufficiency is pharmacological treatment
   (d) A single dose of the anaesthetic agent etomidate results in adrenal suppression
   (e) Production of mineralocorticoids is preserved in patients with secondary adrenal failure

2 Concerning glucocorticoids:
(a) They are cholesterol derivatives produced in the zona glomerulosa of the adrenal cortex
(b) Most cortisol circulates in the unbound physiologically active form
(c) Glucocorticoids mediate their effects through membrane bound, G-protein-linked receptors
(d) Glucocorticoids reduce levels of glucose in blood
(e) Endothelial production of nitric oxide is enhanced by glucocorticoids

3 Concerning adrenal insufficiency in stress:
(a) Hypotension in patients with acute adrenal insufficiency may be refractory to treatment with vasopressors
(b) Patients are usually hypovolaemic
(c) It is useful to perform a short synacthen test while patients are receiving exogenous glucocorticoids
(d) Evidence supports the use of supplemental corticosteroids in patients with septic shock
(e) A patient with rheumatoid arthritis who has been taking 5 mg prednisolone for four years will need supplemental corticosteroids when undergoing minor surgery in addition to their routine dose of prednisolone

Making sense of 'funny thyroid function tests'

1 A 73-year-old gentleman attended his general practitioner's surgery for annual review of his type 2 diabetes, which was complicated by cerebrovascular disease. He was on a number of drugs including aspirin, an angiotensin-converting enzyme inhibitor, and thyroxine.

Results of investigations	*Value*	*(Normal range)*
Level of free thyroxine (FT4) in serum	17.6 pmol/l	(9–20)
Level of thyroid-stimulating hormone (TSH) in serum	16.5 mU/l	(0.4–4)

The most likely explanation for this pattern of TFTs is:
(a) Aspirin-induced interference with measurement of FT4
(b) Autonomous secretion of TSH (TSHoma)
(c) Erratic compliance with thyroxine therapy
(d) Malabsorption of thyroxine
(e) Non-thyroidal illness

2 A 66-year-old man with a past medical history of ischaemic heart disease and polymyalgia rheumatica consulted his general practitioner because of tiredness, lethargy, and weight gain. He had recently been discharged from hospital after an episode of acute dyspnoea and palpitations.

On examination, his pulse was 76 beats per minute sinus rhythm and his blood pressure was 135/80 mmHg. He was clinically euthyroid, with no palpable goitre. Auscultation of the chest revealed a pansystolic murmur, with radiation to the axilla, and bibasal fine inspiratory crepitations. He had mild pedal oedema.

Results of investigations	*Value*	*(Normal range)*
Level of FT4 in serum	15.6 pmol/l	(9–20)
Level of free triiodothyronine (FT3) in serum	3.5 pmol/l	(3–7.5)
Level of TSH in serum	8.9 mU/l	(0.4–4)

The most likely explanation for this pattern of TFTs is:
(a) Treatment with amiodarone
(b) Autonomous secretion of TSH (TSHoma)
(c) Non-thyroidal illness
(d) Treatment with prednisolone
(e) Interference with TSH assay

3 A 23-year-old woman with a strong family history of thyroid disease reported numerous symptoms suggestive of hypothyroidism since the birth of her first child. Her past medical history was unremarkable and she was not taking any drugs regularly.

On examination, her pulse was 66 beats per minute sinus rhythm and her blood pressure was 100/65 mmHg. She had a small symmetrical goitre.

Results of investigations	*Value*	*(Normal range)*
Level of FT4 in serum	12.2 pmol/l	(9–20)
Level of FT3 in serum	3.4 pmol/l	(3–7.5)
Level of TSH in serum	0.6 mU/l	(0.4–4)
Level of antithyroid peroxidase in serum	150 U/l	(<100)

The patient should be advised that she has:
(a) Latent Graves' disease
(b) Normal thyroid function
(c) Partial deficiency of TSH
(d) Postpartum thyroiditis
(e) Subclinical hypothyroidism

Infectious disease

Imported infectious disease emergencies

David A Warrell

□ THE INCREASING RISK OF IMPORTED EXOTIC INFECTIONS

International tourism has grown prodigiously over the last few years. Tourist arrivals in 2007 will increase by 4.1% to 880 million, 30% of which will be to tropical or subtropical developing countries (www.world-tourism.org/). This creates an increasing risk to Western travellers of acquiring an exotic infection in a tropical developing country (Table 1). Admitting physicians should therefore consider a broader range of differential diagnoses, diagnostic tests, and specific treatments. Among the more common infectious disease health risks faced by travellers to developing countries are traveller's diarrhoea, malaria, dengue, acute lower respiratory tract infections, hepatitis A, gonorrhoea, and rabies from animal bites.[1,2]

□ ILLUSTRATIVE CASE HISTORIES

Case 1

A 26-year-old woman was admitted to the Emergency Department of a hospital in the United Kingdom (UK) having had a cardiac arrest. Five days earlier she had

Table 1 Importable, acutely life-threatening, exotic infections.

Viruses
- Hepatitis
- Yellow fever
- Haemorrhagic fevers
- Encephalomyelitis – for example:
  - Arboviral
  - Rabies
  - Nipah

Bacteria
- Enteric fevers
- Melioidosis
- Tularaemia
- Leptospirosis
- Rickettsioses
- Relapsing fevers
- Antibiotic-resistant strains – eg:
  - Extensively drug-resistant *Mycobacterium tuberculosis*
  - *Acinetobacter baumannii*

Fungi
- *Penicillium marneffei*
- *Paracoccidioides brasiliensis*

Protozoa
- Malaria
- Babesiosis
- Kala-azar
- Amoebiasis

Helminths
- *Strongyloides* spp.
- *Trichinella* spp.

begun to complain of tiredness and back pain, and three days earlier she 'seemed to catch her breath when sipping liquids or in a draught'. Two days earlier, she had developed dysphagia, urinary incontinence, pain, diarrhoea, and vomiting. She was experiencing hallucinations and was intermittently agitated and terrified. Her medical attendants diagnosed hysteria, some other kind of mental condition, or anxiety about a possible pregnancy and prescribed tranquilisers.

Travel history

Two months earlier while enjoying 'the holiday of a lifetime' with her husband in Himachal Pradesh, northern India, she had been bitten on her leg by a neighbour's dog. She cleaned the wound with whisky and consulted the doctor in a nearby village, who asked whether the dog was mad. When told that the dog did not seem to be mad, he prescribed an antibiotic and a homeopathic remedy for tetanus. The next day she visited a Red Cross hospital in the local large town, but no tetanus vaccine was available there. One month after the bite, she returned to England, where the unhealed bite wound was dressed daily at the local hospital. After the cardiac arrest that prompted her admission to hospital, she did not recover consciousness and died 36 hours later. Rabies was confirmed at autopsy.[3]

Conclusions

Classic rabies (genotype 1) virus is enzootic in most areas of the world except parts of Western Europe, the Mediterranean, Iceland, Japan, Oceania, and the Antarctic. However, rabies-related bat lyssaviruses are found in parts of Europe and Australia. In humans, they can cause a fatal encephalomyelitis that is indistinguishable from classic rabies. India is the country worst affected by rabies. An estimated 16 million bites from potentially rabid dogs and 20,000 human deaths from rabies occur each year despite the use of 4 million courses of rabies postexposure prophylaxis every year.[4] In the tragic case of the 26-year-old woman, the diagnosis was not made while she was still alive. Although rabies encephalomyelitis is essentially untreatable, diagnosis is important. A treatable diagnosis must be excluded and recognition of rabies should lead to appropriate palliative treatment for the patient and measures to minimise staff exposure. Travellers should be educated about the risk of bites from dogs, cats, monkeys, and other wild mammals in India and other areas in which rabies is endemic. Highly effective pre-exposure vaccination with tissue-culture rabies vaccines should be encouraged. Among the 24 human cases of rabies imported to the UK over the last 100 years, two-thirds were from the Indian subcontinent and none had received pre- or postexposure rabies prophylaxis.

Useful websites

- www.dh.gov.uk/en/Publicationsandstatistics/Publications/Publications PolicyAndGuidance/DH_4010434
- www.hpa.org.uk/infections/topics_az/rabies/menu.htm

- www.cdc.gov/rabies/
- www.who-rabies-bulletin.org/
- www.who.int/rabies/en/

Case 2

A 35-year-old man in respiratory distress with fever, haemoptysis, shock, and confusion was transferred to an intensive care unit. Four days earlier, he had been admitted to an infectious disease ward with a five-day history of tiredness and coryza and three days of fever (up to 39.5°C), chills, and myalgia. On that occasion, the results of all the laboratory tests were normal, except a platelet count of 103×10^9/l. Two malaria films had proved negative and a provisional diagnosis of dengue was made.

Travel history

One week earlier, the man had returned from a three-week trip to a wildlife park in Sabah, Borneo. While in the rainforest, he had walked for miles through wet muddy terrain and had been troubled with blisters on his feet and leech infestations. His pre-travel vaccinations included typhoid, hepatitis A, and hepatitis B. He had taken atovaquone proguanil hydrochloride (Malarone) as prophylaxis for malaria.

Progress

Two days before the patient was transferred to the intensive care unit, his condition had deteriorated. He continued to be feverish, had painful and tender lower limbs, and started to cough up blood. His platelet count was falling, while levels of C-reactive protein, urea, creatinine, bilirubin, transaminases, and creatine kinase were increasing. Eight hours before he was due to be transferred, he became acutely breathless, with frank haemoptysis, confusion, hypotension (85/45 mmHg), tachycardia (120 beats per minute), tachypnoea, and desaturation. He had no rash. During his time in the intensive care unit, he was intubated, ventilated, haemoperfused, and treated for nosocomial pneumonia. Three days after transfer, serological test results confirmed the diagnosis of leptospirosis (immunoglobulin (Ig) M positive on leptospira antibody enzyme-linked immunosorbent assay (ELISA) at 1:2560; microagglutination test positive at 1:5120). He eventually made a complete recovery.

Conclusions

The lack of any rash and the development of acute renal failure made the diagnosis of dengue unlikely (www.cdc.gov/ncidod/dvbid/dengue/). Contact with freshwater-laden, rodent-inhabited environments, especially in South Asia, carries a high risk of leptospirosis. During the 'Eco-Challenge-Sabah 2000 multisport endurance race' (21 August–1 September 2000), 26% of 304 expatriate athletes from a variety of western countries caught leptospirosis.[5] Infection can be acquired through broken skin or intact mucosae. Antibiotic treatment, ideally with benzylpenicillin or doxycycline, is recommended at any stage of the disease, but early treatment is most likely to improve the clinical outcome. Doxycycline 200 mg weekly, or the malaria prophylactic regimen of 100 mg daily, is effective in preventing leptospirosis.[6]

Case 3

A 46-year-old man was admitted to hospital with a one-week history of fever, malaise, cough, prostration, and lumps in the skin. The clinical impression was of septicaemic shock. He had ulcerating papules on his forehead, face, and trunk. He was bisexual and had recently been diagnosed as seropositive for HIV.

Travel history

The patient had travelled extensively in the Far East and, nine months earlier, had visited some bat-infested caves in Yunnan, China.

Diagnosis

Penicillium marneffei was found in and cultured from biopsies of the skin and bone marrow, and the patient was successfully treated with amphotericin B.

Conclusions

This case demonstrates that fungal infection alone, without superimposed bacterial sepsis, should be included in the differential diagnosis of septic shock. *Penicillium marneffei* is proving to be an increasingly important opportunistic infection in immunosuppressed people in Asia.[7,8] It has been reported as an imported infection in patients from many southeast Asian countries. Although *Molluscum contagiosum*-like skin lesions have been regarded as virtually diagnostic of *P. marneffei*, identical appearances can be seen in other disseminated fungal infections, notably histoplasmosis and paracoccidioidomycosis. This infection is important to recognise, as it is eminently treatable with amphotericin B and preventable with itraconazole.[9]

Case 4

A 20-year-old British man was admitted to an intensive care unit with respiratory and circulatory failure and disseminated intravascular coagulation. Three days earlier he had been admitted to a district general hospital with a four-day history of cyclical fevers, headache, malaise, and dark urine. On examination, he had appeared unwell. He was sweating, with tachycardia (96 beats per minute), blood pressure of 115/65 mmHg, and fever (39.9°C). On admission to the hospital, all his blood tests were normal, except for a platelet count of 103×10^9/l. The clinical impression was of malaria.

Travel history

One week before his admission to the hospital, he had returned from four months of relief and reconstruction work in West Africa (Morocco, Mauritania, Burkina

Faso, and Ghana). Pre-travel vaccinations were against typhoid, yellow fever, and meningococcal infection. He was prescribed antimalaria prophylaxis with atovaquone proguanil hydrochloride but had stopped taking it one month before leaving Africa. Fewer than six hours after his admission to the hospital, the laboratory reported *Plasmodium falciparum* in the blood film (0.4% of erythrocytes were parasitised). He was started on oral quinine (600 mg three times a day) and was given intravenous fluids. Eleven hours later, he was switched to intravenous quinine, but his condition deteriorated rapidly over the ensuing 36 hours. His blood pressure fell to 99/51 mmHg, heart rate increased to 130 beats per minute, haemoglobin concentration fell to 9.4 g/l, platelet count decreased to 51×10^9/litre, international normalised ratio (INR) increased to 2.3, activated partial thromboplatin time (APTT) increased to 73 seconds, concentration of D-dimer increased to 6843 ng/ml (normal range <500 ng/ml), albumin concentration decreased to 22 g/l, and parasite count rose to 9.0%. On admission to the intensive treatment unit at the tertiary referral hospital, chest radiographs suggested adult respiratory distress syndrome (ARDS), and the patient was intubated and ventilated. His fever persisted, despite clearance or parasites. His blood pressure was maintained at 115/50 mmHg on noradrenaline (0.5 μg/kg/minute) and his heart rate at 100 beats per minute. Ceftriaxone, vancomycin, and meropenem were prescribed, but the ARDS worsened and required increasing ventilatory pressures. Bilateral pneumothoraces developed and were drained, but the patient died nine days after admission.

Conclusions

Malaria is endemic in most tropical countries, but the epidemiological situation is dynamic. Recently, malaria was reintroduced to Jamaica from Haiti, and some western tourists visiting Goa, India, were infected with falciparum malaria – in one case despite prophylaxis with chloroquine and proguanil. There has been one fatality. Between 1,600 and 2,500 cases of malaria are notified in the UK each year. In 2005, there were 1,754 cases, with 11 fatalities, and, over the last 19 years, there has been an average of eight deaths per year. In 2005, 76% of all cases and all but one death were attributed to *P. falciparum* (www.hpa.org.uk/infections/topics_az/malaria/cases_deaths.htm).

Malaria must be excluded in any patient with an acute fever who has visited an endemic area, especially during the previous few months. The travel history may not be volunteered! Falciparum malaria can evolve rapidly; exceptionally, it can kill within 24 hours of the first symptom. Malaria is commonly misdiagnosed as influenza, traveller's diarrhoea, hepatitis, viral encephalitis, or haemorrhagic fever. Patients with suspected malaria should be admitted to hospital. Chemoprophylaxis for malaria should be stopped (to aid microscopical diagnosis), and thick and thin blood films should be examined daily for at least 72 hours or until an alternative diagnosis is made, but experienced parasitologists are not always available. Rapid malarial antigen detection is an alternative. If features of severe malaria develop, a trial of antimalarial chemotherapy should be started immediately.

In the case described here, oral, and later intravenous, treatment with quinine started five days after the onset of symptoms, six hours after admission to hospital and 30 minutes after confirmation of diagnosis failed to prevent the evolution of fatal falciparum malaria. Intravenous sodium artesunate proved superior to intravenous quinine in a multicentre randomised controlled trial in 1,461 patients with severe falciparum malaria in Bangladesh, India, Myanmar, and Indonesia.[10] Compared with quinine, artesunate reduced the rate of fatal cases by 34.7% (95% confidence interval 18.5% to 47.6%, p=0.0002). Artesunate is not yet licensed in the UK, but its use should be considered on a named-patient basis in severely ill patients and in those who fail to respond to optimal quinine treatment. In August 2007, the Centers for Disease Control and Prevention in the USA received permission from the Food and Drug Administration to provide intravenous artesunate for emergency use in the United States for patients with severe malaria. Travellers must be educated to continue chemoprophylaxis for four weeks after leaving the malarious area (one week when they are taking atovaquone proguanil hydrochloride). If malaria is diagnosed, other members of the family or group who were likely to have shared the same exposure as the index case should be checked.

Useful websites

- www.hpa.org.uk/infections/topics_az/malaria/guidelines.htm
- www.hpa.org.uk/infections/topics_az/malaria/pdf/mal_treat_JoI07.pdf
- www.who.int/malaria/docs/TreatmentGuidelines2006.pdf
- www.cdc.gov/malaria/index.htm

TRAVEL HISTORY

A precise travel history is essential. For example, visits to the islands of Ko Samui and Ko Chang in the Gulf of Thailand expose the traveller to no risk (Ko Samui) or a substantial risk (Ko Chang) of malaria. Other important questions about travel include:

- Was the area visited rural or urban? Was accommodation luxurious or rough? Which daytime and night-time activities were undertaken? These factors determine exposure to vectors such as mosquitoes and to foodborne, waterborne, and some other infections.
- What was the detailed itinerary? Even if the traveller's main destination was not endemic for a particular disease such as malaria, stopovers – or even waiting on a runway in an endemic area – might have exposed them to infection.[11]
- When did the symptoms start? Knowledge of the incubation period may help diagnosis: a fever that develops fewer than seven days after arrival in the endemic area cannot be malaria, while a fever that starts more than 21 days after leaving West Africa cannot be Lassa fever.
- Did anything unusual happen to the patient while they were travelling? Trauma, road traffic accidents, blast injuries, and penetrating or aquatic

injuries may have exposed the traveller to environmental pathogens such as *Acinetobacter baumannii* (explosions), *Vibrio vulnificus* (saltwater), *Aeromonas hydrophila (fresh/brackish water)*, *Leptospira* spp. (fresh water), or *Pasteurella multocida* or rabies (mammal bites or scratches). Bites by mosquitoes, ticks, lice, fleas, and reduviid ('kissing') bugs carry the risk of a variety of infections. A needlestick injury, injection, surgery, or contact with blood products could expose the traveller to HIV, human T-lymphotropic virus (HTLV)-1, hepatitis viruses, malaria, other protozoan infections, and *Clostridia* spp. Casual unprotected sex with a stranger carries the risk of a variety of sexually transmitted diseases, HIV, HTLV-1, hepatitis viruses, and herpes viruses.

□ INDIVIDUAL TRAVELLER'S SPECIAL VULNERABILITIES

Lack of pre-travel vaccinations, failure to take appropriate chemoprophylaxis, and failure to prevent exposure are obvious vulnerabilities. Splenectomy confers susceptibility to malaria, babesiosis, and encapsulated bacterial infections. Pregnancy is a risk factor for severe malaria, visceral leishmaniasis, amoebiasis, and listeriosis. Drugs such as glucocorticoids increase the risk of tuberculosis, hepatitis E virus infection, amoebiasis, melioidosis, and invasive strongyloidiasis, while inhibitors of gastric acid secretion increase the risk of gastrointestinal infections. Some chronic infections (for example, HIV and HTLV-1) and chronic illnesses (diabetes mellitus, alcoholic cirrhosis, chronic renal failure, urinary tract calculi, and sickle cell anaemia) decrease resistance to various infections.

Limitations of blind emergency broad-spectrum antibiotic treatment in returned travellers with severe sepsis

Commonly recommended blind broad-spectrum antibiotic treatment consists of a broad-spectrum antipseudomonal penicillin, such as piperacillin with tazobactam or ticarcillin with clavulanic acid, or a broad-spectrum cephalosporin (ceftazidime or cefotaxime). In either case, an aminoglycoside such as gentamicin commonly is added. Such treatment does not cover any viral infection, miliary tuberculosis, rickettsioses, *Acinetobacter baumannii, Listeria monocytogenes* encephalitis, or any fungal, protozoal, or helminthic infection.

□ SURVEILLANCE: CURRENT EPIDEMICS

It is useful to know which diseases are currently epidemic in the country from which the ill traveller has returned. At the time of the *Horizons in Medicine* conference in February 2007, chikungunya fever was affecting millions of people in South Asia and, subsequently, local transmission has been established in northwest Italy; a few cases of yellow fever had been reported in Togo (West Africa) and Bolivia; extensively drug-resistant tuberculosis (XDR-TB) had been diagnosed in 314 people in Kwazulu Natal, South Africa, causing 214 fatalities; sleeping sickness had returned to Malawi;

an epidemic of Rift Valley fever had killed more than 200 people in Kenya, Somalia, and Tanzania; and there had been 16,000 cases of meningococcal meningitis, with 1,700 fatalities, in the Democratic Republic of the Congo, Sudan, and Uganda.

Useful website

- www.promedmail.org/

REFERENCES

1 Behrens RH, Steffen R. Travel medicine. In: Cook GC, Zumla AI, eds. *Manson's tropical diseases.* Edinburgh: WB Saunders, 2003:533–43.

2 Freedman DO, Weld LH, Kozarsky PE *et al.* Spectrum of disease and relation to place of exposure among ill returned travellers. *N Engl J Med* 2006;354:119–30.

3 Warrell DA. *Rabies – the facts.* Oxford: Oxford University Press, 1986:43–5.

4 Knobel DL, Cleaveland S, Coleman PG *et al.* Re-evaluating the burden of rabies in Africa and Asia. *Bull World Health Organ* 2005;83:360–8.

5 Sejvar J, Bancroft E, Winthrop K *et al.* Leptospirosis in 'Eco-Challenge' athletes, Malaysian Borneo, 2000. *Emerg Infect Dis* 2003;9:702–7.

6 Bharti AR, Nally JE, Ricaldi JN *et al.* Leptospirosis: a zoonotic disease of global importance. *Lancet Infect Dis* 2003;3:757–71.

7 Sirisanthana T, Supparatpinyo K, Perriens J, Nelson KE. Amphotericin B and itraconazole for treatment of disseminated *Penicillium marneffei* infection in human immunodeficiency virus-infected patients. *Clin Infect Dis* 1998;26:1107–10.

8 Vanittanakom N, Cooper CR Jr, Fisher MC, Sirisanthana T. *Penicillium marneffei* infection and recent advances in the epidemiology and molecular biology aspects. *Clin Microbiol Rev* 2006;19:95–110.

9 Supparatpinyo K, Perriens J, Nelson KE, Sirisanthana T. A controlled trial of itraconazole to prevent relapse of *Penicillium marneffei* infection in patients infected with the human immunodeficiency virus. *N Engl J Med* 1998;339:1739–43.

10 Dondorp A, Nosten F, Stepniewska K, Day N, White N. Artesunate versus quinine for treatment of severe falciparum malaria: a randomised trial. *Lancet* 2005;366:717–25.

11 Conlon CP, Berendt AR, Dawson K, Peto TE. Runway malaria. *Lancet* 1990;335:472–3.

Update on HIV

Andrew Freedman, Brendan Healy

□ INTRODUCTION

Just more than 25 years have passed since the first description of the acquired immunodeficiency syndrome (AIDS) in gay men in Los Angeles in 1981. The causative agent, later named the human immunodeficiency virus (HIV), was discovered in 1983. Since that time, a vast amount of research has been undertaken, and this has led to a detailed understanding of the life cycle of the virus and the pathogenesis of infection with HIV. This, in turn, has permitted the development of highly effective antiretroviral therapy (HAART), which, although not a cure, has resulted in infection with HIV being regarded as a chronic treatable disease. Nevertheless, challenges remain, including the potential for serious toxicity from long-term drug treatment, as well as the difficulty in developing an effective vaccine to prevent infection.

This paper will focus on the current epidemiology of infection with HIV (both globally and in the United Kingdom (UK)), co-infection with tuberculosis (TB), current treatment strategies, emerging drug treatments, and approaches to prevention of HIV.

□ EPIDEMIOLOGY

The epidemic of infection with HIV has already killed some 25 million people and continues to spread worldwide. An estimated 39.5 million people were living with HIV at the end of 2006 – more than half of these in subSaharan Africa (Fig 1). In 2006, an estimated 4.3 million people were newly infected and there were 2.9 million deaths.[1] Overall, the global incidence of HIV is thought to have peaked in the late 1990s but continues to increase in some countries. Despite the stable incidence, the total number of people living with HIV continues to rise. This is a result of population growth combined with the life-prolonging effects of treatment with antiretroviral drugs, although access to these remains limited in the countries with the highest prevalences of infection.

At the end of 2005, an estimated 63,500 adults in the UK were living with HIV, 20,100 (32%) of whom were unaware of their diagnosis.[2] The prevalence of infection with HIV continues to rise because of increasing numbers of new diagnoses and a reduction in mortality among individuals already diagnosed (Fig 2).

Men who have sex with men remain the group at greatest risk of acquiring infection with HIV within the UK. No decline in the numbers of new infections in

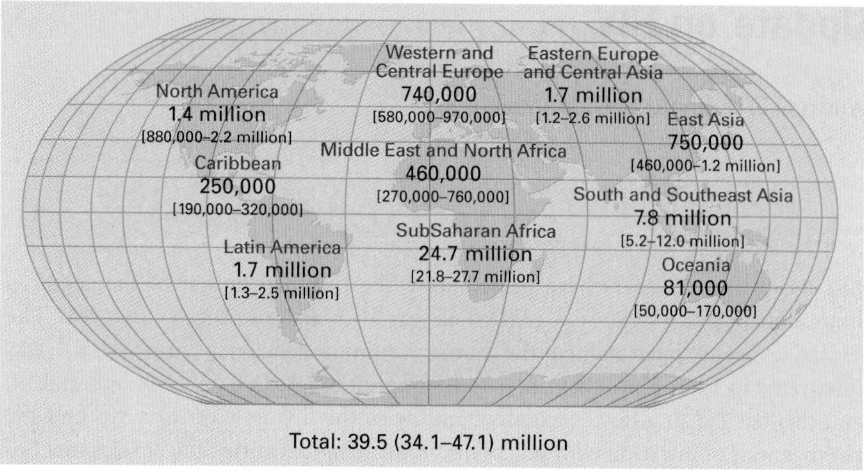

Fig 1 Adults and children estimated to be living with HIV worldwide in 2006. Reproduced with kind permission of UNAIDS.[1]

this group has been seen in recent years; however, the number of heterosexually acquired HIV infections diagnosed in the UK has risen enormously since 1985. Since 1999, there have been more diagnoses of heterosexually acquired infections than infections acquired through sex between men. Most heterosexually acquired infections diagnosed in the UK were acquired abroad (>82%), however, and 72% of these were acquired in Africa.[2] Around 4% of people with heterosexually acquired infections in the UK are infected by a 'high-risk' contact. Around one third of heterosexually acquired infections currently are estimated to be undiagnosed and almost half are diagnosed late in the course of illness – that is, when the CD4 count is <200 cells/mm^3.[2]

□ JOINT UNITED NATIONS PROGRAMME ON HIV/AIDS

The year 2006 saw the tenth anniversary of the Joint United Nations Programme on HIV/AIDS (UNAIDS). The 2006 report from UNAIDS highlighted the many positive aspects of the global response to HIV and emphasised the strong foundations that now exist in most countries. The report noted the significant increases in available resources and public expenditure, the improved access to treatment globally, the improvements in diagnostic capability worldwide (including the screening of blood for transfusion), the improvement in education in schools, and the enhanced prophylactic antiviral coverage of HIV-positive pregnant women.[1]

Considerable weaknesses in the global response to the epidemic still exist, however; particularly the considerable gaps in delivery of programmes for prevention to those most at risk, young people, men who have sex with men, and intravenous drug users. In addition, services to prevent infection of infants with HIV currently are inadequate, with only 9% of pregnant women being covered.[1]

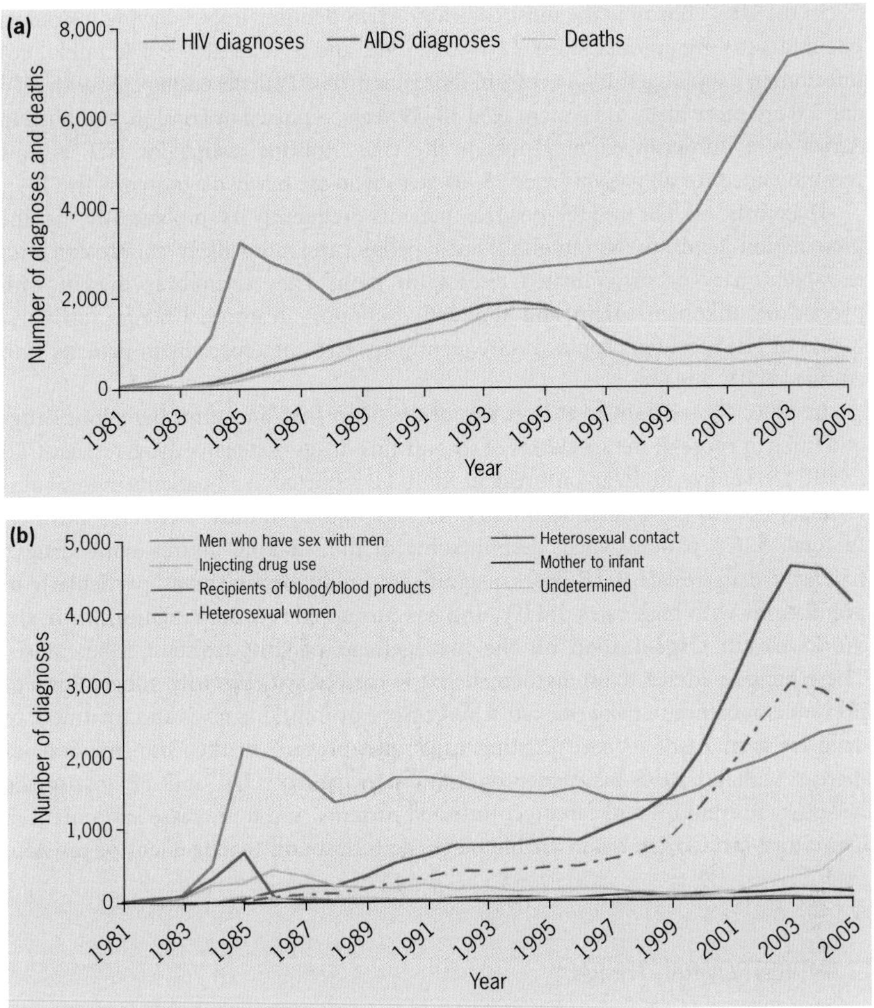

Fig 2 Number of **(a)** HIV and AIDS diagnoses and deaths in HIV-infected people and **(b)** HIV diagnoses by exposure category in the UK between 1981 and 2005. Reproduced with kind permission of Health Protection Agency, Centre for Infections.[2]

□ CO-INFECTION WITH HIV AND TUBERCULOSIS

Tuberculosis (TB) is now the leading cause of death among patients living with HIV worldwide. The estimated 14 million patients who are co-infected worldwide are at increased risk of progressive primary disease (30% risk in HIV-positive people compared with 5–10% in HIV-negative individuals) and reactivation (5–10% risk per year in HIV-positive people). In total, up to 50% of patients living with HIV/AIDS will develop TB; this compares with the 5–10% lifetime risk among HIV-negative people. Human immunodeficiency virus continues to fuel the re-emergence of TB and accounts for 9% of all cases of TB worldwide and more than 30% in Africa.

In the UK, TB is now the most common AIDS-defining illness, having overtaken pneumocystis pneumonia in 2002 (<5% in 1992 and 31% in 2002). The rate of co-infection in people aged 15–64 years in the UK is 3.7%.[3] Patients co-infected with HIV and TB are more likely to be men, aged 30–39 years, reported in London, and born in Africa or a European country outside the UK.[3] Routine testing for HIV is now recommended for all patients aged 15–64 years who are newly diagnosed with TB.

Diagnosis of TB in HIV-positive patients frequently is problematic, as the presentation tends to be 'atypical'. Such people are more likely to present with extrapulmonary or disseminated disease, or both. They commonly present with pyrexia of unknown origin and minimal respiratory features. Changes on chest X-rays of HIV-positive people also frequently are atypical, especially in patients with advanced HIV disease.

In 2006, TB resistant to at least two of the main first-line antituberculous drugs and three or more of the six classes of second-line drugs (extensive drug-resistant TB (XDR-TB)) emerged. In an outbreak of XDR-TB reported in 53 patients in Kwazulu-Natal, South Africa, 44 had been tested for HIV and all of those were HIV-positive. In total, 52/53 patients died, despite some of them taking antiretroviral drugs.[4] Extensive drug-resistant TB poses a significant public health threat, particularly in populations with high rates of HIV, and has prompted recommendations from the World Health Organization on the management of drug-resistant tuberculosis. These include advice to strengthen the basic care of patients with tuberculosis to prevent emergence of drug resistance and ensure prompt diagnosis and treatment of drug-resistant cases to cure existing cases and prevent further transmission; to increase collaboration between programmes to control HIV and TB to provide necessary prevention and care to co-infected patients; and to increase investment in laboratory infrastructures to enable better detection and management of resistant cases.[4]

☐ ANTIRETROVIRAL THERAPY

It is 20 years since the first drug to treat HIV infection, zidovudine (AZT), was licensed and just more than 10 years since the introduction of combination therapy – HAART. The pace of investigations into HIV and the speed of development of treatments for HIV is unrivalled, such that 19 different antiretroviral drugs in four separate drug classes are currently licensed in the UK (Table 1).

Combination treatment with two nucleoside or nucleotide analogue reverse transcriptase inhibitors (NRTIs) and either a non-nucleoside reverse transcriptase inhibitor (NNRTI) or a boosted protease inhibitor (PI) is now established as the preferred first-line regimen.[5] Understanding of potency and toxicity within drug classes has also led to preferential use of certain agents. Lipoatrophy occurs more frequently with thymidine-analogue NRTIs such as stavudine and zidovudine. Hyperlipidaemia and heart disease are more common with the PIs.

Initial treatment responses to HAART have continued to improve year on year since 1996, as judged by the reduced risk of virological failure in the first year of treatment.[6] This is likely to result from a combination of improved treatment

Table 1 Antiretroviral drugs licensed in the UK in March 2007.

NRTIs	NNRTIs	PIs	Fusion inhibitors
• Zidovudine	• Efavirenz	• Indinavir	• Enfuvirtide
• Lamivudine	• Nevirapine	• Ritonavir	
• Didanosine		• Saquinavir	
• Stavudine		• Nelfinavir	
• Abacavir		• Lopinavir	
• Emtricitabine		• Fosamprenavir	
• Tenofovir		• Atazanavir	
		• Tipranavir	
		• Darunavir	

NNRTI = non-nucleoside reverse transcriptase inhibitor; NRTI = nucleoside or nucleotide analogue reverse transcriptase inhibitor; PI = protease inhibitor.

options and strategies that increase adherence. Drug development has also led to a significant reduction in pill burden, such that effective antiretroviral therapy can now be administered as a single pill taken once daily. These simplified regimens improve adherence – a factor associated with improved outcome.

Baseline genotypic resistance testing is now carried out routinely before initiation of antiretroviral therapy in view of the recognised risk of transmitted drug-resistant virus.

When should treatment start?

Initiation of antiretroviral therapy when CD4 counts are >200 mm^3 is of established benefit. The risk of death or disease progression is higher and the efficacy of HAART reduced in patients in whom treatment is delayed until the CD4 count has decreased to below this level. The guidelines of the British HIV Association (BHIVA) have, until now, recommended starting treatment when the CD4 count is <350 mm^3 and >200 mm^3 or if there is symptomatic infection.[5] This range was chosen because the absolute risk of AIDS-related diseases in people with CD4 counts >250 mm^3 is sufficiently low that the potential risks of treatment were considered to outweigh the benefits.

The most appropriate CD4 count at which to start treatment of HIV remains uncertain, however, and has not been investigated in a randomised controlled trial. Treatment regimens are now less toxic and better tolerated and treatment options more extensive than previously. The exact timing of treatment initiation is a compromise between the potential risks of treatment and the potential benefits. The potential risks of early treatment include:

- ☐ drug toxicity (immediate life-threatening side effects, such as hypersensitivity reactions, acute hepatitis, pancreatitis, and lactic acidosis; long-term effects, such as increased risk of myocardial infarction, lipoatrophy, and lipodystrophy; and unpleasant side-effects that impact on quality of life, such as nausea and diarrhoea)

- development of drug resistance
- exhaustion of drug options.

Some of these adverse effects and concerns related to starting antiretroviral therapy early are less pertinent today because of the introduction of well-tolerated, less-toxic regimens that enable good compliance. Our understanding of the long-term effects of antiretroviral therapy has also improved, such that many of these adverse events can be ameliorated or avoided with current drugs.

The potential benefits of starting treatment earlier include:

- preservation of immune function (this may be preferable to immune system restoration)
- decreased risk of transmission
- prolonged disease-free survival
- fewer adverse events
- reduction in mortality because of liver disease and malignancy.[4]

In addition, earlier initiation of treatment for HIV increases the likelihood that CD4 counts will normalise, although the magnitude of the increase is greater when treatment is started at lower levels.[7]

A recently published trial – the strategies for management of antiretroviral therapy (SMART) study[8] – lends some support to starting treatment at higher CD4 counts. It was designed to compare a strategy of episodic treatment – stopped when the CD4 count increased to >350 mm^3 and restarted when it decreased to 250 mm^3 – with continuous treatment in patients (mostly treatment-naive patients) with CD4 counts >350 mm^3. Recruitment to the study stopped after 16 months of follow up because an interim analysis showed increased mortality in the episodic treatment group because of opportunistic disease or death from any cause (hazard ratio 2.6 (95% confidence interval 1.9 to 3.7), p=0.001). Surprisingly, no reduction in drug-related toxicity was seen in the episodic treatment group.[8]

As treatments become safer and better tolerated, there may be a shift towards earlier introduction of HIV treatments in the UK, as advocated by several clinicians.[9] The decision on when to start treatment is likely to be influenced heavily, however, by patient choice and patient readiness to start.

Antiretroviral drugs under development

The life cycle of HIV has been studied extensively, and this has provided numerous potential targets for drug treatment (Fig 3).[10] Enfuvirtide – the first in a new class of antiretroviral drugs (the HIV fusion inhibitors) – was developed in 2003. More recently, work has focused on the development of other entry inhibitors, including chemokine (C-C motif) receptor 5 (CCR5) and chemokine (C-X-C motif) receptor 4 (CXCR4) antagonists, as well as integrase inhibitors. The CCR5 antagonist maraviroc is now available for use on compassionate grounds in the UK. The integrase inhibitor

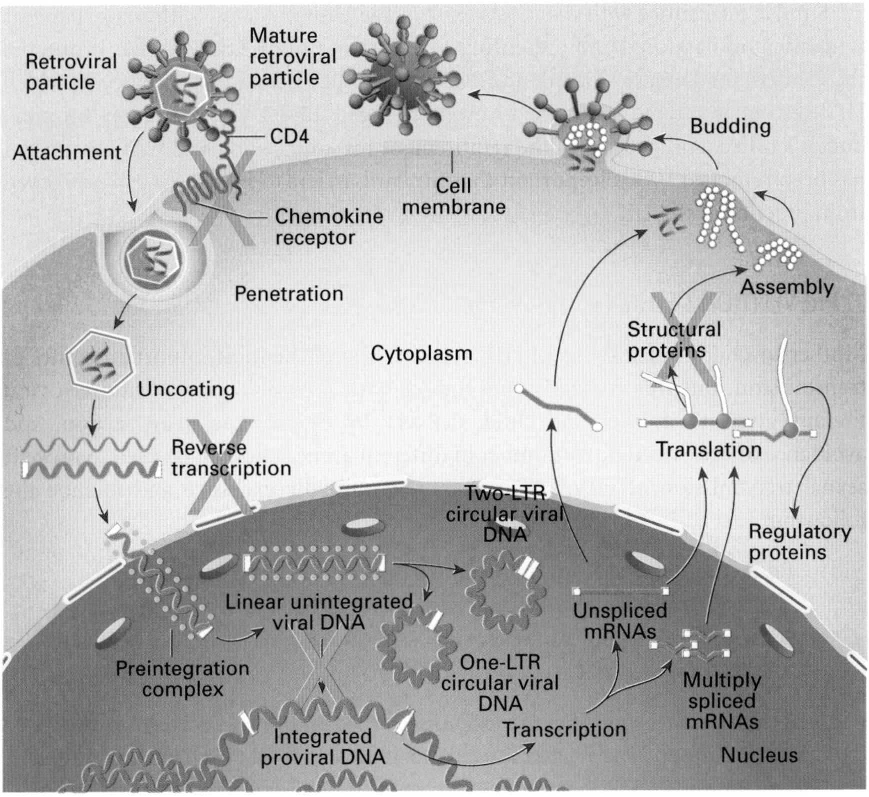

Fig 3 Diagram of the life cycle of HIV, showing target sites for antiretroviral drugs. LTR = long terminal repeat. Adapted from Furtado *et al.*[10]

raltegravir has entered phase II dose-finding trials and has shown rapid and potent HIV suppression in treatment-experienced and treatment-naive patients.

□ LATE DIAGNOSIS

Late diagnosis of HIV remains a significant problem in the UK. An audit undertaken by BHIVA found that 33% of newly diagnosed patients had advanced disease in 2003 compared with 59% in 2001.[11] Although this represented an improvement, opportunities for earlier diagnosis of HIV still were being missed in a significant proportion of patients (17%). These 168 patients had sought medical care from a range of healthcare providers for a wide variety of diseases and conditions associated with HIV in the 12 months before diagnosis; this included 58 hospital admissions, 18 of which were for TB. Of these 168 patients, 160 started antiretroviral therapy at CD4 counts <200 mm^3, which increased their risk of AIDS-related events and death, drug toxicity, and irreversible destruction of immune function.[11] These missed opportunities for diagnosis present a challenge to healthcare providers in the UK. Human immunodeficiency virus is now a chronic treatable condition and patients have a potentially normal life expectancy – as long as diagnosis and treatment are not delayed.

Similar difficulties with diagnosis exist in the United States, with many patients remaining undiagnosed and presenting at a late stage of disease. This has prompted the Centers for Disease Control and Prevention (CDC) to adopt a policy in which HIV testing is offered regularly to everyone aged 13–64 years in every hospital, doctor's office, and clinic and the requirement for counselling and written consent has been removed.[12] It is important that similar barriers to HIV testing are removed from practice in the UK.

□ PREVENTION OF HIV

Mother-to-child transmission of HIV remains one of the most important routes of transmission, but this is largely preventable with a combination of antiretroviral therapy given to mother and child, delivery by elective caesarean section, and avoidance of breastfeeding. A number of different approaches can be used to prevent sexual transmission of HIV.[13] These are not mutually exclusive and include the following:

- □ Education – Education to promote behavioural change, including abstinence and the use of condoms. This approach has been impressively successful in certain countries, such as Uganda, but has been less effective, to date, in many others.
- □ Male circumcision – Three randomised trials in different African countries were all stopped early after interim analyses showed a 50–60% reduction in acquisition of HIV in circumcised men. Circumcision removes the foreskin, which is rich in cells susceptible to infection with HIV (Langerhans cells), and reduces but does not remove completely the risk of acquisition of HIV. It therefore may prove to be a useful adjunctive measure in prevention of HIV.
- □ Vaginal microbicides – A large number of agents are being developed for topical vaginal application to try to block transmission of HIV to women. Although this is a promising approach, two phase III trials recently were halted after early results suggested that one such agent, cellulose phosphate, seemed to increase transmission.
- □ Vaccines – The high rate of mutations and the genetic diversity of HIV means that the development of a preventative vaccine remains a distant goal, although some candidate vaccines are undergoing clinical trials.
- □ Postexposure prophylaxis – The use of a short course of antiretroviral therapy after potential exposure to HIV originally was recommended after needlestick injuries in the healthcare setting. In recent years, it has been used after sexual exposure, although no evidence from randomised trials supports its efficacy.
- □ Pre-exposure prophylaxis – Trials are underway to assess the efficacy of administering the drug tenofovir to individuals at high risk of acquiring HIV infection.

☐ CONCLUSION

The management of HIV has advanced considerably since the virus was discovered in 1981. Drug developments have resulted in a considerable choice of antiretroviral drugs that are effective, well tolerated, and available in once-daily regimens with a low pill burden. The development of antiretroviral therapy has led to a change of emphasis in the challenges that face clinicians in 2007. In the developed world, the challenge is to ensure that all people infected with HIV are diagnosed at the earliest opportunity, so that effective treatment can be initiated at the appropriate time. This requires a lower threshold for testing for HIV in all healthcare settings, so that opportunities for diagnosis are not missed. In the developing world, the challenge is one of logistics – to deliver antiretroviral therapy and education on prevention of HIV to those at greatest risk. The HIV epidemic has contributed to the re-emergence of many diseases, including TB. The development of XDR-TB provides a new global public health problem and individuals positive for antibodies to HIV are particularly susceptible. Despite the huge advances in the care of patients with HIV, many issues remain unresolved and developments in therapeutics continue to evolve.

REFERENCES

1 Joint United Nations Programme on HIV/AIDS. *2006 Report on the global AIDS epidemic. A UNAIDS 10th anniversary special edition.* Geneva: UNAIDS, 2006. Available at: www.unaids.org/en/HIV_data/2006GlobalReport/default.asp (last accessed 9 October 2007).

2 The UK Collaborative Group for HIV and STI Surveillance. *A complex picture – HIV and other sexually transmitted infections in the United Kingdom: 2006.* London: Health Protection Agency, Centre for Infections, 2006.

3 Ahmed AB, Abubakar I, Delpech V *et al.* The growing impact of HIV infection on the epidemiology of tuberculosis in England and Wales. *Thorax* 2007;62:672–6.

4 World Health Organization. *Emergence of XDR-TB. WHO concern over extensive drug resistant TB strains that are virtually untreatable.* Geneva: WHO, 2006. Available at: www.who.int/mediacentre/news/notes/2006/np23/en/index.html (last accessed 9 October 2007).

5 Gazzard B, Bernard AJ, Boffito M *et al.* British HIV Association (BHIVA) guidelines for the treatment of HIV-infected adults with antiretroviral therapy (2006). *HIV Med* 2006;7: 487–503.

6 Lampe FC, Gatell JM, Staszewski S *et al.* Changes over time in risk of initial virological failure of combination antiretroviral therapy: a multicohort analysis, 1996 to 2002. *Arch Intern Med* 2006;166:521–8.

7 Moore RD, Keruly JC. CD4+ cell count 6 years after commencement of highly active antiretroviral therapy in persons with sustained virologic suppression. *Clin Infect Dis* 2007; 44:441–6.

8 El-Sadr WM, Lundgren JD, Neaton JD *et al.* CD4+ count-guided interruption of antiretroviral treatment. *N Engl J Med* 2006;355:2283–96.

9 Phillips AN, Gazzard BG, Clumeck N, Losso MH, Lundgren JD. When should antiretroviral therapy for HIV be started? *BMJ* 2007;334:76–8.

10 Furtado MR, Callaway DS, Phair JP *et al.* Persistence of HIV-1 transcription in peripheral-blood mononuclear cells in patients receiving potent antiretroviral therapy. *N Engl J Med* 1999;340:1614–22.

11 Sullivan AK, Curtis H, Sabin CA, Johnson MA. Newly diagnosed HIV infections: review in UK and Ireland. *BMJ* 2005;330;1301–2.

12 Branson BM, Handsfield HH, Lampe MA *et al.* Revised recommendations for HIV testing of adults, adolescents, and pregnant women in health-care settings. *MMWR Recomm Rep* 2006;55(RR-14):1–17.

13 Anonymous. Newer approaches to HIV prevention. *Lancet* 2007;369:615.

Highly pathogenic avian influenza H5N1 in humans

Iain Stephenson

□ INTRODUCTION

Global pandemics of influenza A have previously emerged at irregular intervals and have resulted in huge societal disruption. During the 20th century, an influenza H1N1 virus in 1918, an H2N2 virus in 1957, and an H3N2 virus in 1968 emerged to cause pandemics. The 'Spanish flu' pandemic of 1918–9 remains the greatest outbreak of an infectious disease in history and accounted for up to 40 million deaths. The World Health Organization (WHO) has declared that the world is as close as ever to the next pandemic. Outbreaks of highly pathogenic avian influenza H5N1 virus among poultry and migratory birds occurred initially in southeast Asia and have spread west into Europe and Africa as the virus seems to have established endemnicity in bird populations. Multiple sublineages of H5N1 have emerged in geographically distinct regions. Sporadic infections with H5N1 in humans have been associated with close contact with infected birds. The high mortality and aggressive clinical course in infected people have alarmed public health authorities. Although no evidence suggests sustained transmission between humans, recombination of H5N1 with circulating human influenza, or mutations within its genome, could generate a virus of pandemic potential with devastating consequences.

□ VIROLOGY

Influenza viruses possess a segmented RNA genome and belong to the *Orthomyxoviridae* family. Influenza A infects a range of mammal and avian species, whereas type B is principally a human pathogen. In humans, influenza A causes frequent, usually annual, outbreaks and occasional pandemics, while influenza B outbreaks occur every few years. Virus surface glycoproteins are critical to pathogenesis. The virus haemagglutinin binds to receptors on the host target cell and facilitates entry into the cell. As the main antigenic determinant, it is the major ingredient of influenza vaccine. Neuraminidase is essential for viral replication and is an important target for antiviral drugs as its activity is conserved across subtypes.

Currently circulating human influenza A/H1 and H3 viruses undergo antigenic variation or 'drift' that necessitates regular updating of vaccine to match the prevalent strain. Inefficient proofreading by RNA polymerase results in multiple transcription errors that may generate antigenic variants capable of evading pre-existing immunity and reinfecting individuals to cause interpandemic outbreaks. The segmented nature of the genome permits a further type of antigenic variation. The simultaneous infection of a cell by two influenza viruses may allow recombination of RNA segments to create a 'reassortant' virus that contains a mixture of genes – so called 'antigenic shift'. Pandemic influenza may arise if a novel virus capable of efficient and sustained replication and transmission among humans emerges to infect a globally susceptible population.

Aquatic birds are the natural reservoir of influenza A viruses, among which a total of 16 haemagglutinin (H1–H16) and nine neuraminidase (N1–N9) subtypes have been identified. In natural hosts, faeco-oral routes of transmission maintain avian influenza viruses, and infection typically causes subclinical gastrointestinal disease. Both H5 and H7 subtypes, however, have the ability to evolve into highly pathogenic forms and cause lethal systemic infection. The molecular determinants that confer virulence of highly pathogenic avian influenza viruses are unclear, but the ease with which the haemagglutinin molecule is cleaved and activated is a key factor. Over the last 30 years, sporadic outbreaks of avian influenza viruses among poultry have caused significant economic damage in many countries across the world.

□ HUMAN PANDEMIC INFLUENZA VIRUSES

The pandemic viruses of 1957 (H2N2) and 1968 (H3N2) were reassortant viruses that contained genes from human and avian influenza strains.[1] In both cases, avian influenza viruses contributed at least the haemagglutinin gene to the pandemic strain. Reconstruction of the 1918 pandemic virus reveals a different origin.[2] All of its genes are related closely to known genes of the avian influenza virus, which indicates that it emerged directly without recombination with human strains. Despite the variety of viruses in the natural reservoir, only a few subtype combinations (H1, H2, H3, N1, and N2) have caused widespread human respiratory disease. The genetic adaptations required to allow influenza viruses to efficiently replicate and transmit between humans are uncertain; however, changes in the RNA polymerase genes and haemagglutinin are implicated. Haemagglutinin binds to sialic acid receptors on the target cell. Human influenza haemagglutinin binds to receptors containing α2,6-galactose linkages, whereas avian haemagglutinin binds to those containing α2,3-galactose linkages. Host specificity of influenza viruses matches the abundance of sialic acid α2,6-galactose linkages on cells in the human upper respiratory tract and α2,3-galactose linkages on avian intestinal cells. Swine respiratory epithelium express both linkages, so pigs can be infected with avian and human influenza viruses. Genetic reassortment between avian and human viruses has been suggested to occur in pigs (or any other intermediate host capable of dual infection) to generate new potentially pandemic strains of influenza. Close association of humans to agriculture, waterfowl, poultry, and pigs has identified Asia as a potential 'mixing bowl' in which new strains of influenza virus could be generated. Molecular characterisation of avian isolates is important to track and identify any changes that might potentially herald the emergence of a pandemic virus.

□ CHRONOLOGY OF AVIAN AND HUMAN INFLUENZA A/H5N1 SINCE 1997

During 1997, outbreaks of highly pathogenic avian influenza H5N1 erupted in the live bird and poultry markets of Hong Kong. The first association of respiratory infection with H5N1 was in May 1997 in a child aged three years; however, pandemic alarms were raised when six deaths among an additional 17 humans occurred towards the end of the year.[3] There was little evidence of secondary spread, and further infections in humans were prevented by the mass culling of poultry. This particular lineage of H5N1 virus (clade 3) has not been isolated since then. Although H5N1 viruses later re-emerged in poultry markets, no further cases were reported in humans until February 2003, when H5N1 viruses were isolated from two severely ill members of a family returning to Hong Kong from China.[4] Around this time, large numbers of waterfowl in Hong Kong died from H5N1 infection. As avian influenza does not typically cause disease in its natural host, this was noteworthy, because it suggested that changes that determine phenotypic virulence had occurred. Subsequently, H5N1 has caused fatal infections in bird species previously unknown to be susceptible, including wild ducks, geese, herons, egrets, and birds of prey. In addition, H5N1 has extended its host range into mammals, with fatal respiratory infections acquired by eating infected carcasses reported in cats, tigers, and leopards.

Between late 2003 and 2005, highly pathogenic avian influenza H5N1 caused unprecedented multiple outbreaks across southeast Asia.[5,6] Huge numbers of backyard poultry flocks, live bird markets, and wildfowl have been infected or destroyed. H5N1 seems to have become established as an endemic virus in this region. Near simultaneous outbreaks across the region pose questions about routes of transmission. Transportation of poultry and products is accepted to have played a major role in dissemination of the virus throughout the region; the contribution of migratory birds is controversial. Notably, Australia remains free of H5N1, despite the fact that migration bird pathways pass through intensely infected H5N1 regions into Australia.

Between April and December 2005, however, the virus seemed to be rapidly jumping long distances westwards through central Asia. Outbreaks of H5N1 in poultry in western China, Kazakhstan, Russia, Azerbaijan, and then Turkey were associated with deaths of wild waterbirds in local lakes. Molecular analysis of isolates of H5N1 from poultry and wild birds affected in Turkey confirmed antigenic similarity to Chinese viruses, which suggested that migratory birds were spreading H5N1.[6] The first fatal human cases outside southeastern Asia were reported among Turkish poultry farmers in early 2006.[6] Since then, the H5N1 virus has continued to progress into countries of the European Union, and outbreaks in commercial poultry farms have occurred in France, Germany, Hungary, and the UK. Multiple introductions by migratory birds have caused outbreaks among wildfowl and geese in countries between Spain and Greece. An outbreak at farm in the UK in January 2007 seems to have been caused by transportation of contaminated poultry products across Europe. The progression of H5N1 into Egypt and subSaharan Africa is a potentially serious cause for concern. Several states in West Africa have reported H5N1 in poultry flocks, and fatal human infections occurred in Nigeria in

January 2007.[6] Surveillance and control of emerging H5N1 viruses in the resource poor settings of Africa will be challenging.

Since the emergence of H5N1 in humans in 1997, molecular surveillance of haemagglutinin H5 and antigenic characterisation of viruses have revealed significant antigenic differences between the viruses isolated from humans in 1997, 2003, and 2005 onwards.[5,6] Most isolates of H5N1 from birds currently fall into two distinct phylogenetic clades. Clade 1 viruses emerged in poultry in Vietnam, Thailand, and Cambodia around 2003 and were responsible for most human infections up to 2005. Viruses continue to circulate in this region and cause infrequent infections in humans. Clade 2 viruses circulated in birds in Indonesia and China during 2003–4 and spread westwards via the Middle East and Turkey into Europe and Africa. They have been responsible for most human infections since 2005, principally in Indonesia and most recently Nigeria. At least three distinct sublineages of the clade 2 viruses have caused human infections in discrete geographical areas. Clade 3 viruses caused the outbreaks in Hong Kong in 1997 and have not been isolated since that time. New clades are potentially emerging in birds in China but have not yet been associated with human infections. Prompt characterisation of emerging antigenic variants is vital to generate well-matched vaccine reference strains.

□ CLINICAL INFECTION WITH H5N1

Since 2003, a total of 274 human cases have been reported to the WHO, with mortality >60%.[6] Human infections have been confirmed in Thailand, Vietnam, Indonesia, Cambodia, China, Turkey, Iraq, Azerbaijan, and Nigeria. Most cases of H5N1 in humans are associated with direct exposure to infected poultry, and, to date, no evidence suggests sustained human-to-human transmission. In humans, infection with H5N1 results in rapid onset of respiratory failure and sepsis, with high mortality compared with epidemic human influenza.[3,4] Identification of sialic acid receptors that contain α2,3-galactose linkages (avian haemagglutinin preferring) on human alveolar tissue may explain high rates of complicating pneumonia. Infection of human macrophages in vitro with H5N1 viruses induces high levels of cytokines, which suggests that the severity of disease may be related to excessive proinflammatory responses that accompany primary H5 infection and viraemia.[4,7] The isolation of H5N1 from throat, cerebrospinal fluid, and stool specimens in several Vietnamese children who presented with severe diarrhoea and encephalopathy indicates extrapulmonary viral replication and suggests the spectrum of disease may be wider than considered, which could mean that numbers of human cases have been underestimated.[8] Although attention has focused on the threat posed by H5N1, other avian influenza subtypes – including H7N7, H7N3, and H9N2 – have caused illness in humans since 1999.

□ VACCINES AGAINST INFLUENZA

Influenza vaccines are the principal form of prophylaxis against influenza. Interpandemic vaccines are trivalent and contain 15 μg haemagglutinin from each of two influenza A (H1N1 and H3N2) strains and one influenza B strain. Licensed inactivated influenza vaccines are produced from reassortment viruses that express the desired surface haemagglutinin and neuraminidase, with the remaining gene segments derived from an attenuated human strain that has the high growth characteristics needed for production. Reassortant viruses for vaccines are grown in embryonated hens' eggs, inactivated, and formulated. Most vaccines are detergent-treated virus particles (split product vaccines) or purified haemagglutinin and neuraminidase (subunit vaccines). Both formulations are well tolerated and have excellent safety profiles. Whole virus vaccine preparations are generally more immunogenic but are associated with increased adverse effects and are little used or unlicensed in most countries. Inactivated influenza vaccines induce an antibody response that is relatively strain specific, display reduced efficacy against antigenically drifted viruses, and are generally ineffective against unrelated strains.

☐ VACCINES FOR INFLUENZA H5N1

As highly pathogenic viruses such as H5 and H7 are lethal to chicken embryos and cannot be grown in sufficient quantities in eggs, vaccines from these viruses cannot be produced by standard methods. Preparation of vaccines requires secure biocontainment to protect production staff who work with highly pathogenic avian strains and to reduce the potential for accidental release and the contamination of nearby susceptible birds and animals. This is unachievable for large-scale production of vaccines grown in eggs. Genetic manipulation can remove the multibasic sequence at the cleavage site of the highly pathogenic haemagglutinin (the principal determinant of virulence) and regenerate an influenza virus that carries a modified haemagglutinin gene. Experienced laboratories can generate an infectious but attenuated antigenically matched H5N1 virus suitable for growing large amounts in eggs within weeks of its isolation. Any attenuated virus derived from a highly pathogenic strain must undergo extensive safety evaluation before it can be brought out of secure biocontainment. Vaccine production work with such 'genetically modified organisms' may require additional regulatory hurdles in relation to the risk of environmental contamination and waste disposal. Intellectual property rights on reverse genetics exist, and licences may need to be granted before commercial vaccine production can begin.

Clinical trials with non-adjuvanted split product vaccines derived from H5N1 viruses attenuated by reverse genetics have shown that this is a very poor immunogen compared with human influenza strains.[9] Two doses of vaccine containing up to 30–45 μg H5 haemagglutinin content induce only limited seroconversion rates.[10,11] This is 4–6 times the standard vaccine dose and is unacceptable for the global vaccine supply that will be needed in a pandemic event. Why is it important to produce low-dose vaccines? The current manufacturing capacity of inactivated spilt product or subunit influenza vaccines can deliver about 300 million doses of trivalent vaccine containing 15 μg haemagglutinin per strain per six months. This is equivalent to 900 million doses of monovalent H5N1 vaccine – enough for 15% of the world's population to receive one dose. As the population will be immunologically naive to a new pandemic strain, however, individuals require at least two injections to achieve seroprotection. If vaccines that contain four times the antigenic dose are formulated, the available production capacity of split product vaccines per six months will be around 100 million doses, which does not cover the population of the member states of the European Union that have vaccine manufacturing facilities. The addition of adjuvant aluminium salts to split product H5N1 vaccines seems to have limited clinical benefit.[11] The most promising pandemic H5 vaccine candidates have been formulations that contain whole virus grown in eggs or cells or split product vaccines adjuvanted with proprietary adjuvants.[9,12] Clinical studies suggest that two doses of vaccines that contain as little as 5 μg H5 haemagglutinin induce acceptable responses; however, most facilities for manufacturing influenza vaccines in the European Union are designed to produce split product interpandemic vaccines and not whole virus preparations and cannot be readily adapted to new methods of production. Although proprietary adjuvants permit significant dose reductions in the antigen content of vaccines, there are limits to manufacturing capacity and they are likely to be unaffordable for many countries. New vaccine approaches, including live attenuated, DNA, recombinant protein or cell-grown vaccines, are likely to offset shortfalls in the future, but these advances are currently unlicensed.

□ CONCLUDING COMMENTS

Some national authorities, including those in the UK, are stockpiling H5N1 vaccines. Although this is a sensible precaution, we cannot predict which, if any, of the circulating subclades will emerge as a pandemic threat and thus which vaccine strains should be stockpiled. Furthermore, we do not know the optimum dose or vaccine schedule in different populations, including healthy adults, children, and elderly people. Pandemic preparedness has focussed attention on H5N1, but it is important to note that other avian subtypes – including H6N1, H7N3, and H9N2 – circulate widely in live bird markets and could emerge to haunt us.

REFERENCES

1 Potter CW. Chronicle of influenza pandemics. In: Nicholson KG, Webster RG, Hay AJ, eds. *Textbook of influenza.* Oxford: Blackwell Science, 1998:3–18.

2 Tumpey TM, Basler CF, Aguilar PV *et al.* Characterization of the reconstructed 1918 Spanish influenza pandemic virus. *Science* 2005;310:77–80.

3 Katz JM, Lim W, Bridges CB *et al.* Antibody responses in individuals infected with avian influenza A (H5N1) viruses and detection of anti-H5 antibody among household and social contacts. *J Infect Dis* 1999;180:1763–70.

4 Peiris JS, Yu WC, Leung CW *et al.* Re-emergence of fatal human influenza A subtype H5N1 disease. *Lancet* 2004;363:617–9.

5 Chen H, Smith GJ, Li KS *et al.* Establishment of multiple sublineages of H5N1 influenza virus in Asia: implications for pandemic control. *Proc Natl Acad Sci USA* 2006;103:2845–50.

6 Cheung CY, Poon LL, Lau AS *et al.* Induction of proinflammatory cytokines in human macrophages by influenza A (H5N1) viruses: a mechanism for the unusual severity of human disease? *Lancet* 2002;360:1831–7.

7 de Jong MD, Bach VC, Phan TQ *et al.* Fatal avian influenza A (H5N1) in a child presenting with diarrhea followed by coma. *N Engl J Med* 2005;352:686–91.

8 Stephenson I, Gust I, Pervikov Y, Kieny MP. Development of vaccines against influenza H5. *Lancet Infect Dis* 2006;6:458–60.

9 Treanor JJ, Campbell JD, Zangwill KM, Rowe T, Wolff M. Safety and immunogenicity of an inactivated subvirion influenza A (H5N1) vaccine. *N Engl J Med* 2006;354:1343–51.

10 Bresson JL, Perronne C, Launay O *et al.* Safety and immunogenicity of an inactivated split-virion influenza A/Vietnam/1194/2004 (H5N1) vaccine: phase I randomised trial. *Lancet* 2006;367:1657–64.

11 Lin J, Zhang J, Dong X *et al.* Safety and immunogenicity of an inactivated adjuvanted whole-virus influenza (H5N1) vaccine: phase I randomised controlled trial. *Lancet* 2006;368:991–7.

☐ INFECTIOUS DISEASE SELF-ASSESSMENT QUESTIONS

Imported infectious disease emergencies

1 Falciparum malaria is often confused with:
   (a) Viral hepatitis
   (b) Infectious mononucleosis
   (c) Measles
   (d) Tuberculous meningitis
   (e) Influenza

2 Regarding malaria in travellers:
   (a) Chemoprophylaxis must be continued for six weeks after a traveller leaves a malarious area
   (b) Chemoprophylaxis should be stopped in a patient with suspected malaria
   (c) Chemoprophylaxis with atovaquone–proguanil (Malarone) can be stopped seven days after a traveller leaves a malarious area
   (d) Diagnosis is excluded by two negative blood smears
   (e) Most cases of falciparum malaria present 3–12 months after a traveller leaves a malarious area

3 Regarding infection with *Penicillium marneffei*:
   (a) It is an increasingly common opportunistic infection in South America
   (b) The rash is diagnostic
   (c) It is treated with antimonial compounds
   (d) It can be prevented with weekly doxycycline
   (e) It can be diagnosed by microscopy of impression smears from skin lesions

4 Regarding leptospirosis:
   (a) *Leptospira* can penetrate broken skin or intact mucosae
   (b) It is a health hazard of marine environments
   (c) It can be prevented by weekly doxycycline
   (d) It is usually diagnosed by finding spirochaetes in thick or thin blood smears
   (e) It can cause pulmonary haemorrhage

Update on HIV

1 With regard to the epidemiology of HIV in the United Kingdom (UK) at the end of 2005:
   (a) An estimated 63,500 adults were living with HIV
   (b) An estimated 3.2% of people positive for antibodies to HIV were unaware of their diagnosis
   (c) The number of diagnosed individuals who were living with HIV in the UK continued to increase
   (d) There were more diagnoses of heterosexually acquired infection than of infections acquired through sex between men
   (e) 80% of those with heterosexually acquired infections were diagnosed with CD4 counts $<200/mm^3$

2 With regard to tuberculosis (TB) and HIV co-infection:
(a) The annual risk of TB reactivation is 5–10 % in people infected with HIV
(b) The risk of progressive primary TB is 10% in people infected with HIV
(c) Tuberculosis is now the most common AIDS-defining illness in the UK
(d) Extrapulmonary disease is more frequent than in people negative for antibodies to HIV
(e) Extensive drug-resistant TB (XDR-TB) remains sensitive to most second-line drugs

3 In relation to initiation of antiretroviral therapy:
(a) Treatment should be started only if the patient is symptomatic or has a CD4 count <200/mm^3
(b) Starting treatment earlier in the course of HIV infection leads to a greater absolute rise in CD4 count
(c) Genotypic resistance testing should be performed before treatment is started
(d) The initial treatment regimen should contain both a non-nucleoside reverse transcriptase inhibitor (NNRTI) and a protease inhibitor (PI)
(e) Episodic treatment is associated with a reduction in drug-related toxicity

4 Evidence from randomised trials supports the use of the following methods for the prevention of HIV transmission:
(a) Vaginal microbicides
(b) Male circumcision
(c) Vaccines
(d) Post-exposure prophylaxis
(e) Pre-exposure prophylaxis

Highly pathogenic avian influenza H5N1 in humans

1 Avian influenza H5N1 is:
(a) Associated with respiratory failure
(b) Easily transmitted between infected people
(c) Localised to southeast Asia
(d) Associated with severe disease in poultry
(e) The only avian strain of influenza to infect humans

2 Seasonal influenza infection is:
(a) Caused by a single circulating virus
(b) Responsible for annual pandemics
(c) Genetically stable
(d) Preventable by a vaccine
(e) Recognises receptors in the upper respiratory tract

3 Most influenza vaccines:
   (a) Are made from viruses grown in eggs
   (b) Contain live virus
   (c) Contain three strains of influenza
   (d) Are able to induce immunity to all known strains of influenza
   (e) Are whole-virus preparations

Hepatology/gastroenterology

Crohn's disease: pathogenic insights from recent genetic advances

Miles Parkes

□ INTRODUCTION

As is the case for most common inflammatory diseases, the pathogenesis of Crohn's disease (CD) is thought to rely on the interaction of as yet undefined environmental triggers with the immune system of a genetically susceptible host. One feature that sets CD apart is the remarkable progress that has been made over the past 10 years, particularly the past year, in defining the nature of the disease susceptibility genes. This promises a quantum leap forward in our understanding of the pathogenesis of CD. Although the data on genetics do not provide absolute answers, they should at least tell us which immunological questions to ask and, by characterising the heterogeneity that undoubtedly exists within CD, greatly facilitate the identification of environmental triggers. This article is intended not as an exhaustive catalogue of suggested genetic associations of CD but rather to illustrate some of the more clear-cut and replicable findings and particularly the exciting progress made over the past year.

Crohn's disease is important because it is common (100–150 per 100,000), mostly affects young adults, and causes substantial morbidity in individuals and substantial costs for the healthcare system. The strong genetic contribution has been recognised for many years from the familial aggregation of cases and the higher concordance in monozygotic compared with dizygotic twin pairs (45% *v* 10%). Until 2006, progress in characterising the genetic variation predisposing to CD was steady rather than spectacular, but substantial strides have been made over the past year. This has reflected the technological shift from candidate gene-based studies and linkage analyses, which generally have lacked statistical power and resolution, to the new technique of high-resolution case–control genome-wide association (GWA) scanning.[1]

□ EARLY SUCCESS IN IDENTIFYING SUSCEPTIBILITY GENES FOR CROHN'S DISEASE

The most notable genetic success achieved using the old methods of linkage analysis and fine mapping came with the identification of the nucleotide-binding oligomerisation domain containing 2 (*NOD2*)/caspase recruitment domain 15 (*CARD15*) gene as a susceptibility gene for CD in 2001. Two groups used complementary strategies to fine-map a 30 Mb region of chromosome 16 to pinpoint this gene: one used classic positional cloning and the other a positional candidate gene approach.[2,3] Within *NOD2*, the three 'common' variants (frequency 1–10%) and many rare variants that predispose to CD cluster around the portion of the gene that encodes a leucine-rich region. This was known to be important in the intracellular binding of muramyl dipeptide (MDP), which is ubiquitous in bacterial cell walls.[4] A person heterozygous for one of these variants has a 1–3-fold increased risk of CD and those who carry two copies have a 17-fold increased risk. The frequency of these mutations among European populations varies, however, and mutations in *NOD2* are not found at all in Japanese CD cohorts.

Among European groups with CD, it is now clear that *NOD2* mutations are specific for ileal CD.[5] The mechanism by which they predispose to this is not clear but most likely reflects a defective modulation of toll-like receptor (TLR) signalling within innate immune pathways. One theory is that this leads to loss of a priming signal regarding bacterial-driven inflammation – and subsequent persistence of inflammation by alternative, possibly adaptive, immune pathways.

The major histocompatibility complex (MHC) region has also shown evidence of linkage to CD. Furthermore, tumour necrosis factor (TNF) promoter polymorphisms and the DRB1*0703 variant that map to this region have shown replicable association with CD. Association mapping is confounded, however, by the strong linkage disequilibrium across this region. The pattern and extent of linkage disequilibrium does vary across the genome, with variable sized 'blocks' of linkage disequilibrium between which haplotypes are seen to be separated by recombination hotspots – genomic segments particularly susceptible to recombination during meiosis. Within the MHC region, linkage disequilibrium is particularly strong and extensive, which means that although an association signal here provides higher resolution than linkage analysis, it does not pinpoint the disease-causing variant as precisely as it would in most other areas of the genome. Functional studies are required to clarify which of the many immunoactive genes within the MHC region confer disease susceptibility.

Another locus of interest identified by linkage studies maps to chromosome 5q and is known as *IBD5*. This was fine mapped by Rioux *et al*, who identified association between CD and a 250 kb 'IBD5 risk haplotype'.[6] This finding subsequently was replicated widely. The association may be due to variants in the organic cation transporter (*OCTN*) gene cluster, which encodes solute transporters, but genetic evidence for this remains equivocal at present, again because of strong linkage disequilibrium across the region.

☐ RECENT PROGRESS FROM GENOME-WIDE ASSOCIATION SCANS

Within the last six months, data have begun to emerge from a number of GWA scans that have been undertaken in large panels of patients with CD. These capitalise on technological advances in high-throughput genotyping, which make possible the analysis of thousands of samples at hundreds of thousands of polymorphic marker loci across the genome. Given knowledge derived from the HapMap project (www.hapmap.org), and careful study design, GWA scans can identify most common disease-predisposing variation across the genome. This technique is currently being applied across the range of complex diseases. One important issue is the choice of threshold for statistical significance. This should be set at or near $p<10^{-6}$ (in the modern era such stringent thresholds should be applied across all genetic association studies including single candidate gene studies to avoid the generation of false positive results) with the additional prerequisite of replication in an independent dataset.

Identification of the gene for the interleukin 23 receptor as a susceptibility gene for Crohn's disease

The first reported GWA scan in CD reassuringly flagged *NOD2* but also identified variants within the gene for the interleukin (IL) 23 receptor (*IL23R*) as being strongly associated with CD ($p=10^{-9}$) in an initial dataset of 547 cases of ileal CD and 500 controls.[7] This result was replicated in two independent panels within the index study and subsequently was replicated by the United Kingdom (UK)'s inflammatory bowel disease (IBD) genetics consortium ($p=10^{-12}$).[8] This clearly is a real effect, and the rapidity with which replication has been seen underlies the power of this technology. One intriguing observation is that the most strongly associated allele that is a non-synonymous coding variant (Arg381Gln) is present in about 2% of cases of CD and 7% of healthy controls – that is, the rare allele is protective against CD or the (very) common allele is the risk allele.

Corroboration of the importance of IL-23 in patients with IBD has come from recent work in mouse models, in which intestinal inflammation can be ameliorated substantially by knocking out the *IL-23* gene or by treating with anti-p19 (IL-23) monoclonal antibody.[9] Interleukin 23 is released by dendritic cells and macrophages and stimulates a unique CD4+ helper T-cell population characterised by the production of IL-17, TNF and IL-6 (Th17 cells). These cells play a central role in driving autoimmune inflammation in a number of animal models: IL-17 induces secretion of proinflammatory mediators and chemokines that promote rapid recruitment of neutrophils. Function of Th17 can be suppressed by IL-12, and it seems that some specific bacterial components such as peptidoglycan exert a differential regulatory effect on antigen-presenting cells by increasing levels of IL-23 but not IL-12. These early regulatory mechanisms are likely to have a substantial impact on the pattern of the inflammatory response. Interleukin 23 is therefore likely to be a key player in the innate and adaptive immune systems. The identification of different roles for IL-12 and IL-23 in the control of immune pathways suggests that IL-23 (and components of its downstream effector pathway) may be a useful 'drugable' target, whose interruption will inhibit IBD while sparing systemic host-protective immunity.

The importance of autophagy in the pathogenesis of CD

Another recently reported CD susceptibility gene is *ATG16L1*. This was identified in a non-synonymous single nucleotide polymorphism scan that looked at a large proportion of the genome's coding variation in three independent panels of patients with CD and was reported by Hampe *et al* in January 2007.[10] This association again was replicated strongly in the panel of 2,000 patients with CD from the UK. This gene seems to play a crucial role in autophagy – the process by which cells in general and macrophages in particular kill intracellular bacteria contained within phagosomes. Defects in this pathway are clearly associated with prolonged survival of, for example, *Mycobacterium tuberculosis* and *Listeria monocytogenes* in mouse models – again implicating defects in one of the early components of the innate immune pathway in the pathogenesis of CD.

A recently published study by the Wellcome Trust Case Control Consortium has identified four more novel CD loci in addition to replicating each of *NOD2*, *IL23R*, and *ATG16L1*. This UK-based GWA scan has genotyped 2,000 patients with CD (together with seven cohorts of other complex diseases) and 3,000 controls at 500,000 markers using the Affymetrix platform. Once again, the results implicate early components of the innate immune pathway – including another autophagy gene (immunity-related GTPase family, *IRGM*) and the *IL12B* gene, which encodes a subunit shared between IL-12 and IL-23. Clearly the consistency of the themes emerging from these studies is a source of major interest.

☐ SUMMARY AND FUTURE PROSPECTS

This evidently is a time of enormous progress in understanding of the genetics of complex diseases in general and of CD in particular. At last we have a molecular genetic technique that – when used in appropriately designed studies and with stringent statistical thresholds – can reliably pinpoint susceptibility genes. For CD, this will allow delineation of the heterogeneity that undoubtedly exists within the CD-affected population, which, in turn, will permit stratification for drug trials and treatment and more accurate prognostication. Importantly, characterisation of the heterogeneity within CD is likely to be a crucial step in understanding the environmental factors that can trigger disease. These, of course, may be separate and specific for the genetically distinct subgroups. Ultimately, the goal is to have sufficient understanding of the pathogenic mechanisms and triggers of CD to permit the development of rational new treatments and possibly target prevention strategies (possibly vaccines) towards genetically susceptible individuals. The challenge ahead is to ensure that the dramatic progress that is being made in the field of molecular genetics is indeed translated to improved management at the bedside.

REFERENCES

1 Cardon LR, Bell JI. Association study designs for complex diseases. *Nat Rev Genet* 2001;2:91–9.

2 Hugot JP, Chamaillard M, Zouali H *et al.* Association of NOD2 leucine-rich repeat variants with susceptibility to Crohn's disease. *Nature* 2001;411:599–603.

3 Ogura Y, Bonen DK, Inohara N *et al.* A frameshift mutation in NOD2 associated with susceptibility to Crohn's disease. *Nature* 2001;411:603–6.

4 Lesage S, Zouali H, Cézard JP *et al.* CARD15/NOD2 mutational analysis and genotype-phenotype correlation in 612 patients with inflammatory bowel disease. *Am J Hum Genet* 2002;70:845–57.

5 Economou M, Trikalinos TA, Loizou KT, Tsianos EV, Ioannidis JPA. Differential effects of NOD2 variants on Crohn's disease risk and phenotype in diverse populations: a metaanalysis. *Am J Gastroenterol* 2004;99:2393–404.

6 Rioux JD, Daly MJ, Silverberg MS *et al.* Genetic variation in the 5q31 cytokine gene cluster confers susceptibility to Crohn disease. *Nat Genet* 2001;29:223–8.

7 Duerr RH, Taylor KD, Brant SR *et al.* A genome-wide association study identifies IL23R as an inflammatory bowel disease gene. *Science* 2006;314:1461–3.

8 Tremelling M, Cummings F, Fisher SA *et al.* IL23R variation determines susceptibility but not disease phenotype in inflammatory bowel disease. *Gastroenterology* 2007;132:1657–64.

9 Hue S, Ahern P, Buonocore S *et al.* Interleukin-23 drives innate and T cell-mediated intestinal inflammation. *J Exp Med* 2006;203:2473–83.

10 Hampe J, Franke A, Rosenstiel P *et al.* A genome-wide association scan of nonsynonymous SNPs identifies a susceptibility variant for Crohn disease in ATG16L1. *Nat Genet* 2007;39:207–11.

11 Parkes M, Barrett J, Prescott N *et al.* Sequence variants in the autophagy gene IRGM and multiple other replicating loci contribute to Crohn's disease susceptibility. *Nat Genet* 2007 Jun 6; epub ahead of print.

Non-alcoholic fatty liver disease

Stephen D Ryder

Non-alcoholic fatty liver disease (NAFLD) was first described in 1980 and is characterised by the histological accumulation of fat within hepatocytes (Fig 1). This histology is identical to that seen with liver disease related to alcohol consumption but, by definition, NAFLD occurs in people with no or only modest consumption of alcohol. The accumulation of fat can be accompanied by inflammation and death of hepatocytes (ballooning degeneration) (non-alcoholic steatohepatitis (NASH)); when this is the case, there is a potential for development of hepatic fibrosis, cirrhosis, and complications of liver disease, including hepatocellular carcinoma. At the time NAFLD was initially described, it was recognised that there was a strong association with features of the metabolic syndrome and that obesity, particularly central obesity, was a major risk factor.

Non-alcoholic fatty liver disease is common. An American study that undertook magnetic resonance imaging spectroscopy of the liver found >5.5% hepatic fat in the livers of 31% of 2,200 apparently healthy people. Of note, 79% of these had normal levels of transaminases, which proved that high levels of transaminases are not a prerequisite for fatty liver disease.[1] These and other epidemiological data suggest that up to 30% of the population and 60–90% of obese people are likely to have fatty liver disease. Probably 2–3% of the population overall and 25% of obese people have NASH and a risk of progressive liver disease. This disease has the potential to be a major health problem in the next few decades as the population gains weight.

Non-alcoholic fatty liver disease is generally detected because of abnormal liver biochemistry, and most patients are asymptomatic at presentation or have non-specific symptoms such as fatigue or right upper abdominal discomfort. In patients who present with increased levels of transaminases, in whom other liver diseases have been excluded as far as possible serologically, NAFLD is by far the most common diagnosis (Fig 2).[2]

The association between NAFLD and metabolic syndrome was noted immediately. Further studies have confirmed that central obesity and insulin resistance are the key drivers for hepatic steatosis. Only 8–12% of patients with NAFLD have a normal body mass index and fewer still have normal hip to waist ratios. In 4,401 apparently healthy Japanese people aged 21–80 years, 812 (18%) had evidence of NAFLD at study onset and 308/3,147 (10%) developed NAFLD over mean follow up of 414 days. The presence of the metabolic syndrome predicted NAFLD with an odds ratio of 4 (95% confidence interval 2.6 to 6.1).[3]

Work from Japan has confirmed that the first change and the primary driver for development of features of the metabolic syndrome is central weight gain. This is

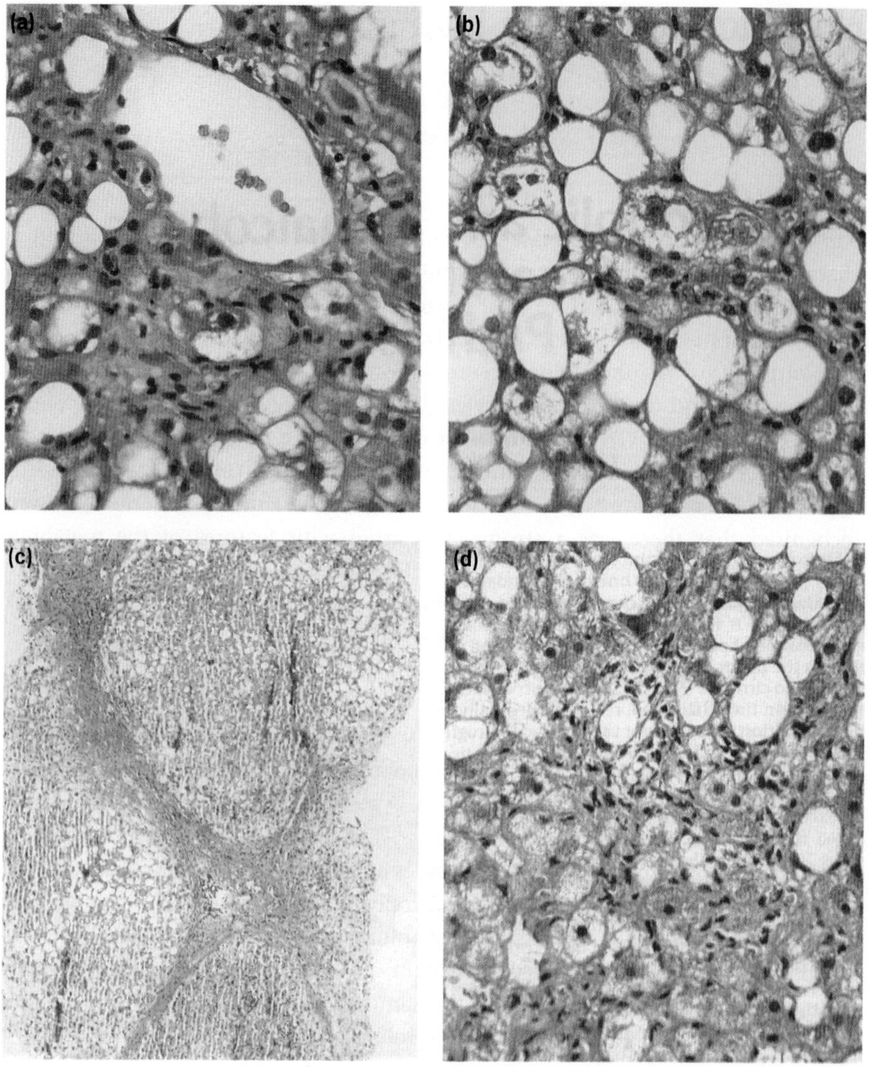

Fig 1 Histological features of non-alcoholic fatty liver disease: **(a)** accumulated fat in hepatocytes with **(b)** Mallory's hyaline and an inflammatory infiltrate, **(c)** cirrhosis, and **(d)** classic pericellular fibrosis.

followed in time by hyertriglyceridaemia, NAFLD, hypertension, and glucose intolerance.[4]

Insulin resistance is the hallmark of NAFLD and directly leads to accumulation of fat within hepatocytes. Hyperinsulinaemia alters metabolism of fat in hepatocytes, which blocks its exit from the cells. Intra-abdominal fat also increases the load of free fatty acid that reaches the liver. Both of these mechanisms are important in the accumulation of lipids within hepatocytes.

Most patients who develop hepatic steatosis do not seem to go on to develop inflammatory liver disease with a risk of fibrosis. Most studies estimate that about

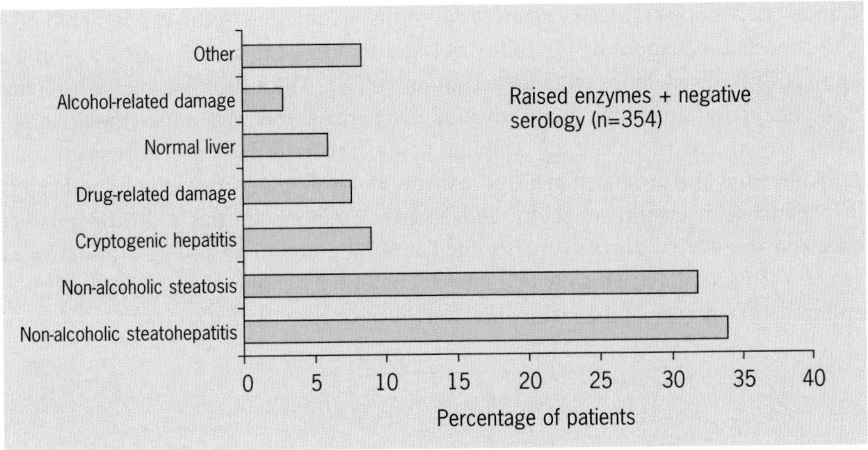

Fig 2 Findings on liver biopsy in a cohort of asymptomatic patients with increased levels of liver enzymes. Reproduced from Skelly *et al* with permission of European Association for the Study of the Liver.[2]

20–30% of patients will develop true NASH, with the remainder having a relatively benign outcome from a hepatological viewpoint. A long-term follow-up study suggested that the risk of cirrhosis 10 years after initial diagnosis of simple fatty liver was 3% compared with progression to cirrhosis in 35% of patients with initial liver biopsies that showed NASH.[5] A long-term follow-up study of a cohort of 129 patients over 13 years showed that mortality was not increased in patients with simple steatosis but that survival of patients with NASH was decreased. In patients with NASH, 15.5% died of cardiovascular disease, 5.6% of extrahepatic cancer, and 2.8% of liver-related diseases. These rates are substantially higher than those in a reference population (7.5% died of cardiovascular disease and 0.2% of liver-related diseases).[6] Patients with NASH are at high risk of both liver and cardiac mortality, presumably because of the severity of their metabolic syndrome. In this study, 41% of patients with NASH showed progression of fibrosis on paired biopsy samples, which suggests that mortality related to liver disease is likely to increase in the future.

Why some patients seem to tolerate fat within their hepatocytes and others go on to develop inflammation and fibrosis currently is unknown. It has been proposed that insulin resistance causes hepatic steatosis but that a second injury to the liver is needed to trigger an inflammatory response. This second injury may be increased levels of bacterial endotoxin in the portal circulation as a consequence of increased bacterial translocation. This phenomenon certainly occurs as liver disease advances, but it is unclear if this is a primary or secondary phenomenon.

The mechanism of the inflammatory cascade in NASH is being elucidated. Levels of tumour necrosis factor (TNF) alpha are increased in the livers of patients with NASH, and this cytokine and its receptor are known to play a significant role in liver injury in patients with NASH. Tumour necrosis factor directly interacts with the insulin receptors in hepatocytes via insulin-receptor substrate 1 and 2, which reduces cellular responses to insulin and therefore contributes to insulin resistance.

Tumour necrosis factor also enhances apoptosis via nuclear factor-kappa B (NFκB). This process is enhanced by instability of lysosomes induced by free fatty acids, and a number of feedback loops enhance activation of TNF. The anti-inflammatory systems that potentially can inhibit this activation are perhaps less well understood. Adipokines, which are produced by adipose tissue, seem to have an important role. Adiponectin is also produced by adipose tissue, and its levels are decreased significantly in patients with insulin resistance and NAFLD. Adiponectin has a downregulatory effect on the TNF pathway – partly mediated by peroxisome proliferator-activated receptor (PPAR) alpha, which is an important potential treatment target. Fig 3 provides an excellent overview of the factors involved in these complex pathways.[7]

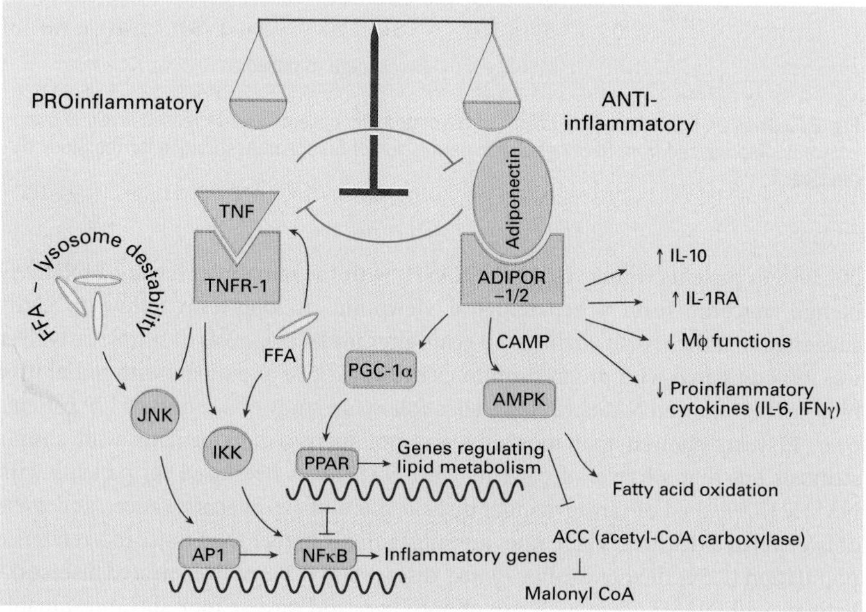

Fig 3 Tumour necrosis factor alpha (TNF-α) and adiponectin interplay in various biological systems, particularly in metabolic homeostasis. Tumour necrosis factor alpha is a key proinflammatory cytokine synthesised by many cell types, including adipocytes, and a pleiotropic mediator of the immune system. Adiponectin is the abundant fat cell-derived product and has important metabolic and immune functions. These two key mediators control each other's synthesis and activity and thereby allow a balanced physiological situation. This could be of key importance in diseases associated with insulin resistance because the critical balance might be impaired, which would lead to chronic inflammation. Such an imbalance might directly lead to insulin resistance. Adiponectin has several anti-inflammatory features other than suppressing TNF-α – for example, it induces other anti-inflammatory cytokines such as interleukin (IL) 10 and IL-1-receptor antagonist (IL-1RA). Adiponectin stimulates use of glucose and oxidation of fatty acids by activating adenosine 5'-monophosphate (AMP)-activated protein kinase (AMPK). It also increases the transcriptional regulator peroxisome proliferator-activated receptor (PPAR) γ coactivator α (PGC-1α) that is required for upregulation of PPAR-α induced by adiponectin. Free fatty acids (FFAs) induce expression of TNF-α and related injury in the liver and lead to lysosomal destabilisation and release of cathepsin B. Lysosomal destabilisation leads to activation of nuclear factor kappa B (NF-κB) and the generation of more TNF-α. In addition, free fatty acids activate the stress and inflammatory kinases Jun N-terminal kinase (JNK) and IκB kinase (IKK) complex. Up arrow indicates upregulation and down arrow indicates suppression. CAMP = cyclic adenosine monophosphate; IFN = interferon. Reproduced from Tilg *et al* with kind permission of the American Gastroenterological Association.[7]

Treatment of NAFLD is directed primarily at reversal of the metabolic syndrome. Strong epidemiological evidence shows that increasing physical activity is an important factor – as is weight loss. A study in women showed a direct negative relation between physical activity and levels of alanine aminotransferase (ALT).[8] These data infer that a modest increase in physical activity is likely to be as effective at reducing fat within the liver as weight loss and that the two factors may be additive. Weight reduction surgery has been shown to reduce fat within the liver, and a number of studies have now shown that non-surgically induced weight loss improves levels of liver enzymes and reduces steatosis within the liver (as assessed by imaging). Weight loss remains the main proved intervention for the management of NAFLD.

A number of drugs are theoretically attractive for the treatment of NAFLD – primarily insulin-sensitising agents, which would be expected to reverse aspects of the metabolic syndrome. In a small study of 14 patients, metformin produced a greater decrease in ALT than diet alone.[9] The thioglitazones, which act via PPAR-α, are another theoretically attractive class of drugs, and initial data suggest they may produce a clinical benefit. A pilot study in 55 patients with type 2 diabetes and NASH confirmed by biopsy were treated with a hypocaloric diet (500 kcal) and randomised to placebo or pioglitazone for six months. Response was assessed by magnetic resonance imaging spectroscopy and biopsy. Significant improvements were seen in the content of liver fat, liver injury, necrosis, and inflammation with pioglitazone.[10] When a number of ongoing trials of these agents in Europe and the United States report in the next year, the role of these agents in the management of NAFLD should become more clear.

REFERENCES

1. Browning JD, Szczepaniak LS, Dobbins R *et al.* Prevalence of hepatic steatosis in an urban population in the United States: impact of ethnicity. *Hepatology* 2004;40:1387–95
2. Skelly MM, James PD, Ryder SD. Findings on liver biopsy to investigate abnormal liver function tests in the absence of diagnostic serology. *J Hepatol* 2001;35:195–9.
3. Hamaguchi M, Kojima T, Takeda N *et al.* The metabolic syndrome as a predictor of nonalcoholic fatty liver disease. *Ann Intern Med* 2005;143:722–8.
4. Suzuki A, Angulo P, Lymp J *et al.* Chronological development of elevated aminotransferases in a non-alcoholic population. *Hepatology* 2005;41:64–71.
5. Teli MR, James OF, Burt AD, Bennett MK, Day CP. The natural history of nonalcoholic fatty liver: a follow-up study. *Hepatology* 1995;22:1714–9.
6. Ekstedt M, Franzen LE, Mathiesen UL *et al.* Long-term follow-up of patients with NAFLD and elevated liver enzymes. *Hepatology* 2006;44:865–73.
7. Tilg H, Hotamisligil GS. Non-alcoholic fatty liver disease: cytokine-adipokine interplay and regulation of insulin resistance. *Gastroenterology* 2006;131:934–45.
8. Lawlor DA, Sattar N, Smith GD, Ebrahim S. The associations of physical activity and adiposity with alanine aminotransferase and gamma-glutamyltransferase. *Am J Epidemiol* 2005;161:1081–8.
9. Marchesini G, Brizi M, Bianchi G *et al.* Metformin in non-alcoholic steatohepatitis. *Lancet* 2001;358:893–4.
10. Belfort R, Harrison SA, Brown K *et al.* A placebo-controlled trial of pioglitazone in subjects with non-alcoholic steatohepatitis. *N Engl J Med* 2006;355:2297–307.

Autoimmune hepatitis

Ye H Oo and David H Adams

☐ INTRODUCTION

Autoimmune hepatitis (AIH), primary biliary cirrhosis (PBC), and primary sclerosing cholangitis (PSC) are the three major autoimmune diseases that affect the liver. Of the three, AIH is the most typical autoimmune disease, being characterised by an infiltrate rich in T cells, high circulating levels of gamma globulins, autoantibodies, human leucocyte antigen (HLA) associations, and links with other autoimmune diseases, and it is the only one of the three diseases that responds consistently to immunosuppressive treatment. Autoimmune hepatitis is caused by dysregulation of the immune system associated with defects in regulatory networks; this allows the emergence of autoreactive T cells that orchestrate a progressive destruction of hepatocytes and, untreated, leads to liver failure. T cells play a major role in the immunopathogenesis, and CD4+ and CD8 T cells are involved, together with effector responses mediated by natural killer (NK) cells and $\gamma\delta$ T cells. A number of triggering factors have been proposed – including viruses, xenobiotics, and drugs – but none have been shown to be involved in pathogenesis.

☐ NATURAL HISTORY

The seminal immunosuppressive trials in autoimmune hepatitis were published more than 25 years ago and showed that untreated AIH has a very poor prognosis but treatment with prednisolone is associated with excellent short- and long-term survival. Up to 30% of adult patients have histological features of cirrhosis at diagnosis, and progression of fibrosis occurs mainly in patients with inflammatory activity despite steroid treatment. The presence of cirrhosis at baseline significantly increases the risk of subsequent death or liver transplantation. The risk of hepatocellular carcinoma (HCC) in patients with autoimmune liver disease is associated with the development of cirrhosis and is no greater than in patients with other non-viral causes of cirrhosis.

☐ PRESENTATION

The prevalence of AIH in developed countries is one in 5,000 to one in 10,000. Overall, 75% of affected people are female, and AIH can affect people from childhood to old age. Presentation is variable. At one extreme, patients present with fulminant hepatitis and liver failure, whereas other patients, particularly the elderly, may be asymptomatic and have an indolent form of the disease. Patients may present with acute hepatitis – with acute onset of jaundice associated with systemic symptoms including arthralgia, anorexia, and fatigue – which symptomatically is identical to acute viral hepatitis. In such patients, liver biopsy shows acute hepatitis without evidence of significant fibrosis or cirrhosis. In others, presentation may be indolent, and in some it may present with symptoms of decompensated cirrhosis, with the diagnosis being made for the first time at the end of the disease process. This pattern of presentation is more frequently seen in older patients. Patients increasingly are being picked up through abnormal liver biochemistry on routine testing for other symptoms or conditions. Autoimmune hepatitis may occur in the presence of other autoimmune diseases, commonly thyroiditis, ulcerative colitis, type 1 diabetes, rheumatoid arthritis, and coeliac disease. Physical examination may be normal or show hepatomegaly, splenomegaly, jaundice, and signs of chronic liver disease. Autoimmune hepatitis first may become evident during pregnancy or in the early postpartum period. Furthermore, postpartum exacerbations may occur in women whose condition improved during pregnancy as a consequence of the natural immunosuppressed state associated with pregnancy.

☐ LABORATORY ABNORMALITIES

Autoimmune hepatitis is characterised by increased levels of transaminases in serum (which reflect liver damage), hypergammaglobulinaemia, and high titres of circulating autoantibodies (which indicate immune activation). It has been classified according to the autoantibodies detected into:

- ☐ type 1 AIH, which is characterised by the presence of anti-smooth muscle antibodies (SMA) and/or anti-nuclear antibodies (ANA) and is the most common form
- ☐ type 2 AIH, which is characterised by anti-liver kidney microsomal (LKM) antibodies and is rare in adults
- ☐ type 3 AIH, which is characterised by antibodies to soluble liver or liver–pancreas antigens.

About 20% of patients will not have any of the above autoantibodies. In other patients, autoantibodies to asialoglycoprotein receptor and anti-neutrophil cytoplasmic antibodies (ANCA) may be found. In Caucasian people, AIH is associated with HLA DRB1*0301 and DRB1*0401, with other susceptibility alleles sharing a similar motif in DR.β71.

Histological findings

Autoimmune hepatitis has no diagnostic features on liver biopsy, and the findings must be interpreted in the context of clinical, biochemical, and immunological features. Characteristic features include portal inflammation with plasma cells, prominent interface hepatitis with ballooning or rosetting of periportal hepatocytes, and a plasma cell-rich lobular infiltrate (Fig 1). Variable degrees of fibrosis or even cirrhosis may be found at presentation.

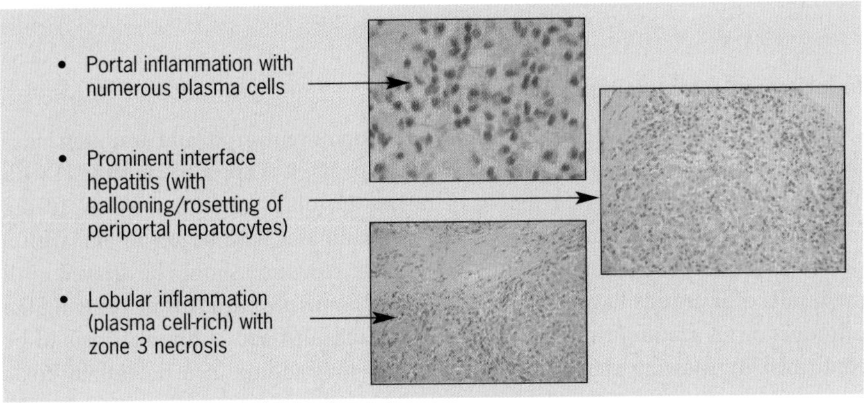

Fig 1 The three characteristic histological features of autoimmune hepatitis are shown. Histological images reproduced courtesy of Professor Stefan Hubscher, Department of Pathology, University of Birmingham.

☐ DIAGNOSIS OF AIH

The International Autoimmune Hepatitis Working Group (IAHG) generated a scoring system on the basis of clinical, serological, and histological criteria.[3] Points in favour of the diagnosis are female sex, increased levels of transaminases, increased levels of immunoglobulin (Ig) G and non-organ-specific antibodies (ANA, SMA, or LKM-1 antibodies), and a family history of autoimmune disease. Supportive features on liver histology include interface hepatitis, lymphoplasmacytic infiltrate, hepatocyte rosetting and the absence of biliary changes, Mallory's hyaline, and steatosis. Points against the diagnosis are male sex, cholestatic enzymes, recent drugs, consumption of >60 g/day alcohol, antimitochondrial antibodies, and markers of viral hepatitis. This scoring system is useful for defining patients in clinical research, but it is not practical for day-to-day use.

☐ TYPES OF AIH

Type 1 AIH – the most common form – can present at any age, and failure of treatment is rare. Type 2 AIH occurs in a younger age group and is a more aggressive disease. Treatment failure is more frequent and relapse after drug withdrawal is almost inevitable, so most patients with type 2 AIH need lifelong immunosuppressive treatment.[3] The putative type 3 autoimmune hepatitis also has been associated with more frequent relapse.

☐ TREATMENT

Standard treatment is based on corticosteroids and azathioprine, with subsequent reduction of prednisolone to a minimum maintenance dose. Autoimmune hepatitis usually responds to immunosuppression and was the first chronic liver disease for which a significant improvement in patient survival was noted after drug treatment.[1] Most patients need long-term treatment with corticosteroids and/or azathioprine.

Inducing and maintaining remission

Corticosteroids are the drug of choice for induction of remission, and azathioprine is the drug of choice for maintenance. In young patients, it is appropriate to start with high doses of prednisolone (1 mg/kg or 60 mg in total) and to reduce by 10 mg increments weekly to 20 mg/day once the transaminases have begun to fall, with a slower subsequent reduction to 10 mg/day. Further reduction should be delayed until the results of liver tests have returned to normal. Some people advocate delaying the introduction of azathioprine for 2–3 weeks, because this allows the diagnosis to be confirmed by showing steroid responsiveness before adding in a potentially toxic immunosuppressive agent and because liver toxicity due to azathioprine can be confused with non-responsiveness if azathioprine is started immediately. In older patients or those who have comorbidities such as hypertension, osteoporosis, or diabetes, in whom the dosage of prednisolone should be kept to a minimum, it is possible to start with a lower dose of 20–30 mg/day together with azathioprine at a dose of 1–2 mg/kg. Maintenance treatment usually involves azathioprine alone or in combination with low-dose prednisolone. For patients who develop decompensated liver disease despite treatment, orthotopic liver transplantation (OLT) is the treatment of choice. The rare patients who present with fulminant autoimmune hepatitis often fail to respond to immunosuppression and require liver transplantation. Although it is worth starting immunosuppressive treatment, it is important not to delay referral to a transplant centre if the patient has evidence of liver failure as shown by the development of encephalopathy, coagulopathy, or renal failure.

Complications of long-term treatment with immunosuppressive drugs should be foreseen – through monitoring of blood pressure, examination of urine for glucose, and monitoring of full blood counts in patients taking azathioprine to detect bone marrow suppression – and treated appropriately. All patients who are taking >7.5 mg/day prednisolone should be advised to take supplements of calcium and vitamin D or bisphosphonate to prevent osteoporosis.

Remission, relapse, and when to stop treatment

Remission is defined as a lack of symptoms, with normal levels of aminotransferases in serum, normal levels of IgG, and inactive liver histology. It is achieved in more than 80% of patients who take prednisolone and azathioprine.[4] The risk of relapse is high after discontinuation of treatment, particularly in patients with type 2 disease positive for LKM antibodies, in whom relapse is almost universal. Most relapses occur within 12 weeks of stopping treatment; however, some relapses may take months or even years to develop, and patients must be monitored closely for at least one year after treatment is stopped. Withdrawal of steroids should not be attempted before 12 months of treatment, and maximisation of the dose of azathioprine to

2 mg/kg/day reduces the risk of reactivation. Full-dose treatment needs to be reintroduced after symptomatic relapse, although induction of a second remission is the usual outcome. A common cause of relapse in adolescent patients is a failure to take treatment, and evidence of non-adherence or psychosocial problems should always be sought in young patients who relapse unexpectedly.

When to repeat liver biopsy

Follow-up biopsies should be considered because the risk of progression to cirrhosis is 5% per year and is much higher in patients with continuing inflammation. Overall, 25% of patients with normal levels of transaminases have inflammatory lesions on biopsy, although normal levels of IgG and transaminases are associated histologically with minimal inflammatory activity in 90% of patients. The other scenario in which repeat biopsy is invaluable is to confirm remission before a trial of treatment withdrawal. Patients in remission with minimal inflammatory activity on biopsy have a higher chance of successful treatment withdrawal.[5] Fig 2 shows an algorithm that outlines the strategy to follow when deciding on the level of immunosuppression in patients with AIH

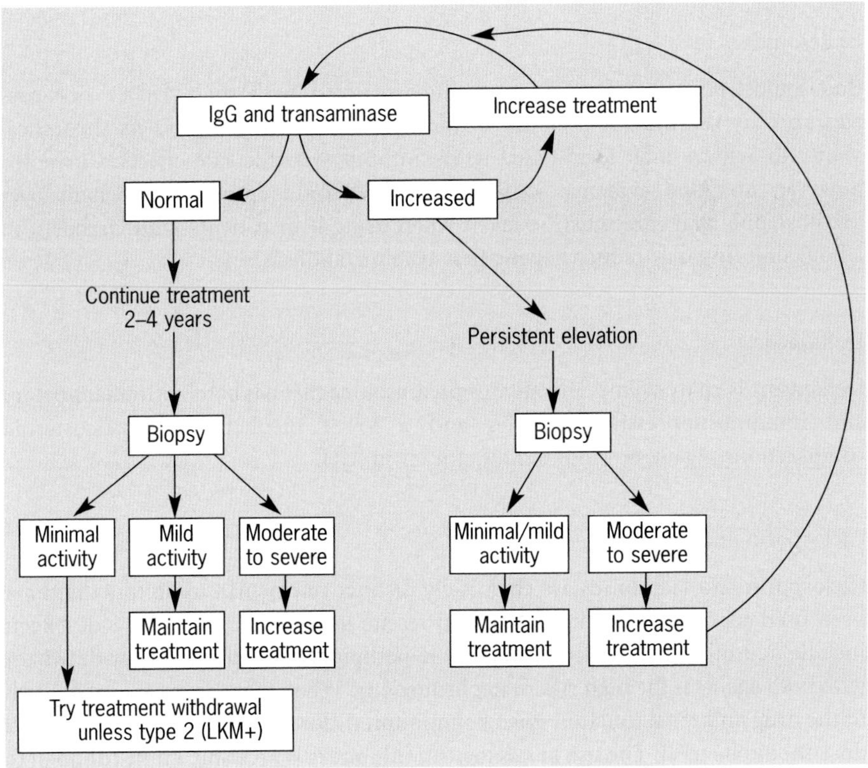

Fig 2 Algorithm for adjusting therapy in patients with autoimmune hepatitis.

Treatment failure and alternative treatments for AIH

As mentioned above, remission will be achieved in more than 80% of patients who take prednisolone and azathioprine.[4] Alternative treatment may be needed because of failure to achieve remission or because of side-effects. Treatment failure may be due to an incorrect diagnosis or non-compliance, and these possibilities must be excluded actively before making a diagnosis of non-responsiveness. Some patients need high doses of corticosteroids to maintain remission or a second cycle of induction treatment. Intolerance of side-effects is the other reason for considering alternative treatment. Long-term use of glucocorticoids is complicated by many side-effects – including diabetes, osteoporosis, and hypertension – and younger patients, in particular, may find the cosmetic side-effects unacceptable. A small number of patients cannot tolerate azathioprine because of symptomatic side-effects, including nausea, rash, abdominal discomfort, and severe and potentially life-threatening complications such as pancreatitis, cholestatic hepatotoxicity, and bone marrow suppression. Several alternative treatments have been tried, but the quality of evidence is poor, being based on a small non-controlled series, with few prospective studies.

Alternative agents used in the treatment of AIH

Some agents proposed as alternatives to standard treatment are described below.

Budesonide

Budesonide is a second-generation glucocorticoid with high (90%) first-pass clearance by the liver. A potential advantage over prednisolone is its theoretical ability to achieve high local tissue levels without systemic side-effects. Currently, however, no good evidence suggests that budesonide provides a benefit over prednisolone, and care must be taken when using it in patients with cirrhosis, in whom shunting may reduce hepatic first-pass metabolism.

Deflazacort

Deflazacort is an oxazoline derivative of prednisolone that has both anti-inflammatory and immunosuppressive activities and a lower incidence of corticosteroid complications. Again, no studies show efficacy in AIH.

Ciclosporin and tacrolimus

Ciclosporin and tacrolimus are chemically distinct calcineurin inhibitors that have been used successfully for induction and rescue in patients with AIH. Side-effects include neurotoxicity, hypertension, and hyperlipidaemia, but the major drawback with both agents is the high risk of nephrotoxicity. When these drugs are used, levels of the drug and renal function must be monitored closely and the minimal effective dose should be used. The use of calcineurin inhibitors is probably safest confined to centres such as transplant units with extensive experience in their use.

Cyclophosphamide

Cyclophosphamide is a cytotoxic agent commonly used to treat vasculitis. Experience in patients with AIH is limited to anecdotal and case reports, which suggest patients may respond. The ability of this drug to inhibit antibody production is of theoretical benefit. Again, the risk of toxicity means its use should be restricted to units with extensive experience of immunosuppressive treatment.

D-penicillamine

D-penicillamine is a modified amino acid with anti-inflammatory activity and metal-chelating properties. Toxicity includes mucocutaneous, gastrointestinal, renal, haematological, pulmonary, and autoimmune complications.

Methotrexate

Methotrexate has been reported to be effective at normalising levels of liver enzymes, improving liver histology, and maintaining remission with a steroid-sparing effect. It is teratogenic in women of child-bearing age, however, and has been associated with liver fibrosis when used to treat psoriasis.

Ursodeoxycholic acid

Ursodeoxycholic acid (UDCA) may improve liver biochemistry, but its use neither permits a reduction in the dose of steroids nor affects clinical outcome or histological activity, so it cannot be recommended routinely.

Mycophenolic acid

Mycophenolic acid is used extensively in the management of patients who have received liver, heart, or kidney transplants without reported hepatotoxicity. Two formulations currently are available: an enteric formulation and an ester. Mycophenolate mofetil (MMF) is an ester prodrug of mycophenolic acid (MPA) and is converted into MPA after oral absorption. Mycophenolic acid is a non-competitive inhibitor of inosine monophosphate dehydrogenase, which blocks the rate-limiting enzymatic steps in de novo purine nucleotide synthesis, thereby arresting replication of DNA in T lymphocytes and B lymphocytes. Mycophenolate mofetil is well tolerated, with leucopenia and diarrhoea being the main side-effects. Unlike the calcineurin inhibitors, MMF does not have neurotoxic or nephrotoxic side-effects. Although effective, MMF is expensive, especially in comparison with corticosteroids and azathioprine; it is also teratogenic, which is an important factor in the choice of treatment for a disease that often affects women of child-bearing years. Mycophenolate has been used in several other autoimmune diseases, such as rheumatoid arthritis and ulcerative colitis, but with limited effect. The only evidence for efficacy in AIH comes from a few retrospective studies in which it was used in patients with refractory disease (Table 1).

Table 1 Treatment strategy for autoimmune hepatitis.

Standard therapy	Alternative treatment*
Induction • Prednisolone 1 mg/kg/day • Weekly reduction (by 10 mg steps) to 20 mg/day over six weeks, then add azathioprine when levels of AST have decreased to 2–3 times the normal range or • Prednisolone 20 mg/day and azathioprine 1 mg/kg/day	• Calcineurin inhibitors (ciclosporin or tacrolimus) • Ciclosporin or tacrolimus • Cyclophosphamide • Budesonide
Maintenance of remission Aim: normal transaminases and normal IgG • Increase azathioprine to 1.5 mg/kg/day • Steroid reduction to <10 mg/day once biochemical remission achieved	• Calcineurin inhibitors (ciclosporin or tacrolimus) • Ciclosporin or tacrolimus • Mycophenolate mofetil • Cyclophosphamide • Methotraxate

AST = aspartate aminotransferase.
*For patients with relapse or failure of standard treatment and those intolerant of steroids or azathioprine.

Richardson and colleagues studied seven patients with type 1 AIH who were intolerant of (n=3) or refractory to (n=4) azathioprine. Patients received MMF (2 g/day) in addition to prednisolone over a median follow up of 46 months. Five of seven patients had normal levels of transaminases after three months of treatment. The prednisolone requirement was reduced from a median of 20 mg/day to 2 mg/day after nine months, with significant improvement in histology. One patient required a reduction in the dose of MMF because of a decrease in white cell count, but no other adverse effects were noted.[6] Devlin reported five patients unresponsive or unable to take azathioprine or corticosteroids, in whom levels of transaminases normalised and the dose of corticosteroids could be reduced after treatment with MMF.[7] A Canadian study reported similar findings in patients with AIH refractory or resistant to corticosteroids or azathioprine, or both.[8] Complete response to MMF was seen in 64% of patients, and the mean dose of prednisolone was reduced from 20 mg/day before treatment to 4.7 mg/day. We analysed data from two large specialised centres and found 25 patients who were switched to MMF, nine of whom (36%) achieved remission defined as levels of aspartate aminotransferase (AST) less than twice the upper limit of normal. The response rate was dependent on the reasons for stopping standard treatment. Of seven patients who failed to respond to azathioprine, only one (14%) reached remission. Results were better for patients who switched to MMF because of intolerance of azathioprine, with 8/18 (44%) achieving remission.

Biological agents in AIH

In theory, immune-modulating biologic agents should be effective in patients with AIH. Anti-B cell treatment has been tried in other autoimmune diseases and theoretically is attractive because of its ability to inhibit production of autoantibodies. Clinical experience with anti-cytokine treatments, particularly anti-tumour necrosis factor alpha (TNF-α), is increasing. No current evidence shows that such drugs are effective in AIH, and given the fact that most patients respond to conventional immunosuppression, it seems unlikely that the current generation of antibody-based treatments will find a place in the management of AIH.

□ AUTOIMMUNE HEPATITIS AND PREGNANCY

Autoimmune hepatitis may present rarely during pregnancy or more commonly after delivery, but because the disease affects young women, it is not uncommon to be faced with a patient with established AIH who wants to become pregnant or has already done so. Whereas most patients with AIH can expect a good outcome, higher complication rates are reported in pregnant women and their fetuses, particularly in those with type 2 or type 3 AIH. In addition, the disease may flare after delivery as the pregnancy-associated immunosuppressive state is lost. There is no reason to council against pregnancy, however, as long as the disease is well controlled at the time of conception. Patients who are cirrhotic need to be monitored carefully to make sure that complications of portal hypertension do not develop during late pregnancy. Fertility used to be claimed to be greatly reduced in women with cirrhosis, but this is not the case – at least for those with compensated cirrhosis – and patients should be advised about contraception. The immunosuppression of pregnancy may lead to autoimmune diseases going into remission during pregnancy; however, this does not mean that immunosuppressive treatment can be omitted. Treatment should be continued. Azathioprine and corticosteroids are relatively safe, but MMF is teratogenic in animals and should be avoided wherever possible. Patients on MMF who plan to get pregnant should be switched to another immunosuppressant or should receive cover with a higher dose of steroids during pregnancy.

□ AUTOIMMUNE HEPATITIS AND LIVER TRANSPLANTATION

End-stage cirrhosis in patients with AIH is an indication for liver transplantation, as is fulminant autoimmune hepatitis. The overall success of liver transplantation is high, but a proportion of patients – up to 25% in some series – are at risk of developing recurrent disease despite maintenance immunosuppression to prevent graft rejection. Recurrent AIH is characterised by the persistence of autoantibodies, increased levels of IgG, and typical features on liver biopsy. It is interesting that an autoimmune disease can recur in the context of allogeneic HLA after transplantation. This has led to the concept that it is, in fact, a form of graft rejection rather than autoimmunity. Autoantigens, however, can be presented by allogeneic HLA, which provides a mechanism for true autoimmune disease to recur. The long-term use of low-dose steroids after transplantation has been claimed to reduce the incidence of recurrent disease.

Patients transplanted for other causes may develop de novo autoimmune hepatitis after transplantation, with classic biochemical, serological, and histological features of AIH. This is more common in children (5–10%). Most affected patients respond to increased levels of immunosuppression, although rare cases have progressed to cirrhosis and graft failure. Again, it is unclear whether the immune response is directed against the graft rather than self antigens, and this might be a form of late cellular rejection rather than true autoimmune disease. In support of this hypothesis, autoantibodies have been described transiently in association with episodes of rejection, and acute rejection has predictive value for the subsequent development of de novo autoimmune hepatitis.

☐ OVERLAP SYNDROMES WITH OTHER AUTOIMMUNE LIVER DISEASES

Overlap syndromes are defined as autoimmune liver diseases that are difficult to classify within a single diagnostic category – that is, PBS, PSC, or AIH – because they have biochemical, immunological, clinical, or histological features suggestive of more than one disease process. The common forms seen are PBC with features of AIH and AIH with biliary features suggestive of PSC. They may occur at the same time (true overlap syndromes) or as sequential syndromes, when the patient presents with features of one disease and subsequently develops the other. The association between AIH and PSC is particularly interesting. Both diseases can be associated with inflammatory bowel disease (IBD), and recent evidence from our laboratory suggests that the liver disease is driven by the recruitment of effector lymphocytes that are activated in the gut. We have shown that long-lived memory lymphocytes arise as a consequence of bowel inflammation and can be recruited to the liver. Such cells recirculate between the liver and gut without causing damage for many years, but subsequent encounters with an antigen in the liver results in activation and the promotion of tissue damage and disease. When lymphocytes are activated in gut-associated lymphoid tissues (GALT), they are not only programmed to respond to antigen but are also imprinted with a homing phenotype that directs their subsequent trafficking back to the gut. After antigen clearance, long-lived memory cells retain gut tropism and thereby provide immune surveillance against the same pathogen entering the gut in the future.

The molecular basis of this tissue-specific homing recently was elucidated. It involves interactions with tissue-specific adhesion molecules and chemotactic cytokines (called chemokines), which are presented on the endothelium that lines the vessels in the target tissue and are recognised by lymphocytes with appropriate receptors. The endothelium in the gut expresses a unique adhesion molecule called mucosal addressin cell adhesion molecule-1 (MADCAM-1) that is absent from other vascular beds and a unique chemokine CCL25 that is restricted to the small bowel. Activation of lymphocytes in the gut imprints the responding lymphocytes with the receptors for these gut-specific molecules – the integrin $\alpha4\beta7$ and the chemokine receptor CCR9, respectively. Overall, 20% of the T cells that infiltrate the liver in patients with AIH and PSC that complicate IBD are $\alpha4\beta7$+CCR9+ cells and thus of gut origin, whereas these cells are found at very low frequencies in patients with other liver diseases. Furthermore, these cells are memory-effector T cells that secrete interferon (IFN) γ, which suggests they are effector cells capable of promoting inflammation of the liver. Both MADCAM1 and CCL25, which are absent from the normal liver, are present on the hepatic endothelium in liver diseases associated with IBD, which provides a mechanism for recruitment of these cells. Some mucosal lymphocytes thus can bind liver endothelium, which allows them to recirculate between the liver and gut to provide immune surveillance across both sites. If these cells are activated by cross-reactive liver antigens or gut antigens that have entered through the portal circulation, however, this leads to their local expansion and the establishment of chronic inflammation in the form of AIH or PSC. The link between AIH and PSC is supported further by observations that they can occur together, particularly in children.

Czaja and Carpenter reported that 20/84 patients with AIH had biliary changes on liver biopsy in the absence of antimitochondrial autoantibodies.[13] In other respects, the disease behaved like AIH and responded to immunosuppressive treatment. Gregorio *et al* reported similar findings serologically but evidence of PSC on cholangiography or liver biopsy in children with AIH,[14] who also showed a good response to corticosteroids (unlike patients with classic PSC). Furthermore, evidence shows that these diseases can occur sequentially, with patients who initially presented with AIH subsequently progressing to a clinical picture dominated by features of PSC. All of the above evidence suggests that in some patients, particularly those with IBD, autoimmune sclerosing cholangitis and autoimmune hepatitis may be part of the same disease process and that AIH can progress to a biliary syndrome that resembles PSC.

REFERENCES

1. Cook GC, Mulligan R, Sherlock S. Controlled prospective trial of corticosteroid therapy in active chronic hepatitis. *Q J Med* 1971;40:159–85.
2. Lohse AW, Gerken G, Mohr H *et al.* Relation between autoimmune liver diseases and viral hepatitis: clinical and serological characteristics in 859 patients. *Z Gastroenterol* 1995;33:527–33.
3. Alvarez F, Berg PA, Bianchi FB *et al.* International Autoimmune Hepatitis Group Report: review of criteria for diagnosis of autoimmune hepatitis. *J Hepatol* 1999;31:929–38.
4. Milkiewicz P, Hubscher SG, Skiba G, Hathaway M, Elias E. Recurrence of autoimmune hepatitis after liver transplantation. *Transplantation* 1999;68:253–6.
5. Czaja AJ, Bianchi FB, Carpenter HA *et al.* Treatment challenges and investigational opportunities in autoimmune hepatitis. *Hepatology* 2005;41:207–15.
6. Richardson PD, James PD, Ryder SD. Mycophenolate mofetil for maintenance of remission in autoimmune hepatitis in patients resistant to or intolerant of azathioprine. *J Hepatol* 2000;33:371–5.
7. Devlin SM, Swain MG, Urbanski SJ, Burak KW. Mycophenolate mofetil for the treatment of autoimmune hepatitis in patients refractory to standard therapy. *Can J Gastroenterol* 2004;18:321–6.
8. Chatur N, Ramji A, Bain VG *et al.* Transplant immunosuppressive agents in non-transplant chronic autoimmune hepatitis: the Canadian Association for the Study of Liver (CASL) experience with mycophenolate mofetil and tacrolimus. *Liver Int* 2005;25:723–7.
9. Mora JR, Iwata M, Eksteen B *et al.* Generation of gut-homing IgA-secreting B cells by intestinal dendritic cells. *Science* 2006;314:1157–60.
10. Adams DH, Eksteen B. Aberrant homing of mucosal T cells and extra-intestinal manifestations of inflammatory bowel disease. *Nat Rev Immunol* 2006;6:244–51.

11 Eksteen B, Grant AJ, Miles A *et al.* Hepatic endothelial CCL25 mediates the recruitment of CCR9+ gut-homing lymphocytes to the liver in primary sclerosing cholangitis. *J Exp Med* 2004;200:1511–7.

12 Vergani D, Mieli-Vergani G. Mechanisms of autoimmune hepatitis. *Pediatr Transplant* 2004;8:589–93.

13 Czaja AJ, Carpenter HA. Autoimmune hepatitis with incidental histologic features of bile duct injury. *Hepatology* 2001;34:659–65.

14 Gregorio GV, Portmann B, Karani J *et al.* Autoimmune hepatitis/sclerosing cholangitis overlap syndrome in childhood: a 16-year prospective study. *Hepatology* 2001;33:544–53.

Selecting cases for liver transplantation

Kathryn L Nash and Alexander Gimson

☐ INTRODUCTION

More than 40 years have passed since the first human liver transplantation was performed. The intervening years have seen dramatic advances in surgical techniques, improved criteria for selecting recipients, and more specifically targeted immunosuppression. These and other advances have led to dramatic improvements in graft and patient survival.[1] Over the same period, the number of people eligible for liver transplantation has increased, principally because of increases in cirrhosis due to hepatitis C, alcoholic and non-alcoholic fatty liver disease, and hepatocellular carcinoma (HCC). Unfortunately, the number of cadaveric organ donors in the United Kingdom (UK) has decreased by 10.6% over the past 10 years, while the number of patients on the transplant waiting list has increased by 115% (Fig 1).[2] As a result, 16% of patients listed for a liver transplant in the UK will not receive an organ because they have died or deteriorated on the waiting list. As well as developing strategies to try to increase the donor pool through the use of split liver donors, non-heart beating donors, and live donor transplantation, transplant centres are now faced with the problem of trying to refine the selection criteria for accepting patients onto the transplant waiting list in order to achieve the maximum benefit from transplantation.

When considering how to allocate a scarce resource, different perspectives can be applied. Firstly, from the recipients' view, organs could be allocated to those with greatest need – that is, those who have the highest predicted mortality without a transplant. This would allow the most severely ill patients a chance of transplantation, but their transplant-related mortality may be high because of the severity of their disease. Alternatively, from the donors' perspective, prioritisation may be performed on the basis of organ utility, such that organs are offered to those predicted to have the best outcome after a transplant. This would allow greater survival of the donor organ but might result in patients being transplanted earlier, when their risk of dying without a transplant is low. Systems of organ prioritisation have attempted to define the benefit of a transplant – that is the difference between survival curves with and without transplantation – to try to combine individual autonomy and organ utility. In the UK, liver transplantation is generally considered when the projected mortality from liver disease without transplantation at one year exceeds 15% and the patient is deemed to have a >50% probability of being alive five years after a transplant with a quality of life that is acceptable to the patient. The difficulty is how to accurately model these risks to allow transplantation of patients

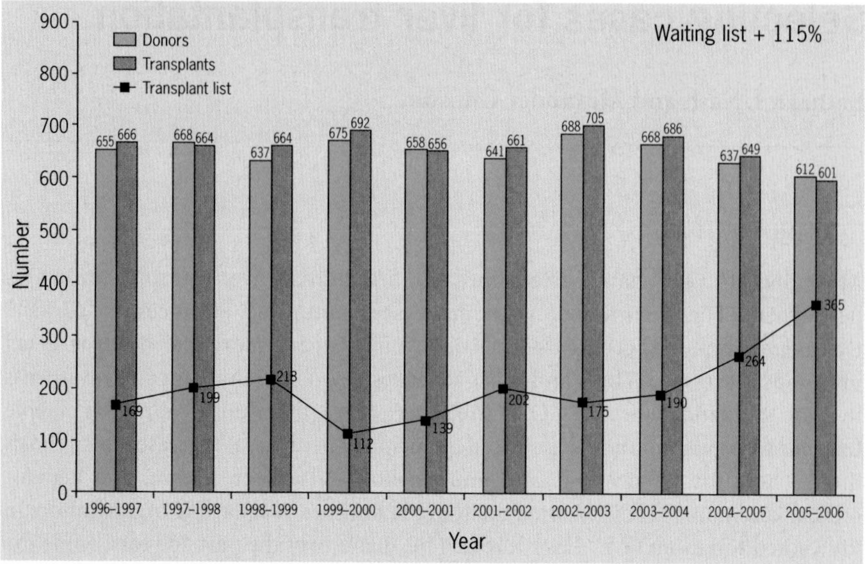

Fig 1 Numbers of donors, transplants, and patients on active transplant list at 31 March in programme for transplantation of livers from deceased people in the UK between 1 April 1996 and 31 March 2006. Data from UK Liver Transplant database. Reproduced with permission of UK Transplant.[2]

from all liver transplant units who are on the waiting list with similar risks of dying according to disease stratification and so achieve equity and justice.

In most cases, liver transplantation is undertaken because of the high risk of death associated with conditions such as fulminant hepatic failure, HCC, and chronic liver disease. The literature on predicting risks and benefits for transplantation in these groups is extensive. In a small minority of patients, transplantation is undertaken when the immediate risk of death is low but there is a window of opportunity such that if transplantation is not undertaken at this time the patient will become too high risk – for example, due to hepatopulmonary syndrome or portopulmonary syndrome. In addition, in patients with conditions such as primary biliary cirrhosis complicated by pruritus or polycystic liver disease complicated by pain or mass symptoms, transplantation may be considered for those with symptoms when the risk of death from the underlying disorder is low but the impact of such symptoms on quality of life is unacceptably high. Finally, liver transplantation may be undertaken in an attempt to cure an underlying disorder such as familial hyperlipidaemia, amyloidosis, or oxalosis when the liver itself is not diseased. In these minority indications for transplantation, risk modelling is much more difficult because of the paucity of data.

□ ACUTE LIVER FAILURE

Acute liver failure is the rapid onset of encephalopathy within eight weeks of the onset of symptoms. In the UK, the main cause is paracetamol-related hepatotoxicity, with other drugs, viruses, and autoimmune diseases the causes in most of the remaining cases. About 14% of the liver transplants performed in the UK are in patients with acute liver failure. The process of selecting appropriate candidates is problematic, as these patients have a very high mortality but the potential for full hepatic recovery. In addition, there is only a short window of opportunity in which to perform the operation.

The guidelines of King's College Hospital are often used, as they are applicable early in the hospital admission and use readily available parameters. These criteria are highly specific at predicting death (positive predictive value 67–100%) but less sensitive (negative predictive value 42–86%).[3,4] The current transplant criteria for super-urgent liver transplantation in the UK, based on these guidelines, also include increases in levels of lactate in serum in patients with paracetamol-related hepatotoxicity and evidence of clinical deterioration, such as increased intracranial pressure or increasing requirements for ventilatory support or inotropes (Table 1). Patients who are listed for super-urgent transplantation take priority over all other patients on the liver transplant waiting list, as their window of opportunity is short. The severity of illness at the time of transplantation means these patients have significantly worse short-term survival compared with those transplanted for chronic liver disease, but their long-term survival is comparable (Fig 2).

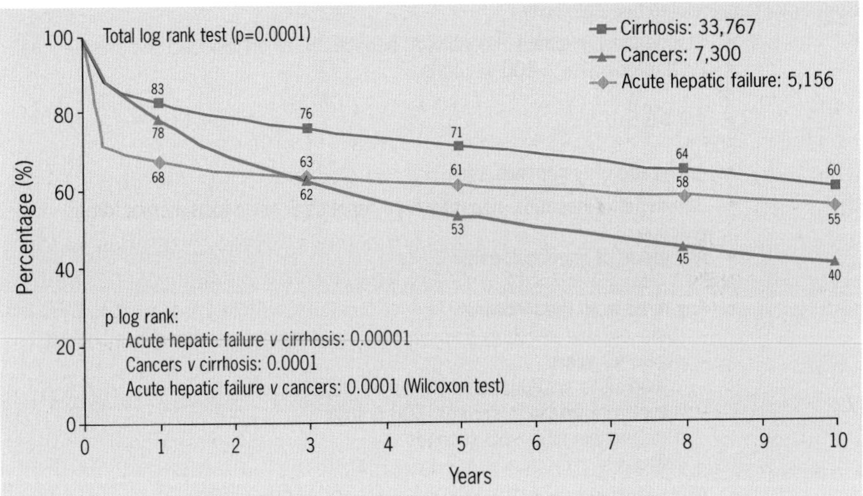

Fig 2 Patient survival according to the first indication of liver transplantation. Data from the European Liver Transplant Registry between January 1988 and December 2005. Reproduced with permission of European Liver Transplant Registry.[1]

☐ HEPATOCELLULAR CARCINOMA

The incidence of HCC is increasing throughout the world. Ninety percent of cases of HCC occur on a background of cirrhosis, and the median survival of cirrhosis-related HCC is six months in untreated patients. In the UK, about 12% of liver transplants are performed in patients with HCC. Transplantation offers the chance of cure for appropriately selected patients; this is in contrast with the alternative

Table 1 UK Transplant's selection criteria for transplantation patients with acute liver failure.

Category	Aetiology
Paracetamol-related hepatotoxicity	
1	• Paracetamol poisoning • pH <7.25 more than 24 hours after overdose and after fluid resuscitation
2	• Paracetamol poisoning • Coexisting prothombin time >100 seconds *or* • INR >6.5 and levels of creatinine in serum >300 µmol/l or anuria *and* • Grade 3–4 encephalopathy
3	• Paracetamol poisoning • Levels of lactate in serum more than 24 hours after overdose >3.5 mmol/l on admission *or* • >3.0 mmol/l after fluid resuscitation
4	• Paracetamol poisoning • Two of the three criteria from category 2 • Clinical evidence of deterioration (for example, increased intracranial pressure, fraction of inspired oxygen (F_iO_2) >50%, increasing inotrope requirements) in the absence of clinical sepsis
Non-paracetamol-related hepatotoxicity	
5	• Seronegative hepatitis, hepatitis A, hepatitis B, or an idiosyncratic drug reaction • Prothrombin time >100 seconds *or* • INR >6.5 *and* • Any grade of encephalopathy
6	• Seronegative hepatitis, hepatitis A or hepatitis B or an idiosyncratic drug reaction • Any grade of encephalopathy *and* • Any three from the following: – Unfavourable aetiology (idiosyncratic drug reaction, seronegative hepatitis) – Age >40 years – Jaundice to encephalopathy time >7 days – Levels of bilirubin in serum >300 µmol/l – Prothrombin time >50 seconds – INR >3.5
7	• Acute presentation of Wilson's disease or Budd-Chiari syndrome • Combination of coagulopathy and any grade of encephalopathy
8	• Hepatic artery thrombosis on days 0–14 after liver transplantation
9	• Early graft dysfunction on days 0–7 after liver transplantation • At least two of the following: – AST >10,000 – INR >3.0 – Levels of lactate in serum >3 mmol/l – Absence of bile production
10	• Any patient who has been a live liver donor who develops severe liver failure within four weeks of the donor operation

INR = international normalised ratio.

treatments – chemotherapy, transarterial chemoembolisation, and radiofrequency ablation – which may improve symptoms and lengthen survival but rarely result in cure. Surgical resection is performed in some patients with compensated cirrhosis, but the frequency of recurrent disease is high, such that liver transplantation is the preferred option.

Considerable evidence shows that tumour size predicts microscopic vascular invasion, tumour grade, and hence the risk of tumour recurrence after transplant.[5] As a result, the guidelines currently used for patients with HCC are the size-based Milan criteria of Mazzaferro *et al,* in which transplantation is indicated for patients with a single tumour ≤5 cm in diameter or ≤3 tumours <3 cm in diameter with no macroscopic vascular invasion seen on pretransplant imaging.[6] With these criteria, recurrence-free survival at four years of 83% can be achieved, with overall post-transplant survival similar to that for other indications.

Others groups have proposed extending the criteria for transplantation to include patients with a single tumour ≤6.5 cm diameter or ≤3 tumours <4.5 cm in diameter with a total tumour size of <8 cm and have reported acceptable 75% survival rates at five years.[7] As expanding the criteria would greatly increase the number of patients eligible for transplantation when there is already a problem of organ shortage, the liver transplant community in the UK have chosen to continue to restrict cases to those who meet the Milan criteria at the current time.

□ CHRONIC LIVER DISEASE

Most liver transplants in the UK are undertaken in patients with chronic liver disease (about 74%). It is in this vastly heterogeneous group of individuals with multiple different disease aetiologies and varying complications that selection of cases for liver transplantation is the most challenging. A variety of difficulties exist in assessing the prognosis in those with chronic liver disease. The rates of disease progression are dependent on the disease aetiology, and this, in turn, is influenced by specific treatments – both prophylactic and therapeutic – as well as the risk of exacerbations in disease activity, such as flares of viral hepatitis or autoimmune liver disease. In addition, the rate of disease progression is dependent on the onset of complications such as bleeding, infection, or ascites. Comorbidities, such as cardiovascular disease and diabetes, are frequent in patients with chronic liver disease and alter patient prognosis before, during, and after liver transplant.

Survival curves after the development of specific complications such as ascites, bacterial peritonitis, variceal haemorrhage, and hepatic encephalopathy can reasonably accurately predict long-term mortality but the confidence intervals tend to be wide in the shorter term. In addition, as many patients do not survive these initial complications, these models are largely unsatisfactory. Aetiology-specific, Cox proportional regression analysis models exist for some disorders such as primary biliary cirrhosis, primary sclerosing cholangitis, autoimmune liver disease, and alcohol-related liver disease, but, again, confidence intervals are wide and no such model exists for many disease aetiologies. Attention therefore has turned to aetiology-independent scoring systems, such as the Child-Pugh score and the Mayo end-stage liver disease (MELD) score. To be of use, such models need to have easily identifiable variables and defined endpoints, and they need to be reproducible in series of similar cases and generalisable to related different series.

The Child-Pugh score initially was designed to predict mortality in patients with cirrhosis who are undergoing surgery (Table 2). It subsequently has been shown to determine prognosis and has been utilised to predict the patients who might benefit from liver transplantation. Its limitations are that it has a wide standard error and a ceiling effect and its ability to make the correct prognosis is limited (*c* statistic of 0.7–0.8).

Table 2 Child-Pugh classification: (a) scores allocated per component and (b) median survival by total score.

(a)	**Score**		
Component	**1**	**2**	**3**
Ascites	None	Mild	Moderate/severe
Encephalopathy	0	I/II	III/IV
Albumin (g/l)	>35	28–35	<28
Bilirubin (μmol/l)	<34	34–51	>51
Prothrombin time (seconds increased)	1–3	4–6	>6

(b)

Total score	**Grade**	**Median survival (months)**
≤6	A	39
7–9	B	32
≥10	C	8

The MELD score was derived more recently in the United States (US) – initially to predict mortality three months after transjugular intrahepatic stent insertion,[8] but this scoring system subsequently has been applied to those awaiting liver transplantation.[9] This model uses the formula below, which is based on the log of levels of bilirubin, the international normalised ratio, and levels of creatinine, where INR = international normalised ratio, Creat = serum creatinine (mg/dl), and Br = serum bilirubin (mg/dl):

$$\text{MELD} = 10 \times [(0.957 \times \ln(\text{Creat})) + (0.378 \times \ln(\text{Br})) + (1.12 \times \ln(\text{INR})) + 0.643]$$

This scoring system has been validated in separate cohorts and has been shown to be an excellent predictor of mortality at three months in those with a high MELD score (Fig 3). Its predictive power at lower scores has been less good, however, and comparisons with the Child-Pugh score have not all shown a benefit. Several difficulties with the MELD score have been raised, including the fact that it was derived from a different cohort and has been transferred to transplant candidates, limited parameters have been involved, and it may prejudice non-cholestatic liver diseases. Additional predictors of prognosis in patients with chronic liver disease have been characterised in the MELD era and have been shown to improve

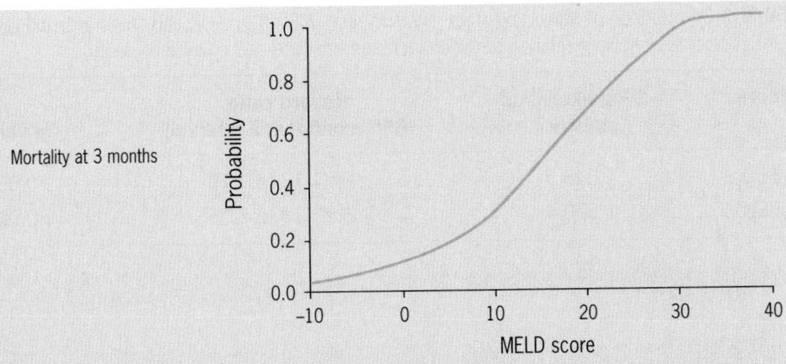

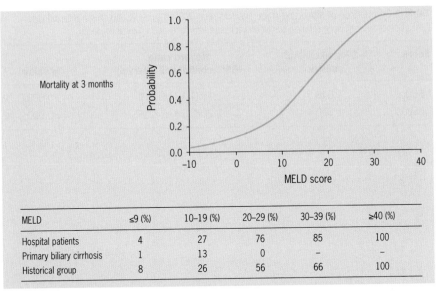

MELD	≤9 (%)	10–19 (%)	20–29 (%)	30–39 (%)	≥40 (%)
Hospital patients	4	27	76	85	100
Primary biliary cirrhosis	1	13	0	–	–
Historical group	8	26	56	66	100

Fig 3 Mayo end-stage liver disease score (MELD).[9]

prediction over and above the MELD score. These include the presence of persistent ascites,[10] hyponatraemia,[10,11] and measurements of portal pressure.[12] In the US, it has been proposed to include levels of sodium in serum to try to improve the predictive ability of MELD, particularly for patients with low MELD scores.

In the UK, a further scoring system – the UK end-stage liver disease (UKELD) score – has been derived. This model uses the formula below, where INR = international normalised ratio, Creat = serum creatinine (μmol/l), Br = serum bilirubin (μmol/l), and Na = serum sodium (mmol/l):

$$\text{UKELD} = 5 \times [(1.5 \times \ln(\text{INR})) + (0.3 \times \ln(\text{Creat})) + (0.6 \times \ln(\text{Br})) - (13 \times \ln(\text{Na})) + 70]$$

This was based on a retrospective assessment of prognostic factors of adult patients registered for their first elective liver transplant between April 2003 and November 2005 and confirmed in a prospective validation of patients between December 2005 and the time of writing. To date, 1,142 patients have been analysed, with the endpoints being death or removal from the transplant list because of deterioration. Four component variables were found to be individually predictive of outcome on a transplant waiting list: INR, levels of bilirubin in serum, levels of creatinine in serum, and levels of sodium in serum, with the latter being the strongest predictor of short-term survival. Cox regression models were then used to estimate weights assigned to these components. Unlike the MELD score, which gives a high weight to levels of creatinine in serum, the UKELD score gives a high weight to levels of sodium in serum and a relatively lower weight to levels of creatinine. Comparisons show that the UKELD score has narrower confidence intervals and increased sensitivity for predicting death than the MELD score, with a one-point increase in the UKELD score increasing the chance of death by 22% compared with 16% for a similar increase in the MELD score (Table 3 and Fig 4).

Table 3 Comparison of Mayo end-stage liver disease (MELD) and UK end-stage liver disease (UKELD) scores showing relation between increase in score and chance of death.

Score	−2 log likelihood statistic	Hazard ratio (95% confidence interval)	p value
MELD	1,648.5	1.16 (1.13 to 1.19)	<0.0001
UKELD	1,600.4	1.22 (1.18 to 1.26)	<0.0001

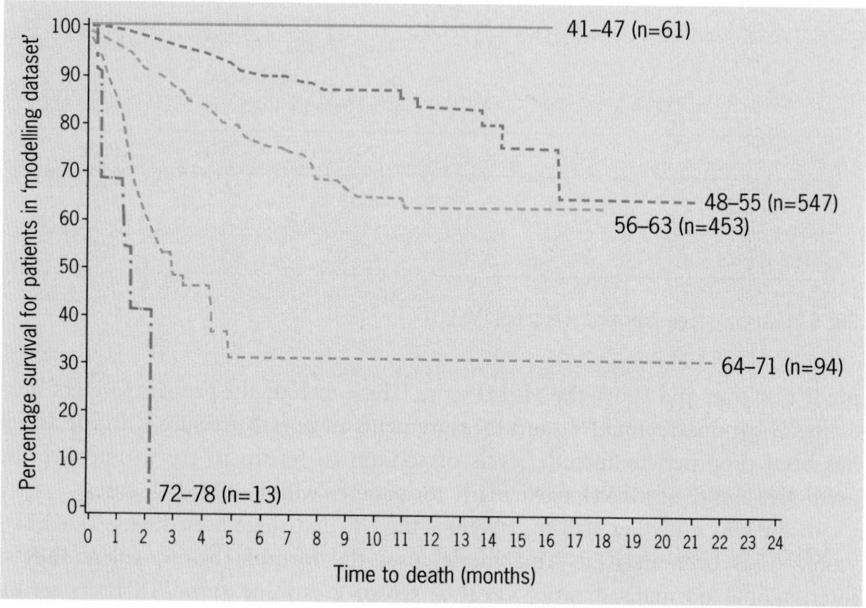

Fig 4 Kaplan-Meier survivor functions for bands of the UK end-stage liver disease score (UKELD).

The liver transplant units in the UK have agreed to select cases for the liver transplant waiting list on a UKELD score predictive of >15% survival at one year (score ≥49). Furthermore, to allow prioritisation of those with the greatest chance of death on the waiting list, cases are ranked with the UKELD, which is the best available prognostic marker of short-term survival. Plans have been made to audit and review the UKELD model regularly and to refine it by looking at the inclusion of other clinical parameters, such as diuretic-resistant ascites, encephalopathy, and the use of transjugular intrahepatic portosystemic shunts (TIPS). As patients with HCC have a high need for transplant but often have lower MELD and UKELD scores, additional weighting may need to be applied to these patients. Furthermore, the exact place of patients with non-fatal liver disease in the modelling system will have to be defined.

☐ CONCLUSIONS

Liver transplantation is a successful treatment for patients with acute liver failure, HCC, and chronic liver disease. The number of recipients awaiting liver transplantation and the length of wait are increasing, so an increasing number of patients are not receiving an organ because of death or deterioration. Greater attention has been focused on taking into account the balance between the individual need for a transplant, organ utility, and overall benefits of transplantation in the criteria for listing patients for transplantation and for allocating organs. Established criteria for transplantation for HCC and acute liver failure due to paracetamol-related and non-paracetamol-related aetiologies may be further refined in the future. Chronic liver disease provides the greatest challenge for selecting appropriate cases for liver transplantation. The UKELD score is a new score that has higher predictive value for prognosis than others and will increasingly be the method of selecting and then prioritising cases with chronic liver disease for transplantation.

REFERENCES

1 European Liver Transplant Registry website. Available at: www.eltr.org/publi/results.php3?id_rubrique=47 (last accessed 22 June 2007.)

2 UK Transplant. *Transplant activity in the UK: 2005–2006.* London: UK Transplant, 2006. Available at: www.uktransplant.org.uk/ukt/statistics/transplant_activity_report/archive_activity_reports/archive_reports.jsp (accessed 11 October 2007).

3 O'Grady JG, Alexander GJ, Hayllar KM, Williams R. Early indicators of prognosis in fulminant hepatic failure. *Gastroenterology* 1989;97:439–45.

4 Shakil AO, Kramer D, Mazariegos GV, Fung JJ, Rakela J. Acute liver failure: clinical features, outcome analysis, and applicability of prognostic criteria. *Liver Transpl* 2000;6;163–9.

5 Pawlik TM, Delman KA, Vauthey JN *et al.* Tumour size predicts vascular invasion and histologic grade: implications for selection of surgical treatment of hepatocellular carcinoma. *Liver Transpl* 2005;11:1086–92.

6 Mazzaferro V, Regalia E, Doci R *et al.* Liver transplantation for the treatment of small hepatocellular carcinomas in patients with cirrhosis. *N Engl J Med* 1996;334:693–9.

7 Yao FY, Ferrell L, Bass NM *et al.* Liver transplantation for hepatocellular carcinoma: expansion of the tumour size limits does not adversely impact survival. *Hepatology* 2001;33: 1394–403.

8 Malinchoc M, Kamath PS, Gordon FD *et al.* A model to predict poor survival in patients undergoing transjugular intrahepatic portosystemic shunts. *Hepatology* 2000;31:864–71.

9 Kamath PS, Wiesner RH, Malinchoc M *et al.* A model to predict survival in patients with end-stage liver disease. *Hepatology* 2001;33:464–70.

10 Heuman DM, Abou-Assi SG, Habib A *et al.* Persistent ascites and low serum sodium identify patients with cirrhosis and low MELD scores who are at high risk for early death. *Hepatology* 2004;40:802–10.

11 Ruf AE, Kremers WK, Chavez LL *et al.* Addition of serum sodium into the MELD score predicts waiting list mortality better than MELD alone. *Liver Transpl* 2005;11:336–43.

12 Ripoll C, Bañares R, Rincón D *et al.* Influence of hepatic venous pressure gradient on the prediction of survival of patients with cirrhosis in the MELD era. *Hepatology* 2005;42:793–801.

□ HEPATOLOGY/GASTROENTEROLOGY SELF-ASSESSMENT QUESTIONS

Crohn's disease and genes

1 Compelling evidence for a genetic contribution to Crohn's disease is provided by epidemiological observation. The following observations provide strong epidemiological evidence for a genetic effect:
(a) Increased concordance for Crohn's disease in affected monozygotic compared with dizygotic twins
(b) Shared extraintestinal manifestations in both Crohn's disease and ulcerative colitis
(c) The presence of multiply affected families with members with ulcerative colitis and Crohn's disease
(d) Similar prevalences for both ulcerative colitis and Crohn's disease
(e) Crohn's disease sub-phenotypes of disease location and behaviour breeding true in multiply affected families

2 Prior to genome-wide association scanning, researchers depended on detailed evaluation of candidate genes implicated by their function or patterns of expression or by fine-mapping within large regions identified in the course of genome-wide linkage scans. Disappointingly, these techniques have led to a large number of false positive associations. Fulfilment of the following criteria can be considered to prove a genetic association:
(a) Adequate case and control sample size
(b) Careful matching of case and control populations
(c) Appropriate statistical thresholds correcting for multiple testing
(d) Statistical methods accounting for known environmental factors
(e) Replication in an adequately powered independent panel

3 The association with IL23R is especially interesting given the recent identification of the importance of its cognate ligand IL23, which was recently shown to have actions distinct from IL-12, with which it shares a subunit. Compelling evidence that IL-23 but not IL-12 is required for intestinal inflammation has been best demonstrated in:
(a) Successful trials of anti-IL23 antibodies in humans
(b) Attenuated inflammation in IL23 –/– knockout but not IL12 –/– knockout mice
(c) Absence of association to IL-12 in candidate gene association studies
(d) The demonstration of IL-23 secretion by activated macrophages
(e) Increased inflammation in animal models given exogenous IL-23

4 A study shows association to a number of markers within IL23R, one of which (Arg381Gln) lies within a coding sequence that alters the resulting protein's amino acid sequence. Many of the other associated variants are either located in non-coding DNA sequences or cause no change to the resulting amino acid sequence and are therefore said to be synonymous. Regarding synonymous single nucleotide polymorphisms (SNPs):

(a) Synonymous SNPs in coding regions may alter protein folding due to different speeds of translation into polypeptide chains
(b) Synonymous SNPs may alter transcription factor binding leading to altered quantities of mRNA and protein
(c) Synonymous SNPs may be associated with a disease due to linkage disequilibrium with a causative marker elsewhere in the gene
(d) Synonymous SNPs may cause disruption of a DNA splice site leading to expression of mRNA (and hence proteins) of abnormal lengths
(e) Synonymous SNPs do not code for amino acid change and therefore cannot alter cellular proteins

Non-alcoholic fatty liver disease

1 Regarding the clinical syndrome of non-alcoholic fatty liver disease (NAFLD):
(a) Waist–hip ratio is the best predictor of NAFLD
(b) 41% of patients with NAFLD will develop histological progression of liver disease in 13 years
(c) Mortality from cardiovascular disease is increased in patients with simple fatty liver
(d) Abnormal transaminases are required for a diagnosis of NAFLD
(e) Women predominate in patients with NAFLD

2 In the liver in NAFLD:
(a) Levels of tumour necrosis factor are decreased
(b) Adiponectin is produced
(c) Gut endotoxin may trigger hepatic fibrosis
(d) Oxidative stress is induced by increased levels of free fatty acids

3 Regarding treatment for NAFLD:
(a) Bariatric surgery has proved benefit in obese patients with NAFLD
(b) Initial pharmacological treatment for patients with type 2 diabetes and NAFLD should be metformin
(c) Weight loss is the best proved treatment for NAFLD
(d) Reductions in dietary fat will directly reduce levels of fat in the liver

Autoimmune hepatitis

1 The following are used to diagnose autoimmune hepatitis or are the most appropriate scoring system:
(a) Clinical signs and symptoms
(b) Histology
(c) Autoantibody test results
(d) Liver histology
(e) International autoimmune hepatitis scoring criteria

2 The typical histological findings of autoimmune hepatitis are:
(a) Mallory's hyaline
(b) Biliary features
(c) Steatohepatitis
(d) Interface hepatitis and lymphoplasmacytic infiltrate
(e) All of the above

3 The following drugs or regimens would be used to achieve induction of remission in patients with autoimmune hepatitis:
(a) Prednisolone 1 mg/kg/day with the dose reduced gradually
(b) Cyclophosphamide induction
(c) Calcineurin inhibitors
(d) Mycophenolate mofetil
(e) Budesonide

4 The complications of long-term steroid treatment are:
(a) Hypertension
(b) Diabetes mellitus
(c) Cosmetic side effects
(d) Osteoporosis
(e) All of the above

5 The following is a second-line immunosuppressive treatment appropriate for young women with treatment failure:
(a) Mycophenolate mofetil
(b) Methotrexate
(c) Tacrolimus
(d) Cyclophosphamide
(e) Penicillamine

6 The following chemokine and adhesion molecule on endothelium in the gut and the following chemokine receptor and integrin on lymphocytes are involved in autoimmune hepatitis or primary sclerosing cholangitis that complicates inflammatory bowel disease:
(a) Chemokine (C-C motif) ligand (CCL) 25, mucosal addressin cell adhesion molecule-1 (MADCAM-1) and CCR9 α4b7
(b) CCL17 and CCR4
(c) CCL28 and CCR10

7 Recurrence of autoimmune hepatitis in the graft after liver transplantation is characterised by:
(a) Persistence of autoantibodies
(b) Increased levels of immunoglobulin G
(c) Typical histological features
(d) The need for long-term use of low doses of steroids after transplantation

Selecting cases for liver transplantation

1 Regarding acute liver failure:
- (a) It is characterised by development of encephalopathy within eight weeks of the onset of symptoms
- (b) In the United Kingdom (UK), it is usually caused by viral hepatitis
- (c) It is universally fatal if a liver transplant is not performed
- (d) The criteria for listing for super-urgent liver transplant differ according to the disease aetiology
- (e) The outcome for patients transplanted for acute liver failure is as good as for those transplanted for chronic liver disease

2 Regarding hepatocellular carcinoma (HCC):
- (a) Liver transplantation is considered when surgical resection is not technically possible
- (b) Liver transplantation for HCC rarely results in a cure but can significantly lengthen life expectancy
- (c) Outcome of liver transplantation is dependent on tumour size
- (d) A patient with five tumours all <1 cm in diameter would be considered suitable for transplantation in the UK
- (e) Patients transplanted for HCC have a better 90-day mortality than those transplanted for acute liver failure

3 Regarding chronic liver disease:
- (a) Patients with chronic liver disease account for most of the patients who undergo transplantation in the UK
- (b) The Child-Pugh score was designed to predict mortality in patients who are on the waiting list for a liver transplant
- (c) The Model for End-Stage Liver Disease (MELD) score most accurately predicts mortality on the liver transplant waiting list when the score is low
- (d) The addition of levels of sodium in serum has improved the predictive power of the MELD score
- (e) The UK End-stage Liver Disease (UKELD) score has higher predictive power than other scores for prognosis while a patient is awaiting a liver transplant

Croonian Lecture

Understanding migraine from bench to bedside

Peter J Goadsby

□ INTRODUCTION

Headache is a common malady and this perhaps partly explains the relative paucity of attention it receives. If common is synonymous with understood or simple, however, neither applies to migraine. It was 220 years before the Croonian lecture addressed the common problem of migraine…and that was from a gastroenterological viewpoint. When the subject was tackled in 1935, Spriggs noted, 'So many headaches were regarded as chronic, recurrent, familial, or due to the nervous make-up of the subject, that they seemed evils to be borne, with such alleviation as a few simple medicines could afford, rather than a field for active inquiry and treatment'.[1] The ensuing 70 years were not altogether happy for headache, but the subject has come of age in the recent past and has become firmly embedded as a brain disorder. Here I will explore current views of the pathophysiology of migraine that have led to the general view of migraine as a disorder of sensory modulation. Endogenous function of the nervous system is episodically deranged with dreadful consequences in terms of disability but wonderful opportunities for clinical scientists to explore mechanisms and provide new avenues for treatment. For more detailed accounts, books cover many aspects of the intriguing problems presented by the headache disorders.[2–4] Some parts of this chapter are modified from recent work.[5]

□ MIGRAINE – THE DISORDER

In essence, migraine is a familial episodic disorder whose key marker is headache with certain associated features.[6] These features give clues to its pathophysiology and ultimately will provide insights that lead to new treatments. The essential elements to be integrated are:

- □ the genetics of migraine
- □ the physiological basis for the aura
- □ the anatomy of head pain, particularly that of the trigeminovascular system
- □ the physiology and pharmacology of activation of the peripheral branches of the ophthalmic branch of the trigeminal nerve

- the physiology and pharmacology of the trigeminal nucleus, particularly its most caudal part – the trigeminocervical complex
- the brainstem and diencephalic modulatory systems that influence trigeminal pain transmission and other sensory modality processing.

Migraine is a form of sensory processing disturbance with wide ramifications within the central nervous system. Although this paper will use pain pathways as an example, it is useful to remember that migraine is not simply a problem of pain.

GENETICS OF MIGRAINE

One of the most important aspects of the pathophysiology of migraine is the inherited nature of the disorder. It is clear from clinical practice that many patients have first-degree relatives who also have migraines.[2,4] Transmission of migraine from parents to children was reported as early as the 17th century, and numerous published studies have reported a positive family history. One important form of migraine – familial hemiplegic migraine (FHM) – deserves some detailed consideration given that a number of causative genes have been identified.

Familial hemiplegic migraine

In about 50% of reported families, FHM has been assigned to chromosome 19p13.[7] Few clinical differences have been found between FHM families linked and not linked with chromosome 19, but the most striking exception is cerebellar ataxia, which occurs in about 50% of families linked to chromosome 19 but none of the unlinked families. Another less striking difference includes the fact that patients from families linked with chromosome 19 are more likely to have attacks that can be triggered by minor head trauma or that are associated with coma.

The biological basis for the linkage to chromosome 19 is mutations[8] that involve the $Ca_v2.1$ (P/Q) type voltage-gated calcium channel *CACNA1A* gene; now known as FHM-I, this mutation is responsible in about 50% of identified families. Mutations in the *ATP1A2* gene[9] have been identified to be responsible in about 20% of FHM families; this gene codes for a Na^+/K^+ ATPase and the mutation results in a smaller electrochemical gradient for sodium ions. One effect of this change is to reduce or inactivate astrocytic glutamate transporters, which leads to a build up of synaptic glutamate. Most recently, the gene for FHM-III has been identified as a mutation in the sodium channel gene *SCN1A*,[10] which would facilitate repetitive high-frequency discharges that, again, might increase synaptic levels of glutamate.

Taken together, the known mutations suggest that migraine, or at least the neurological manifestations currently called the aura, are caused by a channelopathy. The link between the channel disturbance and aura process has shown that human mutations expressed in a knockin mouse produce a reduced threshold for cortical spreading depression (CSD),[11] which has some profound implications for understanding of that process.

□ MIGRAINE AURA

Migraine aura is defined as a focal neurological disturbance manifest as visual, sensory, or motor symptoms.[6] It occurs in about 30% of patients and clearly is neurally driven. The case for the aura being the human equivalent of the CSD of Leao has been well made.[12] What remains in question is whether aura is indeed pain producing.

Several arguments about whether or not the aura process is capable of directly exciting nociceptive afferents have been advanced. The production of plasma protein extravasation by aura has been suggested to support this position,[13] although overwhelming evidence from clinical trials now seems to show that plasma protein extravasation is not pivotal in migraine.[14] Similarly, the effects of migraine preventives in aura have been suggested to provide evidence for a broader role of aura in migraine.[15] On the other hand, topiramate – a proved preventive agent in migraine – also acutely inhibits CSD in cats and rats,[16] although topiramate also inhibits trigeminal neurones activated by nociceptive intracranial afferents[17] but not by a mechanism local to the trigeminocervical complex. Lastly, several clinical questions are unanswered or pose a conundrum for the aura–pain hypothesis:

- □ Aura is clearly not present by clinical criteria in most patients – perhaps it is silent, but it must be very quiet to have avoided detection for four millennia.
- □ Aura can be seen during and even after pain but most importantly in the absence of pain.
- □ Aura can be aborted by ketamine without an effect on the headache.
- □ Aura is not specific to migraine but is also seen in patients with cluster headache, paroxysmal hemicrania, short-lasting unilateral neuralgiform headache with conjunctival injection and tearing (SUNCT), tension type headache, and hemicrania continua.

The issue seems far from resolved.

□ ANATOMY OF HEADACHE

The trigeminal innervation of pain-producing intracranial structures

The large cerebral vessels, pial vessels, large venous sinuses, and dura mater are surrounded by a plexus of largely unmyelinated fibres that arise from the ophthalmic division of the trigeminal ganglion and in the posterior fossa afferents arise from the upper cervical dorsal roots. Trigeminal fibres that innervate cerebral vessels arise from neurones in the trigeminal ganglion that contain substance P and calcitonin gene-related peptide (CGRP),[18] both of which can be released when the trigeminal ganglion is stimulated in humans or cats.[19] Stimulation of the cranial vessels, such as the superior sagittal sinus (SSS), certainly is painful in humans. Human dural nerves that innervate the cranial vessels largely consist of small diameter myelinated and unmyelinated fibres that almost certainly subserve a nociceptive function.

☐ PHYSIOLOGY OF HEADACHE

Peripheral connections

Plasma protein extravasation

Neurogenic plasma protein extravasation can be seen during electrical stimulation of the trigeminal ganglion in rats. Plasma protein extravasation can be blocked by ergot alkaloids, indomethacin, acetylsalicylic acid, and the serotonin-5HT$_{1B/1D}$ agonist sumatriptan.[20] Structural changes in the dura mater, including mast cell degranulation and changes in postcapillary venules such as platelet aggregation, are well described with this stimulus. Although such changes, particularly the initiation of a sterile inflammatory response, are generally accepted to cause pain, it is not clear whether this is sufficient in itself or requires other stimulators or promoters or whether such circumstances particularly occur in migraine. Preclinical studies suggest that CSD may be a sufficient stimulus to activate trigeminal neurones,[13] although this area has been controversial.

Although plasma protein extravasation in the retina (which is blocked by sumatriptan) can be seen after stimulation of the trigeminal ganglion in experimental animals, no changes were seen through retinal angiography during acute attacks of migraine or cluster headache.[21] A limitation of this study was the probable sampling of both retinal and choroidal elements in rats given that choroidal vessels have fenestrated capillaries. Clearly, however, blockade of neurogenic plasma protein extravasation is not completely predictive of antimigraine efficacy in humans, as evidenced by the failure of substance P, neurokinin-1 antagonists, specific plasma protein extravasation blockers, and CP122,288 and 4991w93 (an endothelin antagonist and a neurosteroid) in clinical trials. A more detailed account of these failed developments is available elsewhere.[14]

Sensitisation

Although whether a significant sterile inflammatory response occurs in the dura mater during migraine is unclear, it is obvious that some form of sensitisation takes place during migraine, as pain from non-noxious stimuli (allodynia) is common and has been recognised for many years. About two thirds of patients complain of allodynia. A particularly interesting aspect is that allodynia has been shown in the upper limbs ipsilateral and contralateral to the pain. This finding is consistent with at least third-order neuronal sensitisation, such as sensitisation of thalamic neurones, and firmly places the pathophysiology within the central nervous system. Sensitisation in migraine may be peripheral, with local release of inflammatory markers, which would certainly activate trigeminal nociceptors. More likely is a form of central sensitisation in migraine, which may be classic central sensitisation[22] or a form of disinhibitory sensitisation with dysfunction of descending modulatory pathways.[23,24] Just as dihydroergotamine (DHE) can block trigeminovascular nociceptive transmission,[25] probably at least by a local effect in the trigeminocervical complex,[26] it can block central sensitisation associated with dural stimulation by an inflammatory soup.

Neuropeptide studies

Electrical stimulation of the trigeminal ganglion in humans and cats leads to increases in extracerebral blood flow and local release of CGRP and substance P.[19] In cats, stimulation of the trigeminal ganglion also increases cerebral blood flow by a pathway that traverses the greater superficial petrosal branch of the facial nerve, again releasing a powerful vasodilator peptide (vasoactive intestinal polypeptide (VIP)) (Table 1). Interestingly, VIPergic innervation of the cerebral vessels is predominantly anterior rather than posterior, and this may contribute to this region's vulnerability to spreading depression and explain why aura is so very often seen to start posteriorly. Stimulation of the more specifically vascular pain producing SSS increases cerebral blood flow and levels of CGRP in the jugular vein. Evidence from studies in humans that levels of CGRP are increased in the headache phase of migraine, cluster headache, and chronic paroxysmal hemicrania[27] supports the view that the trigeminovascular system may be activated in a protective role in these conditions, although recent work suggests that these changes are not seen in apparently less affected patients. Moreover, migraine triggered by nitric oxide donors, which effectively represents typical migraine, also results in increased levels of CGRP that can be blocked by sumatriptan – just as in spontaneous migraine. Interestingly, compounds that have not shown activity in migraine, notably CP122,288 (the conformationally restricted analogue of sumatriptan) and 4991w93 (the conformationally restricted analogue of zolmitriptan) both were ineffective inhibitors of release of CGRP after stimulation of the SSS in cats. The recent development of highly specific, non-peptide CGRP antagonists without vascular effects and the announcement of proof-of-concept for a CGRP antagonist in acute migraine[28] firmly establish this as a novel and important new emerging principle for

Table 1 Neuroanatomical processing of vascular head pain.

	Structure	Comments
Target innervation		
Cranial vessels	• Ophthalmic branch of trigeminal nerve	
Dura mater		
First order	• Trigeminal ganglion	• Middle cranial fossa
Second order	• Trigeminal nucleus *(quintothalamic tract)*	• Trigeminal neurone caudalis and C_1/C_2 dorsal horns
Third order	• Thalamus	• Ventrobasal complex • Medial neurone of posterior group • Intralaminar complex
Modulatory	• Midbrain • Hypothalamus	• Periaqueductal grey matter • ?
Final	• Cortex	• Insulae • Frontal cortex • Anterior cingulate cortex • Basal ganglia

acute migraine. At the same time, the lack of any effect of CGRP blockers on plasma protein extravasation explains, in part, why that model has proved inadequate at translating into human therapeutic approaches.

Central connections

The trigeminocervical complex

Fos immunohistochemistry looks at activated cells by plotting the expression of Fos protein. Expression of Fos is noted in the trigeminal nucleus caudalis after meningeal irritation with blood, and Fos-like immunoreactivity is seen in the trigeminal nucleus caudalis and dorsal horn at the C_1 and C_2 levels in cats and monkeys after stimulation of the SSS. These latter findings are in accordance with similar data obtained from measurements of 2-deoxyglucose metabolism when the SSS was stimulated. Similarly, stimulation of a branch of C_2, the greater occipital nerve, increases metabolic activity in the same regions – that is, the trigeminal nucleus caudalis and $C_{1/2}$ dorsal horn. In experimental animals, recordings can be taken directly from the trigeminal neurones, with supratentorial trigeminal input and input from the greater occipital nerve – a branch of the C_2 dorsal root.[29] Stimulation of the greater occipital nerve for five minutes results in substantial increases in responses to supratentorial dural stimulation that can last for longer than one hour.[29] Conversely, stimulation of the middle meningeal artery's dura mater with the C fibre-irritant mustard oil sensitises responses to occipital muscle stimulation.[30] Taken together, these data suggest convergence of cervical and ophthalmic inputs at the level of the second-order neurone. Moreover, stimulation of a lateralised structure, the middle meningeal artery, produces expression of Fos bilaterally in the brains of cats and monkeys. This group of neurones form the superficial laminae of trigeminal nucleus caudalis, and $C_{1/2}$ dorsal horns should be regarded functionally as the trigeminocervical complex.

These data show that trigeminovascular nociceptive information comes by way of the most caudal cells. This concept provides an anatomical explanation for the referral of pain to the back of the head in migraine. Moreover, experimental pharmacological evidence suggests that some abortive antimigraine drugs – such as ergot derivatives, acetylsalicylic acid, sumatriptan, eletriptan, naratriptan, rizatriptan, and zolmitriptan – can have actions at these second-order neurones that reduce cell activity and suggest a further possible site for therapeutic intervention in migraine. This action can be dissected out to involve each of the 5-HT_{1B}, 5-HT_{1D}, and 5-HT_{1F} receptor subtypes[31] and is consistent with the localisation of these receptors on peptidergic nociceptors. Interestingly, triptans also influence the CGRP promoter and regulate CGRP secretion from neurones in culture – as does nitric oxide.[32] Furthermore, the fact that some part of this action is postsynaptic, with either 5-HT_{1B} or 5-HT_{1D} receptors located non-presynatically,[33] offers the prospect of highly anatomically localised treatment options. Data that suggest externalisation of 5-HT_{1D} receptors with stimulation[34] may provide an interesting way to understand why sumatriptan given by injection during migraine aura did not prevent the development of head pain some 20 minutes later.

Higher order processing

After transmission in the caudal brain stem and high cervical spinal cord, information is relayed rostrally.

Thalamus

Processing of vascular nociceptive signals in the thalamus occurs in the ventroposteromedial (VPM) thalamus, medial nucleus of the posterior complex, and intralaminar thalamus. Zagami[35] used application of capsaicin to the SSS to show that trigeminal projections with a high degree of nociceptive input are processed in neurones, particularly in the ventroposteromedial thalamus and in its ventral periphery. These neurones in the VPM can be modulated by activation of $GABA_A$ inhibitory receptors and, perhaps of more direct clinical relevance, by propranolol though a β_1 adrenoceptor mechanism.[36] Remarkably, triptans can also inhibit VPM neurones locally through $5\text{-}HT_{1B/1D}$ mechanisms, as demonstrated by microiontophoretic application,[37] which suggests a hitherto unconsidered locus of action for triptans in acute migraine. Human imaging studies have confirmed activation of thalamus contralateral to pain in acute migraine (Fig 1),[38,39] cluster headache,[40] and SUNCT.[41,42]

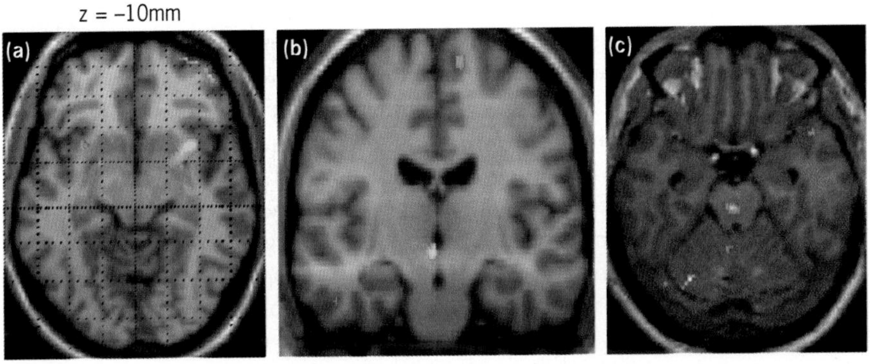

Fig 1 Findings from positron emission tomography in **(a)** experimental head pain, **(b)** cluster headache, and **(c)** migraine. Activation of rostral brainstem structures in migraine and posterior hypothalamic grey matter in cluster headaches seem relatively specific for the syndromes, as neither are seen in experimental ophthalmic (first) division head pain. The findings support the view that primary neurovascular headaches, migraine, and cluster headache fundamentally are disorders of the nervous system. (a) Reproduced from May with permission of Elsevier[61]; (b) Reproduced from May with permission of Elsevier[60]; (c) Reproduced from Bahra with permission of Elsevier.[38]

Activation of modulatory regions

Stimulation of nociceptive afferents by stimulation of the SSS in cats activates neurones in the ventrolateral periaqueductal grey matter (PAG).[43] Activation of PAG in turn feeds back to the trigeminocervical complex with an inhibitory influence,[44,45] and PAG is clearly included in the area of activation seen in studies with positron emission tomography (PET) in people with migraine.[46] This typical negative feedback system will be further considered below as a possible mechanism for the symptomatic manifestations of migraine.

Another potentially modulatory region activated by stimulation of nociceptive trigeminovascular input is the posterior hypothalamic grey.[47] This area is crucially involved in several primary headaches, notably cluster headache, SUNCT,[41] paroxysmal hemicrania,[48] and hemicrania continua.[49] Moreover, the clinical features of the premonitory phase, and other features of the disorder, suggest the involvement of dopamine neurones. Recently, dopamine was shown to inhibit trigeminocervical transmission, probably through predominantly D_2 receptor-mediated mechanisms.[50] Orexin A and B are hypothalamic neuropeptides that bind to two G-protein coupled receptors termed OX_1 and OX_2. Orexins are involved in feeding, the sleep–wake cycle, and regulation of hormones and have been linked with modulation of nociceptive processing. Orexin A inhibits neurogenic dural vasodilation[51] and trigeminocervical neuronal activation from stimulation of trigeminovascular nociceptive afferents.[52] Orexinergic neurones in the posterior hypothalamus can be both pronociceptive and antinociceptive,[24] which offers a further possible region whose dysfunction might involve promotion of the perception of head pain.

□ CENTRAL MODULATION OF TRIGEMINAL PAIN

Brain imaging in humans

Functional brain imaging with positron emission tomography has demonstrated activation of the dorsal midbrain, including the periaqueductal grey (PAG), and the dorsal pons, near the locus coeruleus, in studies during migraine without aura.[46] Dorsolateral pontine activation is seen with PET in spontaneous episodic[39] and chronic migraine[53] and with attacks triggered by glyceryl trinitrate.[38,54] These areas are active immediately after successful treatment of the headache but are not active interictally. The activation corresponds with the brain region that Raskin[55] initially reported and Veloso confirmed causes migraine-like headache when stimulated in patients with electrodes implanted for pain control. Similarly, Welch and colleagues[56] noted excess iron in the PAG of patients with episodic and chronic migraine, and chronic migraine can develop after a bleed into a cavernoma in the region of the PAG or with a lesion of the pons.

Animal experimental studies of sensory modulation

Experiments in animals have shown that stimulation of the nucleus locus coeruleus – the main central noradrenergic nucleus – reduces cerebral blood flow in a frequency dependent manner[57] through a mechanism linked to the α_2 adrenoceptor. This reduction is maximal in the occipital cortex. Although a 25% overall reduction in cerebral blood flow is seen, extracerebral vasodilatation occurs in parallel.[57] The locus coeruleus receives important inputs from orexinergic neurones in the hypothalamus and can affect arousal by altering locus coeruleus neuronal activity. Indeed, neurones of the locus coeruleus are well recognised to modulate arousal states in behaving primates. In addition, the main serotonin-containing nucleus in the brainstem – the midbrain dorsal raphe nucleus – can increase cerebral blood flow when activated. Furthermore, stimulation of PAG will inhibit SSS-evoked trigeminal neuronal activity in cats, but blockade of P/Q type voltage-gated Ca^{2+} channels in the PAG facilitates trigeminovascular nociceptive processing.[23]

Electrophysiology of migraine in humans

Studies of evoked potentials and event-related potentials provide some link between animal studies and human functional imaging. Authors have shown changes in neurophysiological measures of brain activation, but much discussion surrounds interpretation of such changes.[58] Perhaps the most reliable theme is that the migrainous brain does not habituate to signals in a normal way. Similarly, contingent negative variation (CNV), an event-related potential, is abnormal in people with migraine compared with controls.[59] Changes in CNV predict attacks and preventive treatment alter (normalise) such changes.

☐ WHAT IS MIGRAINE?

Migraine is an inherited, episodic disorder involving sensory sensitivity. Patients complain of pain in the head that is throbbing, but there is no reliable relation between vessel diameter and the pain – or its treatment. People with migraine complain of discomfort from normal lights and the unpleasantness of routine sounds. Some mention that otherwise pleasant odours become unpleasant. Normal movement of the head causes pain, and many patients mention a sense of unsteadiness – as if they have just stepped off a boat. How can the perception of so much be so wrong?

Migraine aura cannot be the trigger, as no evidence suggests that it occurs in more than 30% of patients with migraine, aura can be experienced without pain at all, and aura is seen in the other primary headaches. Patients with migraine receive not a photon of extra light than other people, so for that symptom – and for phonophobia and osmophobia – the basis of the problem must be abnormal central processing of a normal signal. Perhaps electrophysiological changes in the brain have been mislabelled as hyperexcitability whereas dyshabituation might be a simpler explanation. If migraine was basically a sensory attentional problem with changes in cortical synchronisation (hypersynchronisation), all of its manifestations could be accounted for in a single overarching pathophysiological hypothesis of a disturbance of sub-cortical sensory modulation systems. Although the trigeminovascular system and its cranial autonomic reflex connections (the trigeminal–autonomic reflex) seems likely to act as a feed forward system to facilitate the acute attack, the fundamental problem in migraine is in the brain. This Croonian lecture should at least signal the development of thought from a gastroenterological perspective to a neurobiological view of migraine. It would be interesting to hear the next lecture on migraine in 70 years to see where the field lies in that period.

REFERENCES

1 Spriggs E. A clinical study of headaches. *Lancet* 1935;ii:63–7.
2 Lance JW, Goadsby PJ. *Mechanism and management of headache.* New York: Elsevier, 2005.
3 Olesen J, Tfelt-Hansen P, Ramadan N, Goadsby PJ, Welch KMA. *The headaches.* Philadelphia: Lippincott, Williams & Wilkins, 2005.

4 Silberstein SD, Lipton RB, Goadsby PJ. *Headache in clinical practice.* London: Martin Dunitz, 2002.

5 Goadsby PJ. Pathophysiology of migraine. In: Lipton RB, Bigal M, eds. *Migraine and other headache disorders.* New York: Marcel Dekker, Taylor & Francis Books, 2006:81–98.

6 Headache Classification Committee of the International Headache Society. The international classification of headache disorders: second edition. *Cephalalgia* 2004;24(Suppl 1):9–160.

7 Ophoff RA, van Eijk R, Sandkuijl LA *et al.* Genetic heterogeneity of familial hemiplegic migraine. *Genomics* 1994;22:21–6.

8 Ophoff RA, Terwindt GM, Vergouwe MN *et al.* Familial hemiplegic migraine and episodic ataxia type-2 are caused by mutations in the Ca2+ channel gene CACNL1A4. *Cell* 1996;87: 543–52.

9 De Fusco M, Marconi R, Silvestri L *et al.* Haploinsufficiency of ATP1A2 encoding the Na+/K+ pump alpha2 subunit associated with familial hemiplegic migraine type 2. *Nat Genet* 2003;33:192–6.

10 Dichgans M, Freilinger T, Eckstein G *et al.* Mutation in the neuronal voltage-gated sodium channel SCN1A in familial hemiplegic migraine. *Lancet* 2005;366:371–7.

11 van den Maagdenberg AM, Pietrobon D, Pizzorusso T *et al.* A Cacnala knockin migraine mouse model with increased susceptibility to cortical spreading depression. *Neuron* 2004;41: 701–10.

12 Lauritzen M. Pathophysiology of the migraine aura. The spreading depression theory. *Brain* 1994;117:199–210.

13 Bolay H, Reuter U, Dunn AK *et al.* Intrinsic brain activity triggers trigeminal meningeal afferents in a migraine model. *Nat Med* 2002;8:136–42.

14 Peroutka SJ. Neurogenic inflammation and migraine: implications for the therapeutics. *Mol Interv* 2005;5:304–11.

15 Ayata C, Jin H, Kudo C, Dalkara T, Moskowitz MA. Suppression of cortical spreading depression in migraine prophylaxis. *Ann Neurol* 2006;59:652–61.

16 Akerman S, Goadsby PJ. Topiramate inhibits cortical spreading depression in rat and cat: a possible contribution to its preventive effect in migraine. *Cephalalgia* 2004;24:783–4.

17 Storer RJ, Goadsby PJ. Topiramate inhibits trigeminovascular neurons in the cat. *Cephalalgia* 2004;24:1049–56.

18 Uddman R, Edvinsson L, Ekman R, Kingman T, McCulloch J. Innervation of the feline cerebral vasculature by nerve fibers containing calcitonin gene-related peptide: trigeminal origin and co-existence with substance P. *Neurosci Lett* 1985;62:131–6.

19 Goadsby PJ, Edvinsson L, Ekman R. Release of vasoactive peptides in the extracerebral circulation of man and the cat during activation of the trigeminovascular system. *Ann Neurol* 1988;23:193–6.

20 Moskowitz MA, Cutrer FM. Sumatriptan: a receptor-targeted treatment for migraine. *Annu Rev Med* 1993;44:145–54.

21 May A, Shepheard S, Knorr M *et al.* Retinal plasma extravasation in animals but not in humans: implications for the pathophysiology of migraine. *Brain* 1998;121:1231–7.

22 Burstein R, Yamamura H, Malick A, Strassman AM. Chemical stimulation of the intracranial dura induces enhanced responses to facial stimulation in brain stem trigeminal neurons. *J Neurophysiol* 1998;79:964–82.

23 Knight YE, Bartsch T, Kaube H, Goadsby PJ. P/Q-type calcium-channel blockade in the periaqueductal gray facilitates trigeminal nociception: a functional genetic link for migraine? *J Neurosci* 2002;22 (RC213):1–6.

24 Bartsch T, Levy MJ, Knight YE, Goadsby PJ. Differential modulation of nociceptive dural input to [hypocretin] orexin A and B receptor activation in the posterior hypothalamic area. *Pain* 2004;109:367–78.

25 Hoskin KL, Kaube H, Goadsby PJ. Central activation of the trigeminovascular pathway in the cat is inhibited by dihydroergotamine. A c-Fos and electrophysiology study. *Brain* 1996; 119:249–56.

26 Storer RJ, Goadsby PJ. Microiontophoretic application of serotonin (5HT)1B/1D agonists inhibits trigeminal cell firing in the cat. *Brain* 1997;120:2171–7.

27 Goadsby PJ. Calcitonin gene-related peptide antagonists as treatments of migraine and other primary headaches. *Drugs* 2005;65:2557–67.

28 Olesen J, Diener HC, Husstedt IW *et al.* Calcitonin gene-related peptide receptor antagonist BIBN 4096 BS for the acute treatment of migraine. *N Engl J Med* 2004;350:1104–10.

29 Bartsch T, Goadsby PJ. Stimulation of the greater occipital nerve induces increased central excitability of dural afferent input. *Brain* 2002;125:1496–509.

30 Bartsch T, Goadsby PJ. Increased responses in trigeminocervical nociceptive neurons to cervical input after stimulation of the dura mater. *Brain* 2003;126:1801–13.

31 Goadsby PJ, Classey JD. Evidence for serotonin (5-HT)1B, 5-HT1D and 5-HT1F receptor inhibitory effects on trigeminal neurons with craniovascular input. *Neuroscience* 2003;122: 491–8.

32 Bellamy J, Bowen EJ, Russo AF, Durham PL. Nitric oxide regulation of calcitonin gene-related peptide gene expression in rat trigeminal ganglia neurons. *Eur J Neurosci* 2006;23:2057–66.

33 Goadsby PJ, Akerman S, Storer RJ. Evidence for postjunctional serotonin (5-HT1) receptors in the trigeminocervical complex. *Ann Neurol* 2001;50:804–7.

34 Ahn AH, Basbaum AI. Tissue injury regulates serotonin 1D receptor expression: implications for the control of migraine and inflammatory pain. *J Neurosci* 2006;26:8332–8.

35 Zagami AS, Lambert GA. Craniovascular application of capsaicin activates nociceptive thalamic neurons in the cat. *Neurosci Lett* 1991;121:187–90.

36 Shields KG, Goadsby PJ. Propranolol modulates trigeminovascular responses in thalamic ventroposteromedial nucleus: a role in migraine? *Brain* 2005;128:86–97.

37 Shields KG, Goadsby PJ. Serotonin receptors modulate trigeminovascular responses in ventroposteromedial nucleus of thalamus: a migraine target? *Neurobiol Dis* 2006;23:491–501.

38 Bahra A, Matharu MS, Buchel C, Frackowiak RS, Goadsby PJ. Brainstem activation specific to migraine headache. *Lancet* 2001;357:1016–7.

39 Afridi SK, Giffin NJ, Kaube H *et al.* A positron emission tomographic study in spontaneous migraine. *Arch Neurol* 2005;62:1270–5.

40 May A, Bahra A, Buchel C, Frackowiak RS, Goadsby PJ. Hypothalamic activation in cluster headache attacks. *Lancet* 1998; 352: 275–8.

41 May A, Bahra A, Büchel C, Turner R, Goadsby PJ. Functional magnetic resonance imaging in spontaneous attacks of SUNCT: short-lasting neuralgiform headache with conjunctival injection and tearing. *Ann Neurol* 1999;46:791–4.

42 Cohen AS. Functional MRI in SUNCT (Short-lasting Unilateral Neuralgiform headache attacks with Conjunctival injection and Tearing) and SUNA (Short-lasting Unilateral Neuralgiform headache attacks with cranial Autonomic symptoms) shows differential hypothalamic activation with increasing pain. *Cephalalgia* 2006;26:1402–3 (Poster 20).

43 Hoskin KL, Bulmer DC, Lasalandra M, Jonkman A, Goadsby PJ. Fos expression in the midbrain periaqueductal grey after trigeminovascular stimulation. *J Anat* 2001;197:29–35.

44 Knight YE, Goadsby PJ. The periaqueductal grey matter modulates trigeminovascular input: a role in migraine? *Neuroscience* 2001;106:793–800.

45 Knight YE, Bartsch T, Goadsby PJ. Trigeminal antinociception induced by bicuculline in the periaqueductal grey (PAG) is not affected by PAG P/Q-type calcium channel blockade in rat. *Neurosci Lett* 2003;336:113–6.

46 Weiller C, May A, Limmroth V *et al.* Brain stem activation in spontaneous human migraine attacks. *Nat Med* 1995;1:658–60.

47 Benjamin L, Levy MJ, Lasalandra MP *et al.* Hypothalamic activation after stimulation of the superior sagittal sinus in the cat: a Fos study. *Neurobiol Dis* 2004;16:500–5.

48 Matharu MS, Cohen AS, Frackowiak RSJ, Goadsby PJ. Posterior hypothalamic activation in paroxysmal hemicrania. *Ann Neurology* 2006;59:535–45.

49 Matharu MS, Cohen AS, McGonigle DJ *et al.* Posterior hypothalamic and brainstem activation in hemicrania continua. *Headache* 2004;44:747–61.

50 Bergerot A, Storer RJ, Goadsby PJ. Dopamine inhibits trigeminovascular transmission in the rat. *Ann Neurol* 2007;61:251–62.

51 Holland PR, Akerman S, Goadsby PJ. Orexin 1 receptor activation attenuates neurogenic dural vasodilation in an animal model of trigeminovascular nociception. *J Pharmacol Exp Ther* 2005;315:1380–5.

52 Holland PR, Akerman S, Goadsby PJ. Modulation of nociceptive dural input to the trigeminal nucleus caudalis via activation of the orexin 1 receptor in the rat. *Eur J Neurosci* 2006;24:2825–33.

53 Matharu MS, Bartsch T, Ward N *et al.* Central neuromodulation in chronic migraine patients with suboccipital stimulators: a PET study. *Brain* 2004;127:220–30.

54 Afridi S, Matharu MS, Lee L *et al.* A PET study exploring the laterality of brainstem activation in migraine using glyceryl trinitrate. *Brain* 2005;128:932–9.

55 Raskin NH, Hosobuchi Y, Lamb S. Headache may arise from perturbation of brain. *Headache* 1987;27:416–20.

56 Welch KM, Nagesh V, Aurora SK, Gelman N. Periaqueductal grey matter dysfunction in migraine: cause or the burden of illness? *Headache* 2001;41:629–37.

57 Goadsby PJ, Lambert GA, Lance JW. Differential effects on the internal and external carotid circulation of the monkey evoked by locus coeruleus stimulation. *Brain Res* 1982;249:247–54.

58 Schoenen J, Ambrosini A, Sándor PS, Maertens de Noordhout A. Evoked potentials and transcranial magnetic stimulation in migraine: published data and viewpoint on their pathophysiologic significance. *Clin Neurophysiol* 2003;114:955–72.

59 Schoenen J, Timsit-Berthier M. Contingent negative variation: methods and potential interest in headache. *Cephalalgia* 1993;13:28–32.

60 May A, Bahra A, Büchel C, Frackowiak RS, Goadsby PJ. Hypothalamic activation in cluster headache attacks. *Lancet* 1998;352:275–8.

61 May A, Kaube H, Büchel C *et al.* Experimental cranial pain elicited by capsaicin: a PET study. *Pain* 1998;74:61–6.

Linacre Lecture

Japanese encephalitis – an exotic Asian virus moving closer to home

Tom Solomon

Japanese encephalitis (JE) is one of the most important causes of viral encephalitis globally, with an estimated 30,000–50,000 cases and 10,000–15,000 deaths per year.[1] In addition, about half the survivors have severe neuropsychiatric sequelae. Although confined to Asia, the disease is spreading. In this paper, which is based on the Linacre Lecture of 2007, I review the Liverpool Brain Infections Group's clinical and pathogenesis research on Japanese encephalitis (www.liv.ac.uk/braininfections), discuss what we know about the virus's geographical spread, and consider how related viruses are moving closer to the United Kingdom (UK). The Linacre Lecture is given in memory of Thomas Linacre, who founded the Royal College of Physicians in 1518, and towards the end of the paper I reflect on what Linacre might have made of the subject were he alive today.

☐ JAPANESE ENCEPHALITIS VIRUS IS AN EMERGING FLAVIVIRUS

Japanese encephalitis virus (JEV) is a single-stranded, positive-sense, RNA virus of the flavivirus genus (family *Flaviviridae*). The genus is named after the yellow fever virus (in Latin, yellow is *flavus*), which was the first virus to be identified in this group, and includes West Nile virus (WNV), dengue virus, and tick-borne encephalitis virus (TBEV). Most flaviviruses are arthropod-borne viruses (arboviruses), being transmitted between vertebrate hosts by mosquitoes or ticks. Many are considered to be emerging, or re-emerging, viruses. A range of factors are thought to contribute to viral emergence, depending on the virus. These include increasing and more rapid travel of humans, increasing human populations and overcrowding, changing agricultural practices, increased transport of farming and agricultural products, and global warming. In addition, we have better diagnostic abilities, greater awareness, and a better ability to communicate our findings, particularly through the internet.

☐ CLINICAL FEATURES OF JAPANESE ENCEPHALITIS REFLECT THE ANATOMICAL LOCALISATION OF DAMAGE

Outbreaks of encephalitis first were described in Japan from the 1870s onwards; Fig 1, which shows the current geographical distribution and the dates of the first big outbreaks or virus isolations, highlights the relentless spread of the disease across Asia. Recent years have seen very large outbreaks in India, and the virus has reached Australia for the first time.

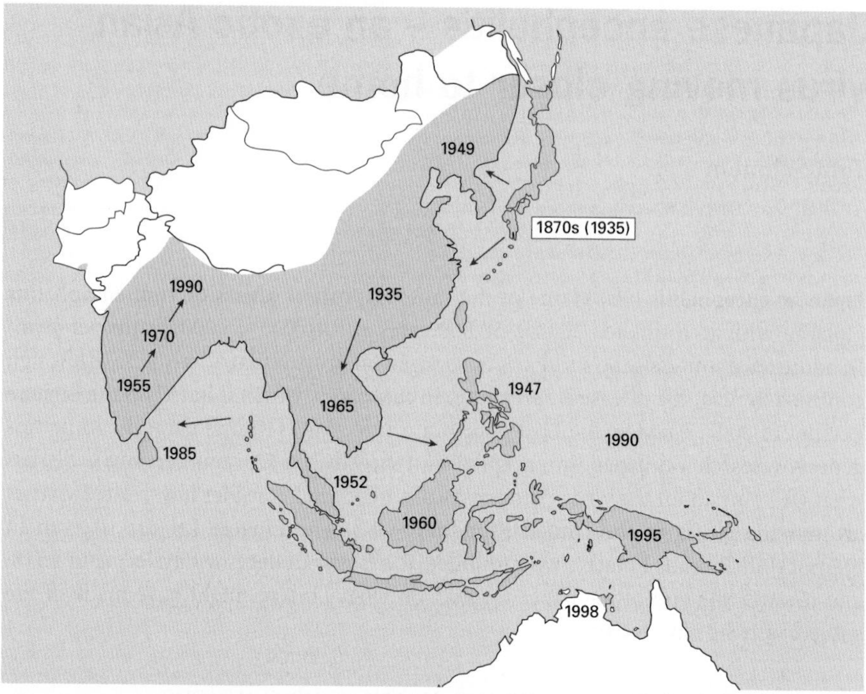

Fig 1 Current distribution of Japanese encephalitis. Epidemics of encephalitis were first described in Japan in the 1870s, and the approximate dates of the first major outbreaks, or first virus isolations, indicate an apparent spread of the disease across Asia from Japan. Newer evidence, however, suggests the virus originated in and spread from the Indonesia–Malaysia region (see Fig 5). Adapted from Solomon *et al* with permission of Springer-Verlag Wien.[2]

Japanese encephalitis virus is transmitted between birds, especially herons, egrets, and other migrating birds, by mosquitoes, particularly *Culex* mosquitoes (Fig 2). Pigs also are infected and become amplifying hosts, increasing the amount of circulating virus. Humans are 'dead-end' hosts, infected coincidentally when bitten by an infected mosquito; however, they do not have prolonged or high viraemia and thus do not usually transmit the virus further.

Because JEV-infected mosquitoes are so ubiquitous across Asia, almost all people who live in rural parts of Asia become infected during childhood, as shown by seroprevalence studies (Fig 3). Most infections are asymptomatic, but a small proportion of infections (one in 300 to one in 1,000) result in clinical features. These may range from a non-specific flu-like illness to a severe meningoencephalitis. Work in the mid-1990s showed that JEV also can present with a poliomyelitis-like acute flaccid paralytic illness.[4] In this series, 50% of patients with acute flaccis paralysis were infected with JEV. A similar presentation has been seen elsewhere in Asia, including India and Japan. Electrophysiological, imaging, and pathological studies in patients infected with JEV and with acute flaccid paralysis indicate that the lower motor neurone cells in the anterior horn of the spinal cord are infected; these are the same motor neurones that are affected by poliomyelitis, which explains the similarity of the clinical syndrome.

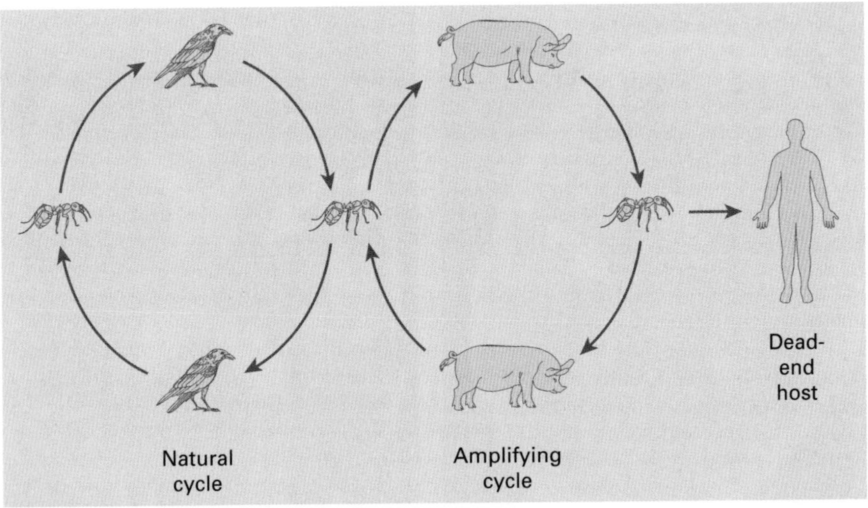

Fig 2 The transmission cycle of Japanese encephalitis virus. The virus is transmitted naturally between aquatic birds by *Culex* mosquitoes. During the rainy season, when there is an increase in the number of mosquitoes, the virus 'overflows' into pigs and other peridomestic animals and then into humans, from whom it is not transmitted further. Reproduced from Solomon with permission of Wiley-Blackwell.[3]

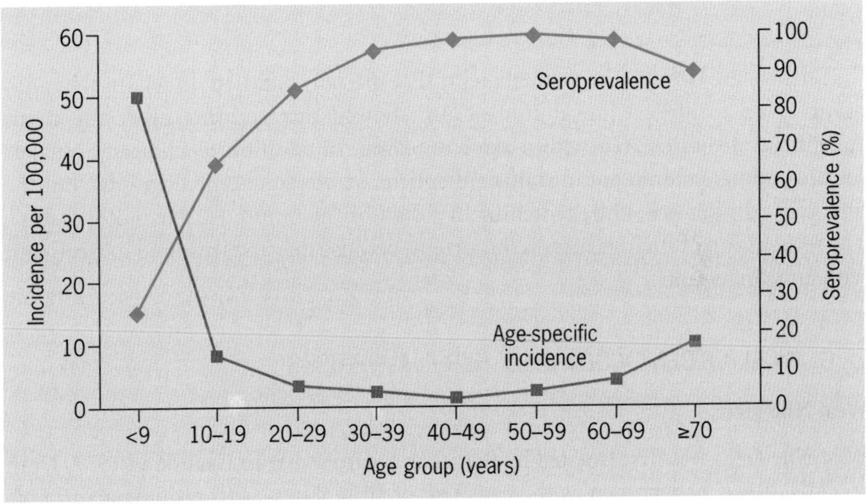

Fig 3 The specific incidence (red) and seroprevalence (blue) of Japanese encephalitis virus in endemic areas of Asia. Adapted from Solomon with permission of the Massachusetts Medical Society.[1]

Not infrequently, patients with JE have tremors, cogwheel rigidity, and mask-like facies – acutely or during convalescence – that are reminiscent of the features of Parkinson's disease. Other movement disorders include orofacial dyskinesias and choreoathetosis. Imaging and pathological studies show the thalamus and other basal ganglia often are targeted in JE, which provides an anatomical correlate for these clinical features (Fig 4). Why the virus targets the basal ganglia and anterior horn cells of the spinal cord is a key unanswered question.

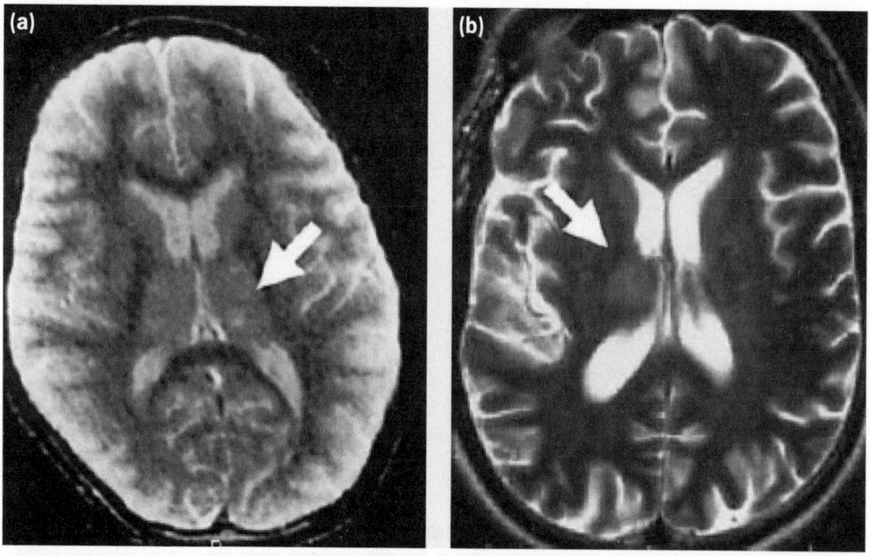

Fig 4 T2-weighted magnetic resonance images showing high signal intensity and swelling in the thalamus (arrows) of patients with **(a)** Japanese encephalitis and **(b)** West Nile encephalitis. (a) Adapted from Solomon with permission of Massachusetts Medical Society.[1] (b) Reproduced from Solomon *et al* with permission of Massachusetts Medical Society.[1]

Seizures are common in patients with JE, especially children, in whom they may occur in up to 90%. Clinical studies also showed that seizures, especially status epilepticus, are associated with a poor outcome. In addition to clinically obvious seizures, some children are in status epilepticus on electroencephalography, but the only clinical signs are subtle twitching of a digit or the mouth (subtle motor status). The recognition of such seizures is important, because they may respond to treatment with anticonvulsants.

□ CLINICAL EPIDEMIOLOGY OF OTHER FLAVIVIRUSES

West Nile virus

West Nile virus was first isolated by British arbovirologists in Uganda in 1937. Until recently, it was best known as the cause of a febrile illness with arthralgia and rash that only occasionally caused disease of the central nervous system. In recent years, however, it has spread to new areas, including southern Europe and the United States (US), where it has caused large epidemics of neurological disease.[5] In these epidemics, elderly people and those with chronic illnesses are more likely to develop neurological disease, which perhaps reflects impaired immunity or defects of the blood–brain barrier – for example, due to cerebrovascular disease.[6] As with JEV, poliomyelitis-like flaccid paralysis and movement disorders sometimes are seen. West Nile virus is also found in southern France, and serological evidence from birds suggests it may have reached the UK, although no virus has ever been isolated here and no endemic cases have been seen.[7]

Tick-borne encephalitis virus

Tick-borne encephalitis virus is found across northern Europe, especially in Scandinavian countries, the former East Germany, Austria, and countries of the former Union of Soviet Socialist Republics (USSR). Different subtypes of the virus exist. In addition to infection after bites from ticks, humans can become infected by drinking infected goat's milk. Tick-borne encephalitis causes a characteristic flaccid paralysis of the upper limbs and also a chronic progressive disease with epilepsia partialis continua (known as Kozhevnikov's epilepsy).[8] Louping ill virus is related to TBEV and is the only flavivirus found naturally in the British Isles, being found in the Scottish Highlands. It is carried by ticks and causes encephalitis in sheep and, very occasionally, in humans.

Dengue virus

Dengue virus is different to the above flaviviruses because humans rather than animals are the natural hosts. Geographically, it is the most widely distributed flavivirus and is also the most common in humans. Virtually every country between the Tropics of Cancer and Capricorn has dengue, and the virus is spreading. It is a common cause of febrile illness in returning travellers – occurring in 6% of hospitalised returning travellers in one series.[9] The virus is best known as a cause of febrile illness with rash or haemorrhagic disease, but it also sometimes causes neurological disease. This occurs as a non-specific complication of haemorrhage and shock, but sometimes is associated with the virus crossing the blood–brain barrier and encephalitis.[10]

□ EMERGENCE AND SPREAD OF FLAVIVIRUSES

How flaviviruses emerge and spread is of major importance. Molecular virological studies of multiple strains of virus suggest that JEV originated from an ancestral strain in the Indonesia–Malaysia region and evolved here into at least four genotypes, the most recent of which have spread to new geographical areas (Fig 5). Migrating birds, particularly egrets, are implicated in the spread of virus to new areas, but windblown mosquitoes may also be important. West Nile virus is also thought to spread principally via north–south migrating birds. How the virus appeared in New York in 1999 is not known. Dengue virus was originally thought to have been a virus of primates, which subsequently adapted to human hosts. This 'crossing of the species barrier' is thought to have occurred in Southeast Asia. The virus now spreads primarily through the travel of viraemic humans.

□ PATHOGENESIS OF FLAVIVIRUS ENCEPHALITIS

Strain virulence determinants are important

The relative contribution of strain virulence determinants and host–defence response in the clinical epidemiology of flaviviruses is the subject of intense study. Certainly for TBEV, the epidemiology suggests that the different subtypes of virus

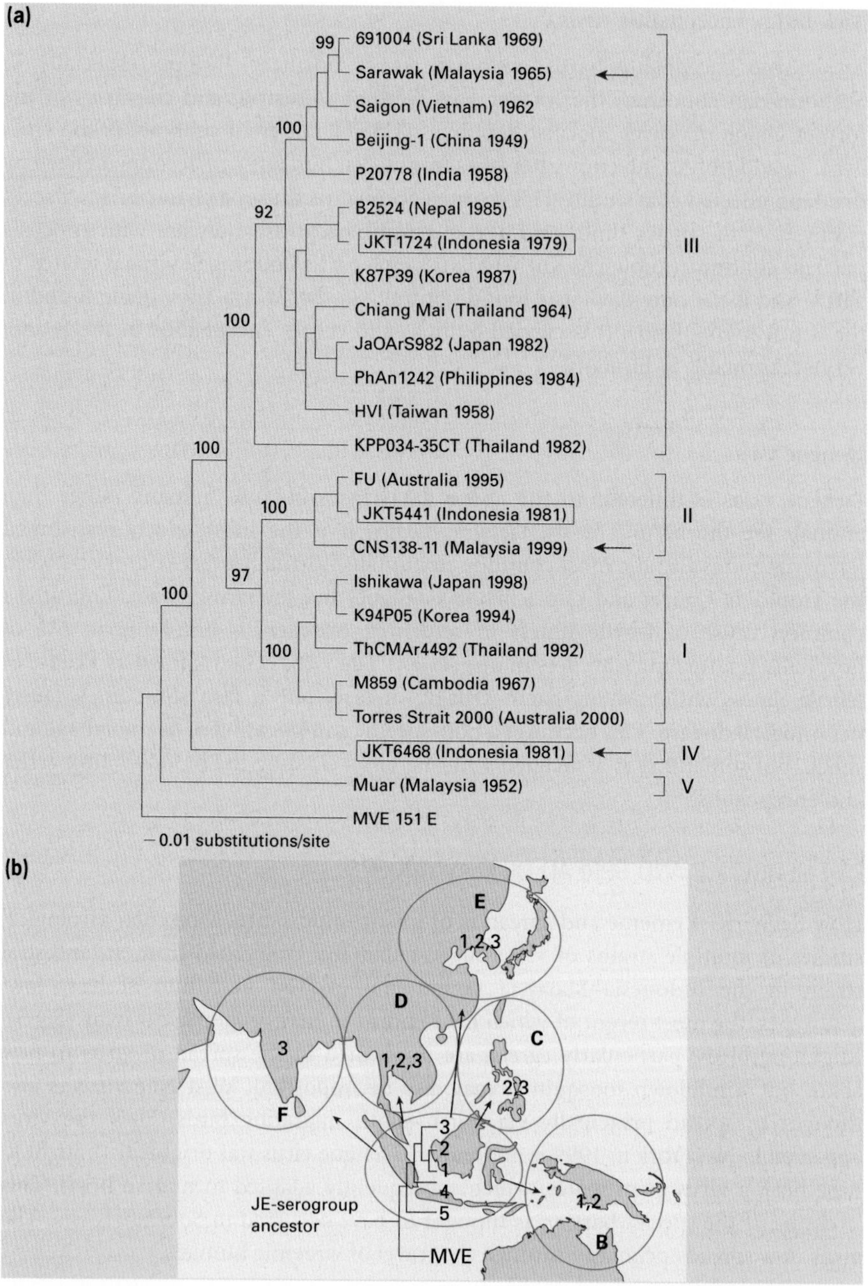

Fig 5 Current beliefs on the origin and distribution of Japanese encephalitis virus (JEV). **(a)** Neighbour-joining phylogenetic tree of envelope protein genes, showing the genetic relation between the different genotypes of virus: genotypes IV and V are thought to represent the oldest lineages. Indonesian strains are boxed, and genotypes are shown. **(b)** Map showing the postulated origin of JEV from a Japanese encephalitis (JE)-serogroup ancestor in the Indonesia–Malaysia region. The ancestral JE strain is believed then to have evolved here into the different genotypes of virus, all of which have been found in this region. Only the more recent genotypes subsequently have spread to new geographical areas. Adapted from Solomon with permission of Springer.[1]

have different virulences. For WNV, the genotype found in America is more virulent in birds and in rodent models than genotypes found in Africa, and this partially may explain the changing epidemiological pattern. For JEV, genotypic differences seem to be associated with viral spread, as indicated above, but whether they also confer differences in virulence in human disease is not clear.

Host response to infection is also critical

For JE, early studies showed that interferon alpha, which is made naturally in response to infections, is effective against the virus *in vitro* and in animal models. Preliminary studies in humans were promising, but a randomised, placebo-controlled trial showed no benefit.[11] Subsequent studies showed that levels of a range of proinflammatory cytokines – including interleukin (IL)-6, tumour necrosis factor alpha, and IL-8 (CXC chemokine ligand 8 (CXCL-8)) – are increased in the cerebrospinal fluid of patients with JE and that these cytokines are associated with fatal outcomes; modestly increased levels of regulated on activation, normally T cell expressed and secreted (RANTES), chemokine (C-C motif) ligand 5 (CCL5)) in the serum are also associated with fatal disease (Table 1).[12]

Interestingly, in one recent study of humans infected with WNV, a defective allele in the chemokine (C-C motif) receptor CCR5 (CCR5Δ32), which is found predominantly in white people, was found to be highly significantly associated with symptomatic infection with West Nile virus in two independent populations in the US.[13]

A strong proinflammatory response to infection with flavivirus has been postulated to possibly contribute to the poor outcome. Pathological studies of humans that died from JE[14] show that perivascular inflammation occurs, sometimes with disruption of the blood–brain barrier and even endovascular necrosis (Fig 6). Similar changes are seen with WNV encephalitis.

□ PREVENTION OF JAPANESE ENCEPHALITIS

The complex ecology of encephalitis caused by flavivirus means that control of mosquitoes and other similar measures are never likely to be fully effective. Vaccines therefore offer the best hope for control. Currently available vaccines against JE include a formalin-inactivated vaccine derived from mouse brain and a live attenuated vaccine. The former has been used in travellers for many years and is safe and efficacious, although it is too expensive for many parts of Asia. At one stage, the vaccine was associated with mucocutaneous allergic-type reactions, and it can also cause very rare neurological adverse events at a rate of about one per million – a similar rate to measles vaccine. It is being replaced with a tissue culture vaccine. Other killed vaccines also are being developed. The live attenuated vaccine is cheap and efficacious, even being used at a single dose in some studies. Until recently, it had not been widely used outside China. The Bill and Melinda Gates Foundation has made £27 million available to support the wider use of vaccines against JE. To help countries decide on the introduction of vaccine, more reliable data on disease burden are needed, which means better detection and diagnosis, as well as more

Table 1 Levels of cytokines, chemokines, nitric oxide (NO), and immunoglobulins on admission in patients who died and survivors.* Values are pg/ml unless otherwise specified. Reproduced from Winter *et al* with permission of Springer-Verlag Wien.

	Median* (interquartile range; range)		
Biomolecule	**Fatal cases (n=13)**	**Survivors (n=105)**	**p value***
In CSF:			
TNF-α	25.3 (11.6–43.7; 0–60)	0 (0–13.0; 0–116.45)	0.093
IL-4	36.5 (14.6 to 72.9; 0–175)	58.3 (0–87.5; 0–218.8)	0.535
IL-6	1377 (418 to 1648; 193–2190)	174.1 (38–849; 0–2821)	0.006
IL-8	1140 (420–1656; 190–3823)	286 (78–799; 0–4714)	0.04
IFN-α	4.4(0.4–13.9; 0–35.6)	0 (0–2.2; 0–53.3)	0.044
IFN-γ	60 (0–240; 0–255)	13 (0–180; 0–320)	0.511
RANTES	32.2 (13–50.1; 3.1–95.4)	18.5 (6–47.6; 0–353.7)	0.486
NO (μmol/l)	97.6 (25.9–67.5; 18–503.5)	54.9 (30.7–69; 14.6–170)	0.875
IgM (units)	60.5 (33.5–60.5; 4–274)	162 (67–229.5; 0–412)	0.035
IgG (units)	5.5(1.5–13; 0–17)	23 (7.5–60; 0–273)	0.003
In plasma:			
TNF-α	0 (0–17.5; 0–180)	0 (0–32.5; 0–3970)	0.91
IL-4	23.9 (0.6–89.6; 0–478.4)	15.9 (0–90.9; 0–1530.4)	0.691
IL-6	1.5 (0–6.5; 0–997.7)	7.4 (0–26.4; 0–2466.2)	0.16
IL-8	29.2 (21.3–92.4; 8–182)	54.0 (16.4–252; 0–5632)	0.506
IFN-α	0 (0–0; 0–31.9)	0 (0–2.6; 0–31.7)	0.201
IFN-γ	0 (0–5; 0–20.1)	0 (0–40; 0–2510)	0.306
RANTES	11312 (8823–15704; 357–17536)	8269 (6158–10113; 1–29224)	0.0314
NO (μmol/l)	79.4 (41–61.5; 3.3–436.5)	119.6 (42.8–93.1; 18.8–631.6)	0.121
In serum:			
IgM (units)	31.5 (12.5–41.5; 2–187)	90.5 (36–148.5; 1–145)	0.009
IgG (units)	10 (4–13; 0–40)	11 (4–28; 0–188)	0.463

IFN = interferon; Ig = immunoglobulin; IL = interleukin; RANTES = regulated on activation, normally T cell expressed and secreted; TNF-α = tumour necrosis factor alpha.
*Mann-Whitney *U* test or *t* test on log transformed data as appropriate.

reliable ways of measuring the outcome in those that survive with sequelae are needed.[15] Because JEV is a zoonotic virus (unlike polio), however, there will always be animal and mosquito reservoirs of virus, and eradication will never be possible. Killed vaccines also are available against TBEV and are used widely in some countries such as Austria. No vaccines are available for dengue or WNV.

□ CONCLUSION

The last decade has seen an extraordinary increase in the activity of emerging viruses, particularly the flaviviruses; this is seen both in the incidence of disease and the amount of interest and concern that the viruses cause. In some ways, however, emerging diseases are nothing new. In Linacre's day, bubonic plague was the most

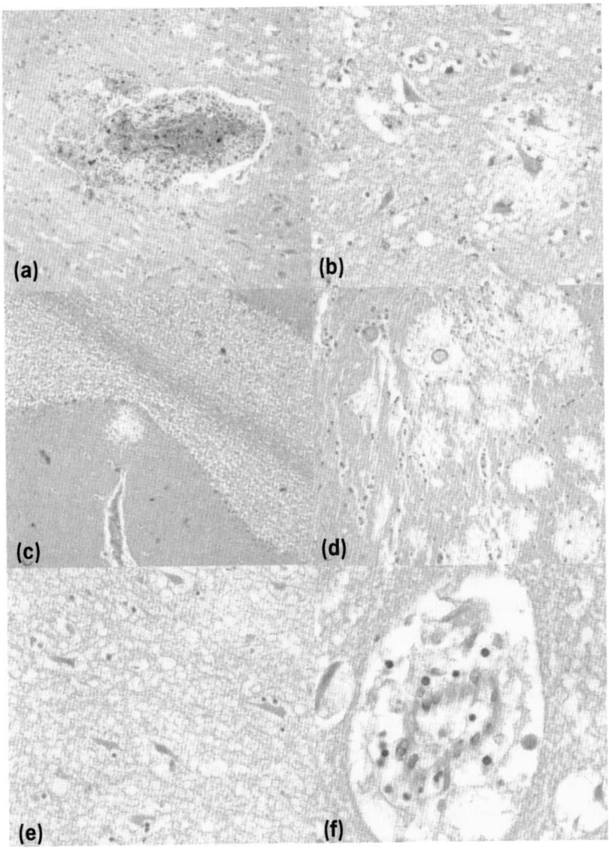

Fig 6 Characteristic histopathology in an 18-year-old man who died of Japanese encephalitis. **(a)** Damaged vein with perivascular infiltrate and necrosis in pontine tissue (original magnification (OM) ≥100). **(b)** Ischaemic, shrunken, damaged neurones in midbrain and thalamus (OM ≥200). **(c)** Cerebellum showing well-preserved Purkinje cells compared with the granular cells – a focal acellular necrotic lesion is visible in the molecular layer associated with an end vessel (OM ≥40). **(d)** Internal capsule showing striking necrotic foci with little peripheral inflammation (OM ≥100). **(e)** Necrotic neurones in subiculum (OM ≥200). **(f)** Damaged vessel with mild lymphocytic infiltrate (OM ≥400). Reproduced from German *et al* with permission of Elsevier.[14]

important emerging infectious disease, and large outbreaks affected London. Indeed, the panic they caused and the associated proliferation of unlicensed 'medical' practitioners were precipitants for the granting of the charter to the Royal College of Physicians in 1518 to better licence and regulate such doctors.

Although louping ill virus is the only flavivirus currently established in the UK, it is a very rare cause of disease. Other flaviviruses, particularly WNV and TBEV, are geographically close to the British Isles and may yet reach our shores. The encephalitis study of the Health Protection Agency in the UK is surveying cases of encephalitis in the northwest and southwest of England, as well as London, with the aim of detecting any such incursions. Meanwhile, dengue virus is an increasing cause of illness in returning travellers. The most deadly flavivirus, JEV, is spreading, but so far seems to be confined to Asia. It continues to be a major cause of neurological disease there, although this may change with the wider use of vaccines.

☐ ACKNOWLEDGEMENTS

I thank my many colleagues in Asia, the US and UK who have supported this work over the last 10 years. Funding has come from the Wellcome Trust, the Medical

Research Council in the UK, and the Gates-funded JE programme of the Program for Appropriate Technology in Health, Seattle.

REFERENCES

1 Solomon T. Flavivirus encephalitis. *N Engl J Med* 2004;351:370–8.

2 Solomon T, Winter PM. Neurovirulence and host factors in flavivirus encephalitis – evidence from clinical epidemiology. *Arch Virol Suppl* 2004;(18):161–70.

3 Solomon T. Encephalitis. In: Gill GV, Beeching NJ, eds, *Lecture notes on tropical medicine*, 5th edition. Oxford: Blackwell Science, 2004:221–5.

4 Solomon T, Kneen R, Dung NM *et al.* Poliomyelitis-like illness due to Japanese encephalitis virus. *Lancet* 1998;351:1094–7.

5 Solomon T, Ooi MH, Beasley DW, Mallewa M. West Nile encephalitis. *BMJ* 2003;326:865–9.

6 Mostashari F, Bunning ML, Kitsutani PT *et al.* Epidemic West Nile encephalitis, New York, 1999: results of a household-based seroepidemiological survey. *Lancet* 2001;358:261–4.

7 Buckley A, Dawson A, Gould EA. Detection of seroconversion to West Nile virus, Usutu virus and Sindbis virus in UK sentinel chickens. *Virol J* 2006;3:71.

8 Gritsun TS, Lashkevich VA, Gould EA. Tick-borne encephalitis. *Antiviral Res* 2003;57:129–46.

9 Stephenson I, Roper J, Fraser M, Nicholson K, Wiselka M. Dengue fever in febrile returning travellers to a UK regional infectious diseases unit. *Travel Med Infect Dis* 2003;1:89–93.

10 Solomon T, Dung NM, Vaughn DW *et al.* Neurological manifestations of dengue infection. *Lancet* 2000;355:1053–9.

11 Solomon T, Dung NM, Wills B *et al.* Interferon alfa-2a in Japanese encephalitis: a randomised double-blind placebo-controlled trial. *Lancet* 2003;361:821–6.

12 Winter PM, Dung NM, Loan HT *et al.* Proinflammatory cytokines and chemokines in humans with Japanese encephalitis. *J Infect Dis* 2004;190:1618–26.

13 Glass WG, McDermott DH, Lim JK *et al.* CCR5 deficiency increases risk of symptomatic West Nile virus infection. *J Exp Med* 2006;203:35–40.

14 German AC, Myint KS, Mai NT *et al.* A preliminary neuropathological study of Japanese encephalitis in humans and a mouse model. *Trans R Soc Trop Med Hyg* 2006;100:1135–45.

15 Solomon T. Control of Japanese encephalitis – within our grasp? *N Engl J Med* 2006;355: 869–71.

Answers to self-assessment questions

☐ CARDIOLOGY

Pulmonary hypertension

1a True	2a True	3a False
b False	b False	b True
c True	c False	c False
d False	d True	d False
e True	e True	e True

Contemporary management of acute myocardial infarction

1a False	2a False	3a False	4a False
b False	b False	b True	b False
c True	c True	c False	c True
d True	d False	d True	d False
e False	e True	e False	e False

☐ RESPIRATORY MEDICINE

New treatments for severe asthma in relation to pathophysiology

1a False	2a True	3a False	4a True
b True	b False	b True	b True
c True	c True	c True	c False
d True	d False	d False	d False
e False	e False	e True	e True

New developments in pleural disease

1a False	2a False	3a True
b False	b False	b False
c True	c True	c False
d False	d False	d False
e False		e True

Emphysema – lung volume reduction and beyond

1a True	2a False	3a True
b False	b False	b False
c True	c False	c True
d True	d True	d True
	e True	e False

☐ MULTI-SYSTEM DISEASE

Systemic amyloidosis

1a True	2a True	3a False
b True	b False	b True
c True	c True	c True
d True	d False	d True
e True	e True	e True

The porphyrias

1a False	2a False	3a False
b False	b True	b False
c False	c False	c True
d False	d False	d False
e True	e False	e False

☐ HAEMATOLOGY

The modern management of chronic myeloid leukaemia

1a False	2a False	3a False	4a True	5a False
b True	b False	b True	b False	b False
c True	c True	c False	c False	c True
d False	d False	d True	d False	d False
e True	e True	e True	e False	e True

The myeloproliferative disorders: management and molecular pathogenesis

1a True	2a True	3a True
b False	b False	b True
c False	c True	c False
d True	d True	d True
e False	e True	e False

☐ SKIN AND BONES

Drug allergies

1a True	2a True	3a False	4a True
b True	b False	b True	b True
c False	c False	c False	c False
d False	d True	d True	d False
e False	e True	e False	e False

Osteoporosis

1a True	2a False	3a True
b False	b True	b True
c True	c True	c False
d True		d False
		e True

Inherited skin diseases: new benefits for patients

1a True	2a False	3a False
b True	b False	b True
c True	c True	c True
d True	d True	d False
e False	e True	e False

☐ RENAL DISEASE

Treatment of antineutrophil cytoplasm antibody-associated systemic vasculitis

1a True	2a True	3a True	4a True	5a False
b True	b True	b True	b True	b False
c True	c True	c True	c True	c False
d False	d True	d True	d True	d False
e False	e True	e True	e True	e False

Polycystic kidney disease – then and now

1a False	2a False	3a False
b True	b False	b True
c True	c True	c False
d False	d False	d True
e True	e True	e True

Acute tubular necrosis – is there any hope of a treatment?

1a False	2a False	3a False
b True	b False	b True
c False	c False	c True
d False	d True	d True
e False	e True	e False

☐ RHEUMATOLOGY

New biologics for rheumatoid arthritis

1a True	2a False	3a True
b True	b False	b False
c True	c True	c False
d False	d False	d False

Systemic lupus erythematosus: a problem with B cells

1a True	2a True	3a True	4a True
b False	b True	b True	b False
c True	c False	c True	c True
d False	d True	d True	d False
e True	e False	e False	e True

New developments in spondyloarthritis

1a True	2a True	3a True
b True	b True	b True
c False	c False	c False
d True	d False	d True
e False	e True	e False

☐ NEUROLOGY

Ion channel disorders

1a True	2a False	3a True	4a False	5a True
b False	b False	b False	b False	b True
c True	c True	c True	c False	c True
d True	d True		d True	d False
	e False			e True

Neurosurgery for movement disorders

1a False	2a False	3a False	4a False
b False	b False	b True	b False
c False	c False	c True	c False
d False	d False	d False	d False
	e True		e True

☐ RADIOLOGY

High-resolution computed tomography and diffuse lung disease – current status

1a True	2a False	3a True
b True	b False	b True
c False	c True	c False
d True	d True	d False
e False	e False	e False

Cancer imaging

1a False	2a True	3a False
b True	b True	b True
c False	c True	c False
d False	d True	d True
e False	e False	e True

Endocrine imaging

1a True	2a True	3a True
b True	b False	b True
c False	c False	c False
d True	d True	d True
e True	e True	e True

☐ ENDOCRINOLOGY

New therapies in the management of type 2 diabetes

1a True	2a False	3a True	4a True
b False	b True	b False	b False
c False	c False	c False	c False
d False	d True	d False	d True
e False	e False		e True

Management of adrenal insufficiency in severe stress and surgery

1a False	2a False	3a True
b False	b False	b True
c True	c False	c False
d True	d False	d True
e True	e False	e False

Making sense of 'funny thyroid function tests'

1a False	2a True	3a False
b False	b False	b True
c True	c False	c False
d False	d False	d False
e False	e False	e False

☐ INFECTIOUS DISEASE

Imported infectious disease emergencies

1a True	2a False	3a False	4a True
b False	b True	b False	b False
c False	c True	c False	c True
d False	d False	d False	d False
e True	e False	e True	e True

Update on HIV

1a True	2a True	3a False	4a False
b False	b False	b False	b True
c True	c True	c True	c False
d True	d True	d False	d False
e False	e False	e False	e False

Highly pathogenic avian influenza H5N1 in humans

1a True	2a False	3a True
b False	b False	b False
c False	c False	c True
d True	d True	d False
e False	e True	e False

☐ HEPATOLOGY/GASTROENTEROLOGY

Crohn's disease: pathogenic insights from recent genetic advances

1a True	2a False	3a False	4a True
b False	b False	b True	b False
c True	c True	c False	c True
d False	d False	d False	d False
e True	e True	e False	e True

Non-alcoholic fatty liver disease

1a True	2a False	3a True
b True	b False	b True
c False	c True	c True
d False	d True	d False
e True		

Autoimmune hepatitis

1a False	2a False	3a True	4a False	5a False
b False	b False	b False	b False	b False
c False	c False	c False	c False	c True
d False	d True	d False	d False	d False
e True	e False	e False	e True	e False

6a True	7a True
b False	b True
c False	c True
	d True

Selecting cases for liver transplantation

1a True	2a False	3a True
b False	b False	b False
c False	c True	c False
d True	d False	d True
e False	e True	e True